T0324897

Clinical Pathology
for Athletic Trainers
Recognizing Systemic Disease

FOURTH EDITION

Clinical Pathology
for Athletic Trainers
Recognizing Systemic Disease

FOURTH EDITION

REHAL A. BHOJANI, MD, CAQSM, FAAFP

Assistant Professor and Fellowship Director
Sports Medicine
UT Health Science Center Houston/IRONMAN Sports Medicine Institute
McGovern Medical School
Department of Orthopedic Surgery
Houston, Texas

DANIEL P. O'CONNOR, PhD, ATC

Interim Dean
College of Liberal Arts and Social Sciences
University of Houston
Houston, Texas

A. LOUISE FINCHER, EdD, ATC, LAT

Dean
School of Health Sciences
Emory & Henry College
Emory, Virginia

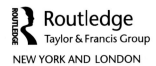

Routledge
Taylor & Francis Group

NEW YORK AND LONDON

Clinical Pathology for Athletic Trainers: Recognizing Systemic Disease, Fourth Edition includes ancillary materials specifically available for faculty use. Included are Test Bank Questions, an Instructor's Manual, and PowerPoint Slides. Please visit http://www.routledge.com/9781630917234 to obtain access.

Cover Artist: Katherine Christie

First published in 2022 by SLACK Incorporated

Published 2024 by Routledge
605 Third Avenue, New York, NY 10158

and by Routledge
4 Park Square, Milton Park, Abingdon, Oxon OX14 4RN

Routledge is an imprint of the Taylor & Francis Group, an informa business

© 2022 Taylor & Francis Group

Drs. Rehal A. Bhojani, Daniel P. O'Connor, and A. Louise Fincher have no financial or proprietary interest in the materials presented herein.

Library of Congress Cataloging-in-Publication Data

Names: O'Connor, Daniel P., author. | Bhojani, Rehal A., author. | Fincher,
  A. Louise, 1961- author.
Title: Clinical pathology for athletic trainers : recognizing systemic
  disease / Rehal A. Bhojani, Daniel P. O'Connor, A. Louise Fincher.
Description: Fourth edition. | Thorofare, NJ : SLACK Incorporated, [2022] |
  Preceded by Clinical pathology for athletic trainers : recognizing
  systemic disease / Daniel P. O'Connor, A. Louise Fincher. 3rd. 2015. |
  Includes bibliographical references and index.
Identifiers: LCCN 2021021742 (print) | ISBN 9781630917234 (hardcover)
Subjects: MESH: Signs and Symptoms | Pathology, Clinical--methods | Sports
  Medicine
Classification: LCC RB127 (print) | NLM WB 143 | DDC
  616/.047--dc23
LC record available at https://lccn.loc.gov/2021021742

ISBN: 9781630917234 (hbk)
ISBN: 9781003523116 (ebk)

DOI: 10.4324/9781003523116

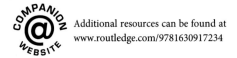

Additional resources can be found at
www.routledge.com/9781630917234

Dedication

For those who got me to where I am, professionally and personally.

—RAB

For Mitzi, always.

—DPO

To my students, past, present, and future.

—ALF

CONTENTS

Clinical Pathology for Athletic Trainers: Recognizing Systemic Disease, Fourth Edition includes ancillary materials specifically available for faculty use. Included are Test Bank Questions, an Instructor's Manual, and PowerPoint Slides. Please visit http://www.routledge.com/9781630917234 to obtain access.

ACKNOWLEDGMENTS

To my family, whom has stood by my side and supported my growth and my aspirations. To the team of athletic trainers who taught me the meaning of Sports Medicine, especially Bob Marley, Kevin Bastin, Brad Brown, Mike Vara, Max Mahaffey. To Lou and Dan, thank you for allowing me to contribute to this project. To Josh Yellen and Mark Knoblauch, who gave me the opportunity to teach aspiring athletic trainers from a physician's perspective.

—*RAB*

A special thanks to Mitzi Laughlin, who (still) has far, far more patience than I deserve. I thank my parents, Dan and Mary, for who I am and what I have. To Michael E. Cooley, ASMI, our talented medical illustrator who has been with us since the first edition: a very special thanks for the figures. To Bill Wissen, Dale Spence, and Allen Eggert, my personal and professional mentors and good friends: thanks for your time and for showing me the way. To Lou: It has been a joy over the many years to work with such a respected, knowledgeable professional and great friend. Your contribution to the second and third editions has improved the value of the book immensely, and my appreciation and admiration for your work is equally immense. Finally, I want to recognize and acknowledge my colleagues and friends in the Greater Houston Athletic Trainers' Society and the Southwest Athletic Trainers' Association (NATA District 6)—the best athletic trainers anywhere.

—*DPO*

To René, thank you for your endless patience and support throughout what, again, seemed like a never-ending project. Thank you to my mentors, Ken Knight and Ken Wright, who were the first to encourage me to write and publish. A special thank you to all of the people at SLACK for their assistance (and patience) with this fourth edition. And lastly, thank you to DanO! As always, it's been an honor to work with you on this project. What a great journey!

—*ALF*

About the Authors

Rehal A. Bhojani, MD, CAQSM, FAAFP is an assistant professor in the Department of Orthopaedic Surgery at the University of Texas Health Science Center, where he serves as the Fellowship Director for the Primary Care Sports Medicine Program. He also served as the Medical Director for the Master of Athletic Training Program at the University of Houston. He serves as Chief Medical Officer for the Houston Dynamo and Houston Dash and is a team physician for the Houston Rockets, University of Houston, and Houston Texans.

Daniel P. O'Connor, PhD, ATC is an associate professor in the Department of Health and Human Performance at the University of Houston, where he also serves on the Executive Board of the Texas Obesity Research Center. His research involves measurement and evaluation of health and health outcomes and has been funded by the National Institutes of Health, the Centers for Disease Control and Prevention, and the National Aeronautics and Space Administration. In addition to the previous editions of *Clinical Pathology for Athletic Trainers*, he has published more than 100 peer-reviewed journal articles and book chapters. Dan has served on many committees in various athletic training professional associations and was President of the Southwest Athletic Trainers' Association (NATA District 6) in 2008-2009.

A. Louise Fincher, EdD, ATC, LAT is Founding Dean of the School of Health Sciences at Emory & Henry College. Lou has more than 30 years of experience as an athletic trainer and an educator. She has spent countless hours developing didactic and clinical education materials both for students and athletic training educators. She also has more than 25 peer-reviewed publications and 50 professional presentations. Lou has served on several National Athletic Trainers' Association (NATA) and Southwest Athletic Trainers' Association committees, including the NATA Executive Committee for Education and NATA Professional Education Committee. As Chair of the NATA Professional Education Committee, Lou oversaw the development of the 5th edition of the *Athletic Training Education Competencies*.

INTRODUCTION

The goal of this fourth edition of *Clinical Pathology for Athletic Trainers: Recognizing Systemic Disease* is to enable athletic trainers and athletic training students to recognize, evaluate, and differentiate common systemic diseases. Our book has been thoroughly updated to align with the fifth edition of the *Athletic Training Education Competencies* and the seventh edition of the *Board of Certification for the Athletic Trainer's Role Delineation Study/Practice Analysis*.[a] We have also incorporated all the relevant current National Athletic Trainers' Association position statements and inter-association consensus statements.

We have made some modifications to the fourth edition that we believe will enhance student learning. All chapters have been updated and expanded using the most current evidence available in the sports medicine literature. We have added information about preparticipation physical examination, screening for cardiovascular disease, traumatic brain injury, obesity, and a number of other medical conditions. The information about differential diagnosis from the final chapter of the second edition has been integrated into Chapter 1, where clinical decision making is discussed. The diagnostic algorithms based on key symptoms from that chapter are now included in the applicable system-specific chapters. Nearly all graphics and photos are now in color. We have continued beginning each chapter with a topical outline that incorporates the chapter's learning objectives and listing the specific Athletic Training Educational Competencies that are addressed.

Clinical Pathology for Athletic Trainers was written by athletic trainers specifically for athletic trainers, acknowledging their unique role in health care. In this edition, a physician was added on to the editorial board to give a different perspective on the vast knowledge base in Sports Medicine. It is intended to be a textbook for athletic training students in athletic training educational programs and a reference book for certified athletic trainers. It emphasizes the clinical recognition and management of non-orthopedic pathology, which allows athletic trainers to recognize systemic illnesses and injuries.

The information in this text was drawn not only from standard medical reference books, but also from research and reviews published in the sports medicine literature. In addition, the comments of many athletic training educators regarding the first, second, and third editions have been incorporated into this fourth edition. Those suggestions were invaluable in revising the book, and we are grateful for that input.

ᵃAvailable online for download:

◊ **Athletic Training Education Competencies (5th ed.)**
  ¤ https://caate.net/wp-content/uploads/2014/06/5th-Edition-Competencies.pdf
◊ **Role Delineation Study/Practice Analysis (7th ed.)—Content Outline**
  ¤ https://bocatc.org/system/document_versions/versions/24/original/boc-pa7-content-outline-20170612.pdf?1497279231

CHAPTER 1

Principles of Clinical Pathology and Decision Making

CHAPTER OUTLINE AND OBJECTIVES

Introduction

◊ Define terminology used to discuss pathology.
  ¤ Pathology in Sports Medicine and Athletic Training
  ¤ Signs and Symptoms
  ¤ Diagnosis
◊ Review the theoretical and scientific bases of clinical pathology.
  ¤ Theories of Disease and Pathogenesis
◊ Discuss the role of the athletic trainer with respect to identifying general medical pathology.
  ¤ Role of Athletic Trainers in Disease Prevention

Diagnostic Reasoning and Clinical Decision Making

◊ Explain the role of clinical reasoning in the clinical decision-making process.

Medical History

◊ Introduce questions included in a medical history relevant to general medical pathology.

Symptoms

◊ Review the behavior and characteristics of symptoms relevant to general medical pathology.

Physical Examination Techniques: Differentiating Normal and Abnormal Responses

◊ Introduce methods of physical examination relevant to general medical pathology.

Bhojani RA, O'Connor DP, Fincher AL. *Clinical Pathology for Athletic Trainers: Recognizing Systemic Disease, Fourth Edition* (pp 1-22). © 2022 Taylor & Francis Group.

Differentiation of Signs and Symptoms

Medical Emergency

◊ Identify signs and symptoms of medical emergencies and explain the associated referral and transport decisions.

Evaluating Seriousness of Condition

◊ Discuss signs and symptoms of systemic pathology that are similar to musculoskeletal pathology.

◊ Describe the process of developing differential diagnoses for pathology involved with each of the major body systems.

Summary

Online Resource

This chapter addresses the following competencies from the *Athletic Training Education Competencies, Fifth Edition*[1]:

Content Area	Competency #
Evidence-Based Practice (EBP)	2
Prevention and Health Promotion (PHP)	9
Clinical Examination and Diagnosis (CE)	13, 16, 17, 18, 20a
Acute Care of Injury and Illness (AC)	5, 41
Healthcare Administration (HA)	22, 23
Clinical Integration Proficiencies (CIP)	5, 6

INTRODUCTION

The practice settings in which athletic trainers work include those in secondary schools, universities, professional sports, hospitals, sports medicine clinics, physicians' offices, the military, and corporate and industrial organizations. Because of the diverse patient populations within these varied practice settings, athletic trainers must be familiar with the common general medical conditions that may occur in these individuals.

Athletic trainers should be aware of the possible origins and/or etiologies of an injury or illness, particularly symptoms that are not associated with a specific traumatic event. Knowledge of pathology and mechanisms of disease will improve athletic trainers' clinical decision-making skills. Certain clinical skills, including taking a medical history, performing a physical examination, analyzing clinical information, and making a medical referral, also depend on this knowledge. Most of the general medical disorders or diseases encountered by the athletic trainer will involve one or more of the body's functional systems (cardiovascular, pulmonary, etc). In most cases, the signs and symptoms will point toward the involvement of a particular organ or system.

This book uses a systems approach for discussing pathology. Each chapter will address the common injuries or illnesses associated with a particular body system.

Pathology in Sports Medicine and Athletic Training

Pathology, a special field of medical science, focuses on the study of the biological causes, effects, and processes of disease.[2] *Pathogenesis* refers to the underlying physiological mechanism causing a disease. *Etiology* is the study of many factors, including pathogenesis, to explain the circumstances under which the disease occurs or develops.[2] For example, the pathogenesis of influenza is infection with a virus from the *Orthomyxoviridae* family; once in the human body, the virus replicates, invades, and damages respiratory tract epithelial cells. The etiology of influenza not only includes viral infection as a necessary component, but also describes how and why people become infected by the virus and how it can be transmitted from person to person; infection typically occurs through contact or inspiration of an infected person's nasal and respiratory secretions, which contain the virus.

Signs and Symptoms

A *sign* is an observable indication of pathology, usually discovered during physical examination. A *symptom* is any abnormal function, appearance, or sensation that is experienced by the patient.[2] Thus, signs are objective and can be measured by the clinician, whereas symptoms are subjective and reported by the patient. Medical conditions often produce characteristic patterns of signs and symptoms.

Each patient's *clinical presentation* is the overall "picture" of signs, symptoms, medical history, and physical examination. This book outlines clinical presentations that are consistent with general medical disease. Standard athletic training and sports medicine texts[3,4] review injuries of bones, joints, and muscles, which are not discussed here.

Diagnosis

The term *diagnosis* refers to the specific injury, illness, disease, or condition a patient has, as determined by a medical examination.[2] The athletic trainer will formulate a clinical diagnosis based on the signs, symptoms, medical history, and physical examination. Often, particularly when dealing with general medical conditions, analysis of this data results in a *differential diagnosis*, or the identification of several conditions that have similar clinical presentations. When this occurs, the athletic trainer will typically consult or refer the patient to a physician, who will perform a medical examination which may also include laboratory or imaging studies to determine the diagnosis.

A disease may affect a person's ability to participate in sports or other physical activities and may require that certain precautions be taken. For example, an athlete with type 1 diabetes mellitus may require a glucose source always be available during practice and competition. Furthermore, *coexisting* or *comorbid conditions* are medical conditions that are already present in addition to the primary problem that can complicate recovery from an injury and/or illness or can require treatment modifications. For instance, hypertension and some of the medications used to treat hypertension limit the type and intensity of exercise the patient may perform. Consequently, hypertension is a comorbid condition that may affect the treatment plan for a muscle or joint injury.

Theories of Disease and Pathogenesis

Several theories provide potential explanations for the origin and nature of disease. The *biomedical* theory of health and illness attributes the cause of disease to abnormal cell, tissue, or organ function. The abnormal function can be caused by anatomical, physiological, or genetic defects, or by factors such as bacteria and viruses. This book uses this type of biomedical model to explain pathogenesis for most conditions.

Psychosocial theories consider the psychological and social effects on the development and progression of illness and disease. Patients who cannot adapt cognitively or socially to a major injury may be more prone to chronic illness and may not respond to treatment as expected. In addition,

Table 1-1. Stages of Disease Prevention

STAGE	PURPOSE	ACTIVITIES AND INTERVENTIONS
Primary	Reduce risk factors	Nutrition, exercise, monitoring of environmental risks, prevention and educational programs
Secondary	Early detection, early intervention, inhibit proliferation	Regular medical checkups, self-examination, early medical treatment
Tertiary	Limit established disease	Medical treatment, supportive and restorative

emotional, academic, financial, or social stressors can cause symptoms that confuse the clinical presentation of an illness. Chapter 14 addresses psychological issues in greater detail.

Last, *genetic* theories focus on factors, such as errors in DNA and RNA replication, that can contribute to pathogenesis, the effectiveness of the immune system's responses, and the rate of tissue healing. Genetic and congenital disorders are commonly identified in pediatric patients (children). Where appropriate, the following chapters discuss specific pediatric concerns. Of note, advances in medicine now may identify factors not known in athlete until adulthood but is beyond the scope of this book.

Role of Athletic Trainers in Disease Prevention

The Board of Certification identifies injury and illness prevention as a major domain of athletic training practice.[5] Table 1-1 summarizes the 3 stages of prevention. *Primary prevention* involves reducing risk of future disease, which may involve nutrition, regular physical activity, and minimizing environmental hazards. *Secondary prevention* includes early detection of illness or disease and preventing or reversing the progression of disease. *Tertiary prevention* attempts to limit the adverse effects of an established disease and restore the highest possible level of function.

Athletic trainers participate in all 3 stages of prevention. With respect to primary prevention, they identify risk factors, monitor the environment, and counsel athletes. Secondary prevention, such as early detection and appropriate referral, is facilitated by knowledge of clinical pathology. Tertiary prevention provides medical treatment for an injury or illness and continues through return to work, competition, or participation in usual daily activities.

DIAGNOSTIC REASONING AND CLINICAL DECISION MAKING

Diagnostic Reasoning

Medical treatment begins with diagnosis. *Diagnostic reasoning* is how a physician *differentiates* (ie, sorts and interprets) signs and symptoms to determine a diagnosis. The diagnostic processes include *triage* (determining the urgency of a medical condition), medical history, physical examination, laboratory tests, and imaging studies.[6] A physician's diagnosis leads to actions such as prescription of medications, surgery, referral to medical specialists, or referral to allied health services.

Table 1-2. Clinical Reasoning Versus Diagnostic Reasoning

	CLINICAL DECISION MAKING	DIAGNOSTIC REASONING
CLINICIAN	Athletic trainer	Physician
PURPOSE	Determine a potential diagnosis and course of action	Determine a diagnosis and course of medical treatment
PROCESSES	History, physical examination, differential diagnosis, reassessment (evaluate progress)	History, physical exam, forming hypothesis, confirming hypothesis (with laboratory and imaging tests)
RESULTING ACTIONS (CLINICAL)	Emergency transport, first aid, treatment plan, rehabilitation, referral to other health care professionals, modify activity	Medication prescription, surgery, referral to health care professionals, treatment plan, return to play guidance

Table 1-3. Purposes of the Medical History

Determine potential pathogenesis

Identify coexisting medical conditions

Determine the stage and/or severity of the injury or illness

Identify contraindications to treatment

Clinical Decision Making

Athletic trainers use *clinical reasoning*, a process similar to physicians' diagnostic reasoning, to differentiate the subjective and objective data gathered through the medical history and physical examination of their patients. Athletic trainers' clinical reasoning and problem-solving skills guide their *clinical decision making* as they formulate a differential diagnosis and course of action for a particular patient (Table 1-2). Through clinical reasoning and decision making, the athletic trainer's diagnosis may lead to actions such as first aid, emergency transport, treatment and rehabilitation, reassessment, activity modification, or referral to other health care specialists. Recognizing characteristic patterns of signs and symptoms such as those described in this book can help to determine the appropriate course of action.

MEDICAL HISTORY

A *medical history* is "an account of the events" related to a patient's state of health.[6] Table 1-3 gives the purposes for the medical history. All illnesses and injuries contain a medical history, which is collected by interviewing the patient. The scope and extent of the interview should be appropriate to the situation. For instance, primary assessment of a traumatic injury need not include a full family medical history. However, a person reporting vague or unusual symptoms in the athletic training room or outpatient clinic needs more extensive questioning.[7] Information from the medical history directs the subsequent physical examination and assists clinical decision making. In a lot of cases, the medical history will significantly guide the clinical decision making.

Table 1-4. Components of a Medical History

Chief complaint
Description and course/history of present illness
Personal medical history
Family medical history
Review of organ systems

Taking a Medical History

The components of the medical history are listed in Table 1-4.[6] Details that are potentially relevant to subsequent physical examination, treatment, or outcome are recorded in the patient's chart or record. A proper medical history focuses on the patient's current issues and establishes a rapport (trust) between the clinician and the patient.[7] Conducting a medical history requires practice to obtain complete and correct information. The clinical presentation is built from information in the medical history.

Participants in organized competitive athletics usually receive a *preparticipation examination*.[8] The preparticipation examination includes a physical screening examination, a survey of personal and family medical history, and a review of the major organ systems. This preseason survey of an athlete's medical history can identify existing pathology that may prevent or limit participation in specific sports. This preliminary record should also be consulted when evaluating injuries and illnesses incurred during the season. In the event that the athletic trainer is unfamiliar with the patient, such as in a clinic, the personal and family medical history is collected during the initial evaluation.

Chief Complaints

The *chief complaints* are the symptoms or functional limitations that cause a patient to seek medical attention.[6] Common chief complaints include pain and disability (inability to perform) in sport, work, or social-familial duties. The athletic trainer uses the chief complaints to guide the evaluation, to evaluate effects of injury or illness, to monitor recovery, and to focus attention on the patient's goals.

Description and Course of Present Illness

The core of the medical history is the course of the present illness, including the patient's description of onset of symptoms, progression of symptoms since onset, and the nature of the problem. Table 1-5 lists some common questions asked during the history of the present illness. Inquiring whether the condition is "getting better, not changing, or getting worse" indicates the progression of the disease. The patient should rate their symptoms numerically using visual analog scales (Figure 1-1) or verbal numerical ratings (eg, "What is your pain on a scale of 0 to 10, with 0 being no pain and 10 being unbearable?"). These ratings can be repeated each day to evaluate recovery.

At the conclusion of the history of present illness, the clinician should have a good description of the patient's condition possibly to form a differential diagnosis. How did it begin and how has it changed? What are the frequency, intensity, and duration of symptoms? What makes the condition better or worse? Information from the history should guide the physical examination and subsequently the clinical decision making.

Personal and Family Medical History

The *personal (or past) medical history* and *family medical history* review the previous medical conditions or illnesses experienced by the patient and immediate family members (Table 1-6).

Table 1-5. Questions for the History of Present Illness

When did your condition start?

What makes your condition better (alleviating factors)? What makes it worse (exacerbating factors)?

Is your condition better or worse in the morning? Is your condition better or worse or at night?

Is your condition better or worse with breathing, eating, urination, excitement or stress, during activity or at rest, or with certain body positions?

Have you had any X-rays, ultrasound, magnetic resonance imaging scans, or computed tomography scans for this condition?

Have you had any other medical tests for this condition?

Have you tried to treat this condition? If so, what treatments have you tried?

What treatment have you received for this condition based on what others have told you?

Is your condition getting better, getting worse, or not changing?

Have you ever had any symptoms or condition like this before?

Is there anything else I need to know about you or your condition?

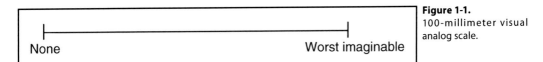

None   Worst imaginable

Figure 1-1. 100-millimeter visual analog scale.

Reports of minor surgeries or health problems should lead the athletic trainer to ask more specific questions. A coexisting condition may require modification of evaluation or treatment techniques. A family history of disease may be relevant if the clinical presentation suggests similar pathology.

Review of Systems

The *review of systems* screens for major organ system disease by asking about specific symptoms by interview or questionnaire (Table 1-7). When any of these symptoms are present, questions specific to the respective systems are indicated. The following chapters will review these specific questions.

Medical Tests

Medical tests for the current condition, such as imaging studies and laboratory tests, and when those tests were performed should be documented. For example, blood and urine tests are often used to inform the diagnostic process for many systemic pathologies. Examples of normal values for blood and urine tests are provided in a table in the back of the book. In addition, prescription and nonprescription medications for all current and coexisting conditions should be recorded. Many medications have side effects or require treatment precautions. Chapter 3 provides an overview of pharmacology and, where applicable, the individual system chapters provide information on the common medications used to treat the conditions within that system.

General Health Information

Additional questions related to the person's health may be necessary (Table 1-8). Poor or declining recent health may indicate *occult* (undetected) or progressive pathology. Sport-specific demands, work environment, or regular physical activity (or inactivity) may be related to pathogenesis and may affect treatment, *prognosis* (predicted outcome of disease), and recovery. Age, gender, race, or occupation may also be relevant to pathogenesis.[7] Other important information to collect

Table 1-6. Past and Family Medical History

Have you or any immediate family member had any of the following major health problems?

• Heart disease	• Cancer	• Diabetes	• High blood
• Stroke	• Kidney disease	• Liver disease	pressure
• Digestive	• Breathing	• Headaches	• Recurrent infections
problems	problems	• Depression/	• Anemia
• Arthritis/joint Pains	• Nerve problems	anxiety	• Substance abuse

How has your current health been over the past few months?

Do you currently have any other injuries or medical conditions?

Have you ever been admitted to a hospital?

Have you ever had surgery?

includes regular physical stresses (eg, prolonged sitting, driving, frequent lifting), psychoemotional stress, exposure to toxins (including smoke, alcohol, caffeine, and other drugs), and usual routine and schedule (does the person "have time" for good nutrition, physical activity, medical treatment, appointments, etc?).[7]

SYMPTOMS

Behavior and Characteristics

Qualities of various symptoms can reveal the nature of the disorder.[7] Table 1-9 compares several qualities of systemic (non-musculoskeletal) and musculoskeletal symptoms. Pain of systemic origin is usually constant, unchanged by movement or posture, most intense at night, and present during function of the affected system(s). Musculoskeletal pain is usually intermittent, changes with body position or posture, decreases at night, and is unaffected by internal organ functions. Table 1-10 lists words patients often use to describe symptoms suggesting systemic pathology.

Anatomical location of symptoms also provides additional clues. The patient can either draw their symptom pattern on a body diagram (Figure 1-2) or simply point to their symptomatic areas. Each organ and system has a characteristic pain referral pattern, as is shown in subsequent chapters. Symptoms that match these visceral (organ) patterns should prompt investigation for other signs.

Acute and Chronic Pain

The term *acute pain* describes pain of sudden onset with high intensity and relatively short duration (hours or days). *Chronic pain* appears gradually with lower intensity and a longer duration (weeks or months). To physicians, chronic pain is typically defined by greater than 6 months. Acute pain that appears without trauma, chronic pain that returns in predictable cycles ("comes and goes"), or chronic pain that progresses in intensity suggests systemic pathology.

Local and Referred Pain

Local pain stays in a specific region or area of the body. *Referred pain* occurs in a region that is distant from the source of the pain. Referred pain is more common in systemic pathology or in areas where the nerve distribution is different, although it can also occur with certain musculoskeletal conditions.

Table 1-7. Review of Systems by Signs and Symptoms

GENERAL SIGNS AND SYMPTOMS	POTENTIAL CONDITION OR SYSTEM OF ORIGIN
Fever, chills, sweats	Infection, cancer; immune system
Severe night pain	Cancer; cardiovascular or gastrointestinal system; growing pain (pediatrics)
Unexplained weight change	Depression, eating disorder, infection, cancer; gastrointestinal or metabolic systems
Unusual fatigue, malaise	Depression, infection, diabetes, anemia, rheumatoid arthritis, eating disorder, cancer; endocrine system
KEY SYSTEM-SPECIFIC SIGNS AND SYMPTOMS	
Chest pain or palpitations	Cardiovascular system
Shortness of breath	Cardiovascular or pulmonary system
Dizziness, light-headedness, fainting	Medications; cardiovascular, metabolic, or neurological system
Nausea, vomiting	Pregnancy, cancer, drug toxicity; gastrointestinal system; medication or substance side effect
Change of bowel movement, diarrhea	Gastrointestinal system
Difficulty, bleeding, or pain while urinating	Infection; urogenital system
Sexual function problems	Psychological; urogenital or neurological system
Visual disturbances	Neurological or cardiovascular system
Numbness, weakness, burning, tingling	Neurological system
Difficulty swallowing, hoarseness	Neoplasm (tumor); neurological or gastrointestinal system

Table 1-8. Recent General Health Status

Have you lost more than 5 to 10 pounds in the past month?

What types of physical stresses does your job involve?

- Sitting
- Deskwork
- Standing
- Large equipment
- Walking
- Small equipment
- Lifting
- Chemical exposure
- Bending
- Climbing

Are you on a diet?

Do you use any tobacco products?

How many drinks of alcohol do you have in 1 week?

How many caffeinated drinks do you have in 1 day?

Are you taking any supplements?

Are you using any illicit drugs? CBD oil?

Table 1-9. General Character and Behavior of Systemic and Musculoskeletal Symptoms

SYSTEMIC	MUSCULOSKELETAL
Constant	Intermittent
No change with movement or posture	Consistent change with movement or posture
No change or worse at rest	Relief with rest
Worse at night	Relief at night
Worse with organ function	Unaffected by organ function

Table 1-10. Pain Descriptors by Possible Systemic Origin of Pathology

SYSTEM	DESCRIPTOR
Vascular	Pulsing, throbbing, pounding, cramping, quivering
Neurogenic	Shooting, stabbing, drilling, sharp, cutting, pinching, pressing, pulling, burning, tingling, stinging
Musculoskeletal	Dull, sore, hurting, aching, heavy
Emotional lability (psychoemotional)	Splitting, exhausting, sickening, cruel, vicious, killing, unbearable, radiating, tight, cold, nagging

Adapted from Melzack R. The McGill Pain Questionnaire: Major Properties and Scoring Methods. *Pain*. 1975;1:277-299.

Constant and Intermittent Pain

Constant pain is always present, although the intensity may vary over time. Patients describe *intermittent pain* as something that "comes and goes." With either constant or intermittent pain, if the intensity varies with certain movements or body position, an acute musculoskeletal injury may be suspected. Conversely, if intensity increases at night, with organ function (eg, digestion, breathing), or does not change at all, the pain may be systemic in origin.

Causes of Pain

Mechanical, chemical, and perceptual mechanisms cause different types of pain, although they can occur in combination with one another.

Mechanical Causes

Anatomical structures under abnormal physical loads or stress can produce pain. Most commonly, musculoskeletal injuries cause this type of pain. Pain caused by mechanical factors is more likely intermittent, related to movement or position, and relieved by removing the offending stress. This type of pain appears only in the injured structure.

Chemical Causes

Biochemical substances released with tissue injury can produce pain. These substances irritate innervated tissues and cause inflammation, as reviewed in Chapter 2. Pain of chemical origin is constant, although intensity may change, and cannot be relieved by movement or position, although it may worsen with such changes. Medication addresses chemical causes and thus nearly always

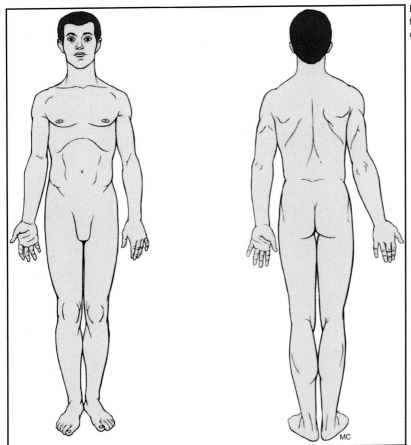

Figure 1-2. Body diagram for documenting location of pain or other symptoms.

decreases this type of pain. Pain caused by chemical irritation is poorly localized and may refer to other locations if nerves or adjacent anatomical structures are affected.

Perceptual Causes

Pain is itself a perception, so all pain has perceptual aspects. An individual's response to pain is affected by their cultural, social, and personal experiences. It is also possible for the physical (mechanical and chemical) origin of pain to be "healed" while the perception of pain remains. If athletic trainers recognize this situation, they should report their observations to the supervising physician and support any subsequently prescribed treatment.

Pain-Generating Tissues

Different tissues also produce different types of pain. Skin and subcutaneous tissues generate *cutaneous* pain, localized to the area of tissue damage. *Deep somatic* pain originates in bones, nerves, muscles, tendons, ligaments, arteries, or joints. Deep somatic pain may also cause autonomic reactions such as sweating, pallor, nausea, and syncope. The internal organs of the cardiovascular, hematological, pulmonary, digestive, urogenital, endocrine, and reproductive systems can produce *visceral* pain. Visceral pain receptors (*nociceptors*) relay a diffuse signal and referred pain to associated dermatomes, as shown in Figure 13-4 (see Chapter 13), or may produce a deep, gnawing ache in the thorax or abdomen.

Table 1-11. Components of the Physical Examination		
Inspection/observation	Neurological exam	Percussion
Vital signs	Smell/odor	Auscultation
Palpation		

PHYSICAL EXAMINATION TECHNIQUES: DIFFERENTIATING NORMAL AND ABNORMAL RESPONSES

Physical examination for systemic pathology has several components (Table 1-11). The physical examination is modified according to suspected pathogenesis, the patient's symptoms, and the urgency of the patient's condition.

Inspection

Inspection involves observing general appearance, eyes, skin, hair, fingernails, obvious deformities, use of assistive devices or supports, behavior, gait, and coordination. Many systemic conditions cause "classic" signs that can be readily observed. It is imperative that these be observed during the entire examination as patients are best observed in their natural state. At times, patients may change their appearance if they feel they are being observed.

Vital Signs

The *vital signs* are heart rate, respiration rate, blood pressure, and body temperature. Vital signs should be assessed in emergencies and when systemic symptoms are reported (see Table 1-7). If a patient's medical history includes hypertension, cardiac pathology, recent infection, chronic illness, or cancer, vital signs should be recorded as an indicator of present health status and to provide a baseline to monitor health status throughout treatment. The common changes in vital signs that might be found with specific injuries and illnesses are discussed throughout this book. In addition, there are other vital signs that can be recorded, including height, weight, body mass index, and oxygen saturation. In some cases, pain scale is also considered a vital sign. This is important to note as these are recorded during preparticipation physicals and in certain disease states (as discussed in various chapters in this book).

Percussion and Palpation

Percussion (striking to cause vibration) over bones may increase the pain of a fracture or bone tumor. Percussion over the abdomen vibrates the internal organs, which increases pain if they are injured or inflamed. Percussion over the thorax can reveal side-to-side differences that might suggest specific pathology (accumulation of fluid or punctured lung). Superficial *palpation* (manual touch) can assess the temperature, texture, moisture, and turgidity (stiffness) of the skin and is used to examine lymph nodes and vascular pulses. Detection of abnormal masses, abdominal rigidity (see Chapter 8), and tenderness is achieved through deep palpation. Chapters 6 and 7 describe percussion and palpation techniques in more detail.

Auscultation

Auscultation is typically performed with a stethoscope to examine cardiac, pulmonary, vascular, abdominal, and bowel sounds. Specific auscultation techniques will be discussed in Chapters 6, 7, and 8. Of note, during your observation of the patient, the clinician may also hear sounds without the stethoscope that may give clues to the diagnosis.

Smell

Unusual odor of the breath or perspiration suggests exhalation of metabolic substances, which can indicate disease, poisoning, or drug abuse. Foul-smelling sputum or other body fluids can indicate infection or endocrine malfunction.

Neurological Screening Examination

Any patient reporting radiating pain, sensory abnormalities, weakness, or recent head injury should receive a neurological screening examination of the cranial nerves, reflexes, sensation, and motor function.

Cranial Nerves and Reflexes

Cranial nerves control smell, vision and eye control, hearing, swallowing, facial sensation and motor control, and tongue control. Cranial nerve tests are reviewed in Chapter 13.

The *deep tendon reflexes* that can be clinically tested include biceps (C5), brachioradialis (C6), triceps (C7), patella (L4), and ankle (S1).[9] The *Babinski sign* is an abnormal reflex that appears when the motor tracts from the brain to the limbs are disrupted, which occurs with spinal cord injury or a severe head injury.

Sensory Testing

Sensation should be tested bilaterally along dermatomal and peripheral nerve distributions. Light touch, which is transmitted to the brain through neural pathways on both sides of the spinal cord, is tested first. If sensation of light touch is impaired, sharp (or temperature) sensation and vibration tests should be performed. Sharp sensation tests the spinal cord columns opposite (contralateral) to the limb being tested and is assessed with a sharp object such as a pin. Vibration sense tests spinal cord columns on the same (ipsilateral) side and is assessed using a tuning fork. Two-point discrimination testing may be useful in dermatomes that are less sensitive to light touch to help differentiate nerve injuries.

Motor Testing

Manual muscle tests may differentiate between *myotomal* (nerve root), peripheral nerve, or muscle lesions. Injured or inflamed nerve roots result in weakness in all the muscles that they innervate. Peripheral nerve damage affects the specific muscles supplied by that nerve, whereas traumatic muscle injuries weaken only one muscle. Nerve injuries may not cause significant pain, but do cause substantial weakness. Muscle injuries usually cause both weakness and pain. Injuries and illnesses involving the nervous system are discussed in Chapter 13.

DIFFERENTIATION OF SIGNS AND SYMPTOMS

This section presents a basic scheme for triage, differentiating a medical emergency from less severe illnesses, and differentiating musculoskeletal injury from systemic illness or disease. Conditions or situations that constitute a medical emergency are reviewed first. These conditions determine the clinical course of action (activating emergency medical services) and thus supersede the need to differentiate the system of origin. It next provides an approach to evaluating illness or

Table 1-12. Medical Emergencies: Immediately Activate Emergency Medical Services

CONDITION	SIGNS AND SYMPTOMS	MANAGEMENT (AFTER ACTIVATING EMS)
Rapid changes (within minutes) in vital signs	Significant changes in blood pressure, heart rate, respiration rate, body temperature	Monitor circulation, airway, breathing (circulation, airway, breathing [CAB]), monitor vital signs
Shock	Systolic blood pressure < 90 mm Hg, tachycardia and hyperpnea, pallor, diaphoresis, cyanosis, altered cognition, lethargy	Elevate feet, CAB, monitor vital signs
Nontraumatic syncope or loss of consciousness	Complete loss of consciousness lasting more than 30 seconds	CAB, monitor vital signs, mental and neurological tests if wakens (urgent referral if reported by subject but not observed by examiner)
Profuse bleeding or bleeding from mucous membranes or orifices	Uncontrolled bleeding that persists longer than 1 or 2 minutes	Treat for shock, apply pressure points if applicable
Abdominal rigidity or severe pain	Tenderness to palpation, unusual distention that is firm, palpable organs/mass	Assess for other systemic signs; monitor vital signs
Prolonged or unexplained severe vomiting or diarrhea	Accompanied by syncope, hematemesis, fever	Prevent dehydration, treat for shock, monitor vital signs
Seizure	No known history of epilepsy or previous seizure	Protect head, awakening and breathing coordination, remove to quiet area after seizure

injury by the relative seriousness of the condition. Last, several tables list conditions of the various organ systems that may produce signs and symptoms similar to musculoskeletal conditions.

MEDICAL EMERGENCY

Several conditions, listed in Table 1-12, constitute a medical emergency, thus requiring emergency medical services (EMS) and immediate transport to a medical facility. Delay of appropriate treatment may cause permanent tissue damage, disability, or death. The role of the athletic trainer in these situations, after recognizing the emergency, is to provide life support or basic first aid until EMS arrives. Monitoring vital signs, treating for shock, splinting suspected fractures, and controlling severe bleeding are examples of appropriate actions once EMS is activated. Noting the time of

Table 1-13. Symptoms Requiring Urgent Referral to a Physician: "Red Flags"

Constant or refractory pain	Unexplained weight loss	Pulsating or severe cramping pain (colic)
Heart palpitations/flutter	Insomnia	Difficult or painful urination
Fainting (syncope)	Inability to tolerate oral intake of food or liquid	Blood or red color in urine
Night pain or night sweats	Incapacitating pain	Severe or progressive dizziness
Difficult or painful swallowing	Severe dyspnea	Malaise, fatigue
Visual problems	Recurrent nausea, vomiting	New onset headaches

Table 1-14. Psychological Red Flags

Disorientation	Permanent or rapidly alternating changes in affect (mood)	Violent behavior
Debilitating apathy or lethargy		Confusion
Sudden cognitive deficit	Behavior is dangerous to themselves or others	Antisocial or avoidance behavior
Acquired memory deficit	Hallucination	Expressive aphasia
	Severe agitation	

Require urgent (within 1 day) or emergency medical referral.

the incident and any known mechanism or circumstances of the injury may also be useful to EMS and medical personnel. A facility or institution's written emergency action plans should be established and reviewed regularly by the athletic training staff and other personnel.

Red Flags

Certain signs and symptoms alert the athletic trainer to serious pathology (Table 1-13). These "red flags" require immediate medical attention. Some red flags are obvious emergencies, but others, such as recurrent fevers, night pain, malaise, and unexplained weight loss, may be discovered during the medical history. Symptoms that are poorly localized, have no known incident associated with their onset, have been relentlessly worsening over time, and are unresponsive to treatment are unlikely to be caused by a musculoskeletal condition. Table 1-14 lists psychological red flags that require urgent medical evaluation.

EVALUATING SERIOUSNESS OF CONDITION

This section presents a framework for triage assessment to determine the relative severity of a condition, thus facilitating clinical decision making (ie, referral to emergency, urgent, or standard/routine medical care). The section is organized from most to least serious situation and assumes the medical emergencies in Table 1-12 have been excluded during the primary assessment. Table 1-15 summarizes the assessment process when determining the seriousness of the condition.

The first and most serious pathological signs are abnormalities of the major life-sustaining functions, such as breathing and maintaining circulation. Heart rate, respiration rate, blood pressure, or body temperature (vital signs) outside the normal ranges, either high or low (Table 1-16),

Table 1-15. Hierarchy of Assessment in Descending Order of Seriousness/Urgency of Condition

1. VITAL SIGNS	Changes in heart rate, respiration rate, blood pressure, body temperature
2. BRAINSTEM AND NEUROMOTOR	Smell, vision, hearing, taste, swallowing, speech, tactile sensation, reflexes, coordination, balance
3. ENDOCRINE AND METABOLIC	Dehydration, lethargy, fatigue, altered cognition, edema, loss or gain in body weight
4. DAILY FUNCTIONS	Sleep, eating, urination, defecation, sexual function

Table 1-16. Abnormally High and Low Values for Vital Signs in Adults

VITAL SIGN	HIGH	NORMAL	LOW
Heart rate (at rest)	> 100 bpm	60 to 100 bpm	< 60 bpm
Respiration rate (at rest)	> 20 breaths/min	12 to 20 breaths/min	< 12 breaths/min
Blood pressure	> 130 systolic > 85 diastolic	90 to 130 systolic 60 to 85 diastolic	< 90 systolic < 60 diastolic
Body temperature	> 100.4°F (38°C)	97°F to 99°F (36.1°C to 37.2°C)	< 96°F (35.5°C)
bpm = beats per minute.			

require prompt medical referral. Baseline preseason values should be documented during preparticipation examination for athletes. Significant changes from these baseline values demand medical explanation. Noticeable changes (ie, steady increase or decrease) over several minutes or hours may indicate rapidly progressing pathology. Many pathological conditions eventually affect these vital body functions, making them useful indicators of potentially serious pathology.

Next, evaluation of brainstem (smell, vision, facial sensation and movement, hearing, taste, speech, and swallowing) and neurological function (reflexes, coordination, ataxia, balance, sensation) is conducted. The brain and nervous system, like the heart and lungs, are very sensitive to changes in the internal environment of the body. Thus, impairment of neurological status usually indicates a significant pathological process. Furthermore, the neurological system allows perception and interaction with the environment. If these functions are impaired, the person may be unable to walk, drive, or perform other tasks safely. Rapid changes (minutes to hours) in neurological function suggests a serious medical condition.

At the next level of severity, signs of endocrine or metabolic disorders are often subtle and therefore require careful examination. Fortunately, most endocrine-metabolic conditions develop more slowly than cardiopulmonary or neurological disorders. Potential indicators include gradual and unexplained changes in body temperature, signs of dehydration (dry tongue, decreased skin turgor, tachycardia, postural hypotension), lethargy or fatigue, altered cognition, peripheral neuropathies (sensory or motor, usually bilaterally distributed), presence of edema, or a greater than 3-5% loss or gain in body weight. Certain metabolic conditions constitute a medical emergency,

Table 1-17. Cardiovascular and Pulmonary Disorders

CONDITION	CONFOUNDING SYMPTOM[a]	DIFFERENTIATING SIGNS AND SYMPTOMS
Cardiac ischemia or valve stenosis	Left arm pain	Chest pain that worsens with activity; dyspnea, diaphoresis, or syncope; over age 35 years
Sickle cell anemia	Leg pain	Abdominal pain, enlarged abdominal organs, nosebleeds, fever, headache; Black male
Thoracic outlet syndrome or vascular occlusive disorder	Arm (or leg) pain	Pain worsens during activity and is relieved by rest; edema, paresthesia, fatigue in limb with exercise, distal cyanosis
Aortic aneurysm	Sudden severe or intermittent moderate back pain	Pain with mild activity or at rest; palpable, pulsating mass in abdomen; auscultated bruit in abdomen; nausea, cough, or paresthesia
Pneumothorax	Back or trunk pain	History of chest trauma, chest pain, severe dyspnea, tachypnea, hyperresonance upon percussion of thorax, absent breath sounds
Spleen injury	Left shoulder pain (Kehr's sign)	Painful or rigid LUQ to palpation, nausea, history of left thorax or abdominal trauma

[a] "confounding symptom" is one that may be confused with a musculoskeletal injury or condition. LUQ = left upper abdominal quadrant.

such as diabetic ketoacidosis (see Chapter 10), but most develop slowly over several days. However, if untreated, the long-term health consequences can be debilitating and permanent.

Last, changes in the regulation or pattern of "normal" day-to-day functions, such as sleep (insomnia, hypersomnia, or frequent sleep disruption), eating (loss of appetite or sudden polyphagia), urination or defecation (frequency and volume), and social and sexual functioning are yet more subtle and difficult to detect. A pathological condition, if serious enough, affects daily life. These effects may be the earliest indicators of a slowly developing chronic disease (eg, cancer, degenerative neurological disorders), but are difficult to observe because of their insidious and personal nature. A careful medical history is required to obtain this information accurately. Any change in these activities that a patient mentions is significant, particularly if accompanied by other systemic signs and symptoms.

Tables 1-17 through 1-21 list pathological conditions by organ system that present signs or symptoms similar to musculoskeletal conditions. Table 1-22 provides possible pathology by body region of symptoms, which could lead to confusion when differentiating musculoskeletal from systemic conditions.

Table 1-18. Gastrointestinal and Hepatic Disorders

CONDITION	CONFOUNDING SYMPTOM[a]	DIFFERENTIATING SIGNS AND SYMPTOMS
Peptic ulcer	Thoracic, chest, or neck pain	Pain changes after eating, pain worse at night, loss of appetite or vomiting may occur; history of NSAID use, alcohol abuse, tobacco use, caffeine use, or psychological stress
Appendicitis	Back or right hip pain	Progressive worsening of condition, nausea, may have fever or fatigue, rebound tenderness of RLQ, decreased appetite,
Hernia	Anterior hip or thigh pain	Pain worse with activity, Valsalva maneuver, or certain postures; tenderness or palpable mass at inguinal or femoral canal
Liver injury	Right shoulder pain	Painful or rigid RUQ to palpation, nausea, vomiting, history of right trauma to thorax or abdomen
Gallstones (cholelithiasis)	Right shoulder pain	Painful or rigid RUQ to palpation, nausea, vomiting, history of intolerance to fatty foods

[a] "confounding symptom" is one that may be confused with a musculoskeletal injury or condition.

NSAID = nonsteroidal anti-inflammatory drug; RLQ = right lower abdominal quadrant; RUQ = right upper abdominal quadrant.

SUMMARY

Athletic trainers use clinical reasoning and clinical decision making to evaluate possible pathogenesis. This process includes taking an appropriate medical history, evaluating symptom patterns, and performing a focused physical examination. The medical history provides information regarding the onset, nature, and course of the condition. The physical examination tests for signs that confirm the history and reported symptoms and completes the clinical presentation. The goal of the examination process is to determine the patient's likely diagnosis—the medical condition that is causing the patient's symptoms.

Table 1-19. Renal, Urogenital, and Endocrine Disorders

CONDITION	CONFOUNDING SYMPTOM[a]	DIFFERENTIATING SIGNS AND SYMPTOMS
Kidney injury	Back or flank pain	History of trauma to abdomen or back, hematuria, painful percussion at CVA, edema of flank
Kidney stone (urolithiasis)	Back or groin pain	Nausea and vomiting, pallor, tachycardia, stable vital signs, positive family history
Prostatitis	Back pain	Pain unchanged by posture; nocturia, increased urgency and frequency of urination, difficulty initiating urine stream, male over age 50 years
Endometriosis	Back pain	Painful and heavy menstruation, painful sexual intercourse, female over age 30 years
Pregnancy	Back (or joint) pain	Amenorrhea, abdominal pain, recurrent nausea, weight gain, distal extremity edema, female beyond menarche; shock if ruptured ectopic pregnancy
Endocrine disorders	Widespread myalgia and arthralgia (depending on gland and hormone affected)	Weakness and atrophy, spasms, tachycardia/bradycardia, fatigue, paresthesias, dry or diaphoretic skin, slow healing

[a] "confounding symptom" is one that may be confused with a musculoskeletal injury or condition.

CVA = costovertebral angle.

Table 1-20. Neurological and Psychological Disorders

CONDITION	CONFOUNDING SYMPTOM[a]	DIFFERENTIATING SIGNS AND SYMPTOMS
Spina bifida occulta	Back pain	Patch of hair over spine, absent spinous process on palpation, normal neurological tests
Multiple sclerosis	Weakness or incoordination	Intermittent sensory and reflex changes, visual disturbance, unusual fatigue (particularly in heat); over age 20 years
Reflex sympathetic dystrophy	Severe localized pain	History of injury with joint immobilization, edema, decreased range of motion, skin and nail changes, increased skin temperature
Amyotrophic lateral sclerosis	Weakness	Bilaterally symmetric weakness, hyperactive reflexes, over age 30
Guillain-Barré syndrome	Leg and back weakness and pain	Rapid progression (hours), headache, fever, history of recent viral infection, loss of reflexes
Myasthenia gravis	Sudden severe muscle fatigue	Rapid progression (hours), diplopia, dysarthria, dysphagia, dyspnea, normal reflexes; over age 20 years
Muscular dystrophy	Hip and shoulder weakness	Slowly progressive (years), frequent falls, difficulty rising from ground or with stairs, waddling gait; age 8 to 12 years at onset
Child abuse	Multiple skin wounds, frequent unexplained injury, or multiple injuries in various stages of healing	Inconsistent or unreasonable history of injury, behavioral problems, difficulty interacting with peers, avoidance behaviors by child and family, substance abuse in family

[a] "confounding symptom" is one that may be confused with a musculoskeletal injury or condition.

Table 1-21. Infections, Immune Disorders, and Cancer

CONDITION	CONFOUNDING SYMPTOM[a]	DIFFERENTIATING SIGNS AND SYMPTOMS
Meningitis	Severe neck pain	Headache, fever, neck rigidity, history of recent URI, vomiting, skin rash on head, altered mental status, rapid progression (hours)
Septic arthrosis and osteomyelitis	Joint or localized bone pain	Signs of acute inflammation, history of recent injury or surgery in the body region, fever (osteomyelitis), rapid progression (septic arthrosis)
RA/JRA	Bilateral hand or foot pain	Mild inflammation of affected joints, morning stiffness; adolescent age (JRA)
Urogenital cancers	Back or hip pain	Mild systemic signs, abdominal pain, abnormal urinary or sexual function (or menstruation in females); palpable mass (testicular or breast), testicular, male 15 to 35 years; prostate male over 50 years; cervical, ovarian, uterine female over 45 years; breast female over 45 years
Lung cancer	Shoulder, arm, or neck pain	History of smoking, dyspnea, hemoptysis, pneumonia, over age 35 years
Leukemia or lymphoma	Deep bone pain	Frequent bleeding episodes, systemic signs, recurrent infection, anemia, lymphadenopathy, vomiting; most over age 10 years
Bone cancers	Dull, aching bone pain or tender bone mass	Impaired or painful joint function, signs of local inflammation, or systemic signs

[a] "confounding symptom" is one that may be confused with a musculoskeletal injury or condition.

JRA = juvenile rheumatoid arthritis; RA = rheumatoid arthritis; URI = upper respiratory infection.

Table 1-22. Possible Systemic Pathology by Body Region

LOCATION OF SYMPTOMS	POSSIBLE SYSTEMIC PATHOLOGY
Arm pain (left)	Cardiac ischemia, spleen injury, lung cancer
Arm pain (right)	Liver injury, gallbladder disorder, lung cancer
Leg or groin pain	Sickle-cell anemia, appendicitis (right hip), hernia
Back or thoracic pain	Aortic aneurysm, pneumothorax, peptic ulcer, appendicitis, kidney disorder, prostatitis, endometriosis, pregnancy, spina bifida occulta, urogenital cancer
Neck pain	Meningitis, lung cancer
Multiple joints or sites	Endocrine disorder, child (or domestic) abuse, rheumatoid arthritis
Weakness or fatigue	Multiple sclerosis, amyotrophic lateral sclerosis, Guillain-Barré syndrome, myasthenia gravis, muscular dystrophy

References

1. National Athletic Trainers' Association. *Athletic Training Education Competencies*. 5th ed. The Commission on Accreditation of Athletic Training Education; 2011.
2. Hensyl WR, ed. *Stedman's Pocket Medical Dictionary*. Williams & Wilkins; 1987.
3. Prentice WE. *Arnheim's Principles of Athletic Training: A Competency-Based Approach*. 14th ed. McGraw Hill; 2010.
4. Anderson MK, Parr GP, Hall SJ. *Foundations of Athletic Training: Prevention, Assessment, and Management*. 4th ed. Lippincott, Williams & Wilkins; 2009.
5. Board of Certification. *Role Delineation Study/Practice Analysis*. 6th ed. Board of Certification for the Athletic Trainer; 2010.
6. LeBlond RF, Brown DD, DeGowin RL. *DeGowin's Diagnostic Examination*. 9th ed. McGraw Hill; 2009.
7. Bickley LS, Szilagyi PG. *Bates' Guide to Physical Examination and History Taking*. 10th ed. Lippincott, Williams & Wilkins; 2009.
8. American Academy of Family Physicians, American Academy of Pediatrics, American Medical Society for Sports Medicine, American Orthopaedic Society for Sports Medicine, American Osteopathic Academy of Sports Medicine. *PPE Preparticipation Physical Evaluation*. 5th ed. McGraw Hill; 2019.
9. Hoppenfeld S. *Physical Examination of the Spine and Extremities*. Appleton & Lange; 1976.

Online Resource

◊ **Medline Plus (U.S. National Library of Medicine, National Institutes of Health)**

  ¤ http://www.nlm.nih.gov/medlineplus/

CHAPTER 2

Pathophysiology

CHAPTER OUTLINE AND OBJECTIVES

Introduction

◊ Explain the concept of homeostasis.
  ¤ Homeostasis
  ¤ Pathophysiology
◊ Describe cellular components and their functions.
◊ Describe cellular adaptations to disease.
  ¤ The Cell
  ¤ Tissue Healing
◊ Discuss the inflammatory process.
  ¤ Inflammation
  ¤ Infection

Cellular Physiology and Pathophysiology: Response to Cell Damage

◊ Explain tissue responses to disease.
◊ Review pathophysiology by tissue type.
  ¤ Bone
  ¤ Connective Tissue, Epithelium, and Endothelium
  ¤ Muscle and Nerve
  ¤ Specialized Cells and Tissues

Summary

Online Resources

Bhojani RA, O'Connor DP, Fincher AL. *Clinical Pathology for Athletic Trainers: Recognizing Systemic Disease, Fourth Edition* (pp 23-34).
© 2022 Taylor & Francis Group.

This chapter addresses the following knowledge and skills from the *Athletic Training Education Competencies, Fifth Edition*[1]:

Content Area	Competency #
Clinical Examination and Diagnosis (CE)	1, 2
Therapeutic Interventions (TI)	1, 5

INTRODUCTION

This chapter reviews normal physiology and introduces the concepts of *pathophysiology*, physiology related to disease. Basic physiology provides a basis for discussion in subsequent chapters. This chapter is not intended to replace more extensive formal study of cell structure and physiology. Many excellent clinical physiology and pathophysiology textbooks are available for greater detail.[2-5]

Homeostasis

Homeostasis is the control of biochemical equilibrium within the body. Many physiological processes are always active to regulate fluid, chemical, and energy balance in the cells, tissues, organs, and systems. This biological balance is dynamic, constantly responding to changes in the internal and external environment. For example, blood glucose concentration increases immediately after eating a meal. In response, cells in the pancreas release insulin, a hormone that helps to move glucose from the blood into the liver and muscles. Once blood glucose concentration has returned to normal, the pancreas stops releasing insulin, which prevents blood glucose concentration from becoming too low. These types of stimulus-response cycles are necessary in all major organ systems to maintain health.

The healthy state can vary somewhat depending on the individual. Thus, "normal," or reference values for physiological indicators, such as blood test results and vital signs, are described as a range of values that depends on age, gender, and other factors. A healthy person's values would be expected to be within this range, and deviation of a person's values outside the reference range may indicate injury or illness. However, a person's values may exceed this range as an adaptation to stress to maintain organ-system function and health. For instance, people living at a high altitude have more red blood cells in circulation as an adaptation to the lower concentration of atmospheric oxygen. This adaptation allows the blood to hold an adequate amount of oxygen for physiological functioning. Athletic trainers should understand the reference ranges and consult their physicians if there are changes in the patient's values.

Pathophysiology

Many diseases disrupt homeostasis, causing deviation from the balanced biochemical state. Pathophysiology is a term that describes the cellular mechanisms of disease and their functional systemic consequences.[2] Signs and symptoms are a result of the functional systemic consequences of pathology. Understanding the healthy physiology of the body's organ systems assists in the discussion of the effects of disease as variance from the healthy state. Study of physiology begins with the basic unit of the body's tissues: the cell.

The Cell

All living cells contain typical structures, including cytoplasm, a nucleus, lysosomes, mitochondria, and a cell membrane. Each structure serves a particular purpose (Table 2-1).[5]

Cells can be damaged by physical trauma, toxins, infection, genetic abnormalities, malnutrition, dehydration, hypoxia, or combinations of these factors.[2-4] Cell damage impairs one or more cell

Table 2-1. Cell Structures and Their Functions

STRUCTURE	FUNCTION
Nucleus	Contains the genetic material of the cell (DNA and RNA)
	Controls cell division and synthesis of protein
Cytoplasm	Provides fluid internal environment of the cell
	Supports all internal cell structures
Lysosomes	Contains catabolic enzymes within the cell
	Disposes cell waste and foreign substances
Mitochondria	Converts carbohydrate, protein, and fat to energy
Cell membrane	A complex, semipermeable phospholipid and protein structure
	Provides the physical border of the cell
	Allows and prevents exchange of molecules and other substances between the internal and external environment of the cell

structures, which affects the respective tissue and organ function, which in turn can affect function of the associated system(s). Cells in other tissues and organs can be affected as the effects spread to surrounding tissues, thus disrupting homeostasis. Some effects of cell damage initiate tissue, organ, and systemic responses that attempt to limit the disease process, to initiate cell repair, and to restore homeostasis.

Once cell damage occurs, the cell either adapts by healing, altering its structure/function, or it dies. Adaptation and repair can occur if the nucleus' function is maintained.[2-4] Extreme adaptations may affect the function of the cell to the extent that they cause subsequent problems in the tissue or organ. Cells may also respond to environmental influences and effects by adapting before cell damage occurs.

Cells adapt in several ways.[2] Cells may shrink and become less active in response to decreased metabolic demands, a process called *atrophy*. Cells may also grow and become more active in response to increased demands, which is called *hypertrophy*. Atrophy is generally caused by disuse due to injury, immobilization, or by impaired cellular metabolism such as malnutrition. Some aspects of aging are due to atrophic cellular adaptation caused by multiple factors, including cell damage caused by exposure to metabolic and environmental toxins over a lifetime. Conversely, hypertrophy increases cell size as an adaptation to chronically increased metabolic or physical demands, such as occurs in muscle tissue with resistance training.

Cells may also adapt by changing their number, type, or morphology (structure). *Hyperplasia* is an increase in the number of cells in a tissue without a change in the rate of cell division or cell function. Hyperplasia occurs as an adaptation to increased metabolic demands, genetic abnormalities, or hormonal imbalances. *Metaplasia* is a replacement of cells of one type by cells of another type, often in response to physical or chemical irritants. These "new" cells do not display changes in rate of division or function, but they may change the relative proportion of one cell type to another within a particular tissue.

When cellular adaptation causes a change into an abnormal cell type that has an increased rate of division, resulting in increased cell numbers, the process is called *dysplasia*. Formation of neoplasms or tumors involves dysplasia. Malignant dysplasia produces neoplasms in a process called *cancer* (rapid proliferation of undifferentiated, non-specific cell types).

Early cell death, or *necrosis*, occurs when cell resources cannot meet the metabolic (ie, oxygen and energy) demands of the nucleus. Necrosis is distinct from *apoptosis*, the process of naturally occurring cell death that occurs at a controlled rate in many tissues (usually programmed within the cell structure). A large number of necrotic cells impair organ function and disable the associated body system, potentially leading to disease or death of the organ.

Most typical cellular adaptations, such as callus formation (hyperplasia) or menstruation (hyperplasia and metaplasia), are temporary physiological responses to maintain homeostasis. Other adaptations to cell damage produce general chemical and physical responses to stimulate repair of tissue structure and function. An example of such a general response is inflammation, discussed later. Other normal and abnormal effects are caused by tissue-specific adaptations, such as the hypertrophy of muscle tissue when regularly exposed to load. When these general and specific effects become pathological and impair organ function, they cause signs and symptoms in the respective system.

Tissue Healing

Damaged tissue is capable of healing in one of 2 ways. First, organ and tissue cells may be regenerated, essentially rebuilding the injured tissue. Second, the damaged cells may be replaced by connective tissue, a process that forms a scar. Scarred tissue may restore structural integrity to the organ but does not function like the original tissue. If a significant amount of scarring occurs, the function of the organ may be permanently impaired. Scarring occurs in response to cellular damage in tissues and organs that cannot regenerate functional cells.

Tissue healing generally progresses in 3 stages: inflammatory, proliferative, and remodeling. The time course of each stage varies by tissue type (Table 2-2). The *inflammatory phase* begins at the moment of tissue injury and includes a vascular response and a cellular response. The vascular response, called *hemostasis*, involves immediate vasoconstriction and platelet activation to control blood loss. After a period of vasoconstriction, the vessels dilate and become more permeable. This permeability allows plasma and other blood compounds to exit the vessel and enter the damaged tissue, causing edema. Some of these compounds are also signals to initiate the cellular response during which various types of white blood cells move into the area to remove bacteria and dead cells. Some of these cells also release growth factors that stimulate cell growth, stimulate revascularization, and attract cells called fibroblasts that function in the proliferative stage. The inflammatory phase typically lasts only days after injury but can be prolonged as long as cells continue to undergo damage.

The *proliferative stage* serves to close the tissue wound. Fibroblasts secrete collagen, a complex protein that binds to itself and other structures to create a scar. In some tissues, the scar eventually becomes vascularized and new functional tissue cells are regenerated beginning at the periphery of the injured region. Fibroblasts continue to secrete collagen until the wound is closed, which may take several weeks. The deposition of collagen stimulates the third stage of tissue healing: remodeling. During this phase, patients may be allowed to start range of motion activities and progress to strengthening.

The *remodeling stage* overlaps with the proliferative stage, and some tissue remodeling occurs while collagen is still being deposited. Remodeling involves a continuous process of simultaneous breakdown and redeposition of collagen. This allows the final collagen structure to form in response to forces experienced by the tissue during this stage. The remodeling stage stops when the structure is restored, although the tissue strength typically does not return to its normal, uninjured state. In tissues that are able to regenerate new functional cells, remodeling involves the creation of the new tissue and restoration of organ function. The remodeling stage continues for many months until the integrity and function of the tissue and organ are restored. Clinicians, as seen in Table 2-2, typically allow patients to return to activity during the remodeling phase.

Table 2-2. Stages of Healing, Associated Time Frames, and Treatment by Tissue Type

TISSUE	STAGE	TIME	TREATMENT OR ACTION
Ligament	Inflammatory	48 to 72 hours	Protect; splint in approximation
	Proliferative	6 to 8 weeks	Active mobilization within limits and activity
	Remodeling	12 to 30 months	Activity as tolerated
Tendon	Inflammatory	48 to 72 hours	Protect; splint in approximation
	Proliferative	4 to 6 weeks	Active and passive mobilization within limits
	Remodeling	12 to 20 weeks	Strengthening and activity as tolerated
Muscle	Inflammatory	48 to 72 hours	Protect; gentle passive or active-assisted mobilization
	Proliferative	4 to 8 weeks	Active muscle recruitment, passive mobilization
	Remodeling	12 weeks	Strengthening and accommodation to load
Bone	Inflammatory	48 to 72 hours	Strict immobilization or surgical fixation; approximation is critical
	Proliferative	3 to 6 weeks[a]	Continue immobilization or fixation until union (or longer), then begin gentle range of motion (no-load bearing)
	Remodeling	6 to 24 weeks[b]	After consolidation, begin load-bearing activity as tolerated
Articular cartilage	Inflammatory	48 to 72 hours	Weight bearing as tolerated; maintain muscular function
	Proliferative	6 months	Controlled weight-bearing activity to stimulate fibrocartilage.
	Remodeling	2 years	Activity as tolerated
Nerve	Inflammatory	2 to 7 days	Medical evaluation; splinting may be needed to stabilize
	Proliferative	1 inch per month	Monitor; periodic sensory and motor testing
	Remodeling	Up to 1 year	Return to normal use; may need strengthening or other therapy

[a] Time for union, not for callus formation or consolidation. The lower extremity generally takes twice as long as the upper extremity.

[b] Time for hard callus formation and consolidation; lower extremity bones generally take twice as long.

Inflammation

Every tissue of the body responds to cellular injury or infection with inflammation. The inflammatory response may be limited only to the affected tissue, producing localized symptoms, or be generalized, causing the systemic symptoms described in Chapter 1. Consequently, diseases of many organ systems can cause similar systemic signs and symptoms, making diagnosis more challenging.

Acute Inflammation

Damaged cells release chemicals (eg, histamine, bradykinin, prostaglandins) that cause local capillaries to dilate and become more permeable. This reaction increases blood flow to the area and allows proteins and plasma fluid to enter the *interstitial space*, the space between cells. Proteins in the blood interact with fibrin and begin to form a collagen clot at the damaged site. The chemicals released by the damaged cells also attract *leukocytes* from the blood. Some leukocytes act as phagocytes and others prolong the inflammatory response. *Phagocytes* dissolve and absorb damaged cell structures, invading microbes, and other debris.

As inflammation continues, excess interstitial fluid causes tissue pressure to increase relative to pressure in the nearby capillaries. Blood flow in the area consequently decreases, producing ischemic damage in otherwise healthy cells and increasing tissue damage. This ischemic secondary tissue damage is greatest near the site of primary cell injury.

These mechanisms cause the characteristic signs and symptoms of inflammation. Pain results from tissue damage (primary and secondary), the inflammatory chemicals, and ischemia. Swelling, erythema (redness), and heat are effects of increased regional blood flow and plasma fluid in the interstitial space. *Ecchymosis* (dark red, blue, or black discoloration) from red blood cells in the tissues may occur. Pain causes local muscle spasm to guard the damaged tissue, thus causing loss of movement and function. The acute phase of inflammation somewhat depends on the extent of cellular damage, but generally lasts from 48 to 72 hours.

Chronic Inflammation

Chronic inflammation, which also can occur in any tissue, is usually a result of long-term chemical irritation or mechanical stress. Chronic inflammation is destructive to the cells and tissues because the chemical action and leukocyte activity is prolonged. In addition, chronic inflammation produces more fibrin and collagen to protect the undamaged tissue or isolate the offending substance. Thus, chronic inflammation can prevent or inhibit tissue healing.

The signs and symptoms of chronic inflammation are the same as acute inflammation, but less intense. Chronic inflammation produces aching pain, pitting edema, mild to moderate muscle spasms, and increased local tissue temperature. Chronic inflammation persists until the cause of cellular damage is removed.

Infection

The response to infection is essentially a specialized inflammatory response. Cell damage caused by the infectious organism causes inflammation. In addition, activation of the immune system in response to infection can also stimulate a generalized inflammatory response. This response is more widespread than occurs with a local tissue wound. Activated leukocytes in the blood affect neurons in the medulla, which causes an increase in body temperature. Involuntary shivering ("chills"), widespread vasoconstriction, and lying down and flexing the body all occur to increase body temperature to a new level. This process is called *fever*, and is defined as temperature greater than 100.4°F.

The presence of fever significantly increases metabolic demands. This causes *hyperpnea* (rapid respiration) and *tachycardia* (rapid heart rate), as well as *catabolism* (breakdown) of muscle and other tissues (except fat) to obtain energy. The effects of fever are unusual fatigue, *malaise* ("feeling bad"), weakness, and loss of appetite. Once the microorganism has been contained and/or eliminated, the fever "breaks." To reduce body temperature, the person exhibits *diaphoresis* (sweating), *lethargy* (extreme drowsiness), and extension of the body in supine. In addition, appetite returns to replace energy stores that were drained during the course of the fever. The duration of fever depends on the extent of infection and the type of infecting organism.

CELLULAR PHYSIOLOGY AND PATHOPHYSIOLOGY: RESPONSE TO CELL DAMAGE

Bone

Normal Morphology and Physiology

Bone provides a framework for the body, levers for muscle, and protection for internal organs (heart, lungs, kidneys, liver, spleen, brain, spinal cord). Mature bone cells are called *osteocytes*, which are produced by cells called *osteoblasts* and resorbed by cells called *osteoclasts*.[2] Bone tissue is being constantly resorbed and rebuilt, maintaining a homeostatic balance. When this balance is disrupted by pathology, bone mass and density can be affected. For example, in the disease process of osteoporosis more bone is resorbed than is rebuilt, resulting in an overall decrease in bone mass and density and, consequently, structural weakening of the bone. *Osteopenia* is the term used for this decrease in bone mass and density and can further deteriorate into osteoporosis. There are also diseases that cause the bone to lose its mineral content, which affects the mechanical properties of bone, or cause an excess growth of bone tissue. In each of these diseases, the normal homeostatic process has been disrupted, leading to deformity or injury in affected bones.

Each bone is covered by *periosteum*, an innervated and vascular structure that provides nutrition to the cortical (compact) bone. Cancellous bone has its own blood supply and contains the bone marrow, which is either yellow (fatty) or red. The red marrow, a critical organ, produces blood cells. In children, most bones contain red marrow, whereas adults have red marrow only in their flat bones (cranium, ribs, pelvis, vertebrae).

Bones articulate to form joints. Joint surfaces are covered with articular cartilage, which decreases the friction between the opposing bones. Articular cartilage is avascular, has no nervous supply, and has very few *chondrocytes* (living cartilage cells) within its tissue.

Pathological Processes

Fracture is physical damage to the structure of a bone and can occur across an entire bone, involving both cortical and cancellous bone, or can occur only in the cortical bone (eg, greenstick and stress fractures). A fracture that penetrates the skin, called a compound (open) fracture, is particularly prone to infection because the bone and other deep tissues are exposed to the environment. Bone infection causes osteomyelitis, an inflammation of bone and bone marrow (see Chapter 4), which destroys healthy bone cells and deforms the bone. Many genetic and metabolic abnormalities of bone, such as osteogenesis imperfecta and osteoporosis, can produce severe deformity and disability. Toxic damage, such as exposure to high-dosage radiation, is another possible source of pathology. Articular cartilage can be damaged by physical trauma (osteochondritis dissecans), inflammation (osteoarthritis, rheumatoid arthritis), or infection.

Response to Injury or Disease

Fractured bone can heal, given the appropriate environment: alignment and approximation of the bone fragments, stability, sterility, and nutrition. In fractured bone, the inflammatory stage includes bleeding (hematoma formation) and muscle guarding. The proliferative stage begins as the hematoma resolves and a fibrin clot forms; osteoblast activity increases to produce new bone cells. Fibrocartilage forms around the fracture and is then gradually replaced by a bony *callus*, or mass of osteocytes in various stages of formation. Once the bony callus is complete, the bone is stable and can bear weight. This process takes approximately 4 to 6 weeks in children and 8 to 12 weeks in adults.[2] The remodeling stage lasts for 1 to 2 years following the fracture as the bone remodels in response to the demands placed on it.

Bone infections heal by a similar mechanism once the infection is eliminated, which often involves surgical resection of necrotic tissue and stabilization with surgical implants. Some genetic and metabolic bone disorders, such as osteogenesis imperfecta or osteoporosis (see Chapter 9), may not allow bone to heal completely.

Articular cartilage has no blood supply. When damaged, it is either replaced by fibrocartilage, which is not as smooth, or not replaced at all. Because articular cartilage also has no nerve supply, pain does not occur unless the underlying (subchondral) bone or synovial tissue is involved. Articular cartilage injuries are relatively permanent, although function may be preserved with replacement by fibrocartilage. Articular cartilage injuries are usually accompanied by subtle joint instability and synovial (joint capsule) inflammation, a clinical syndrome known as arthritis. Significant damage to the articular cartilage, subchondral bone, and synovium may require surgical replacement with an artificial joint.

Connective Tissue, Epithelium, and Endothelium

Normal Morphology and Physiology

Connective tissue consists of collagen and elastin. Connective tissue attaches body structures, such as organs, bones, and muscles, to one another. A higher proportion of collagen indicates relatively greater tensile strength but less flexibility, whereas the opposite is true for a higher proportion of elastin. Connective tissue, although highly vascular and innervated, usually has only a few living cells interspersed in the tissue. There are several types of connective tissue.

Epithelium lines the interior and exterior surfaces of the body, including the skin, the gastrointestinal tract, and the pulmonary system. Epithelium provides a barrier to the external environment. Endothelium lines the cardiovascular system, including the heart, arteries, veins, and lymphatics. Endothelium regulates the exchange of substances between the blood and other organs, including nutrients, metabolic waste products, gases, infectious microorganisms, and toxins. Both epithelium and endothelium have several specialized cell subtypes and exist in various cell thicknesses throughout the body. The rate of replication for these cells is very high. Thus, as a function of homeostasis, relatively new cells are constantly replacing cells that may have been exposed to potentially toxic, infectious, or damaging substances. By constantly replacing cells that have been exposed to the environment, the body can protect itself by always presenting fresh cells as the first line of defense against potential pathogens.

Pathological Processes

Physical damage or infection can damage connective tissue cells. Metabolic diseases (eg, rheumatoid arthritis, gout, vasculitis) are also relatively common in connective tissue causing chronic inflammation, tissue destruction, and scarring. Epithelium and endothelium are prone to cancer and toxic damage because of their constant exposure to the environment (indirectly through the blood in the case of endothelium). Damage to epithelium or endothelium cells causes changes in tissue permeability, which either allow substances that usually do not enter the cell to enter or keep substances that usually move into the cell from doing so. This disruption in cellular exchange affects the function of the cell and the underlying organ, thus disrupting homeostasis.

Response to Injury or Disease

Connective, epithelial, and endothelial tissues follow the typical tissue healing stages previously outlined. Connective tissue heals with collagen only. Hence, any tissue that has elastin as a primary component loses flexibility after injury and healing. This effect may also interfere with normal organ

Table 2-3. Muscle Cell Types, Location, and Function

TYPE	BODY SYSTEM	FUNCTION
Skeletal	Musculoskeletal	Move the bones and body through space
Cardiac	Heart	Maintain blood flow to body
Smooth	Vascular and gastrointestinal	Move blood and food through the respective system

function. For instance, scarring in the abdomen following surgery can sometimes cause a stricture, or narrowing of the intestinal passageway, thus restricting the passage of food. Similarly, scarring in the connective tissues of the thorax may restrict chest expansion or gas exchange in the lungs.

Collagen scar tissue usually provides approximately the same tensile strength as the original connective tissue within 6 to 8 weeks, provided the optimal healing environment (nutrients and oxygen from the blood) is present and the tissue is protected from reinjury. Remodeling of the collagen tissue to arrange fiber alignment consistent with the original structure, however, may take 6 to 12 months. Since collagen aligns along lines of consistent tissue stretch, thus providing higher tensile strength, appropriate functional demands should be placed on the tissue through this period. Again, the elastic qualities of the tissue are not restored by the remodeled collagen, so the healed tissue's properties are somewhat different from the original tissue.

Injured epithelium and endothelium can be replaced with healthy, functional cells provided the damage does not extend through all cell layers and the DNA replication mechanism of the tissue is not impaired. The healing process takes a few days to close the wound, a few weeks to return to full strength, and several months to remodel completely. Function of the resulting scar depends on the extent of the injury. A larger injury, resulting in a larger scar, will have a greater impairment of tissue function. If all cell layers are damaged, the tissue is replaced by collagen scar (metaplasia). If the DNA replication mechanism is affected, a cancerous lesion forms (dysplasia). Replacement of living cells with inflexible collagen not only leads to possible restrictions or obstructions, as previously noted, but also causes the tissue to be nonpermeable, preventing normal cellular exchange. Cancerous changes can also cause obstructions and interfere with normal tissue function.

Muscle and Nerve

Normal Morphology and Physiology

Muscle tissue has 3 types: skeletal, cardiac, and smooth (Table 2-3). The principal function of muscle is contraction, which moves the skeleton, circulates the blood, or moves food through the bowels.

Nerve cells transmit electrical signals that are initiated by external or internal stimuli. These signals control the movement, cognitive, and regulatory systems of the body. Nerve cells within the brain and associated structures can be highly specialized, whereas the structure of nerve cells in the peripheral nervous system tends to be very similar to one another. All nerve cells contain a cell body, dendrites (projections that receive signals from other cells), and axons (projections that send signals to other cells). Chemical processes form the electrical impulses within (primarily via sodium ion exchanges) and between (via neurotransmitters) cells.

Pathological Processes

Skeletal muscle is most commonly affected by physical trauma (contusion or strain) or infection (eg, tetanus), although genetic and metabolic diseases also occur (eg, muscular dystrophy, myasthenia gravis). Cardiac and smooth muscle are more commonly affected by metabolic states (ischemia) and infection. Toxins can also affect the various types of muscle, nervous tissue, or the neuromuscular junction and interrupt function. Interruption of muscle function causes a loss of contraction; depending on the muscle type and location, the effect can be disabling (eg, skeletal muscle) or fatal (cardiac muscle).

Nerve cells are fragile and easily damaged by physical trauma, toxins, infections, and metabolic imbalances. Many pathological processes directly or indirectly affect the nervous system. Thus, signs of nervous system impairment are often early indications of systemic disease. In addition, some diseases affect the biochemical mechanisms that propagate electrical impulse. In such instances, cell structure is maintained although cell function is impaired. Loss of neural function implies a loss of the ability to propagate the electrical signal; the location and type of nerve determines the functional effects of nerve injury.

Response to Injury or Disease

The response of muscle cells to damage is similar to that of connective tissue. Damaged cells are replaced by collagen rather than normal contractile muscle tissue. Depending on the severity and extent of injury, a large noncontractile scar within a muscle can be disabling. If a relatively small proportion of skeletal muscle tissue is damaged, resistance training of the remaining muscle tissue can compensate for the loss of functional motor units. If a significant proportion of the smooth muscle of internal organs or cardiac muscle is damaged, severe impairment or complete loss of function occurs in the associated organ. Extensive damage to cardiac muscle can be fatal.

Damage to the cell body of a nerve cell is permanent. A nerve cell cannot be replaced or regenerated, resulting in permanent loss of the functions associated with that nerve cell. Damage to any portion of the nerve cell (dendrite, axon, or body) in the central nervous system (brain and spinal cord) is also permanent. However, if an axon is damaged in the peripheral nervous system, then it can regenerate provided the myelin (lipoprotein) sheath surrounding the axon is preserved. The axon first degenerates distal to the point of injury (a process called Wallerian degeneration) and then regenerates inside the myelin sheath at a rate of approximately one-quarter inch per month.

Specialized Cells and Tissues

Normal Morphology and Physiology

Cells of the blood, gastrointestinal system, liver, kidneys, and endocrine glands are highly specialized to perform specific tasks (Table 2-4). Most of the functions are integral to larger systems or to homeostasis in general. Thus, abnormal function in one of the systems usually affects one or more of the other systems and often produces the systemic signs described in Chapter 1.

Pathological Processes

Pathology of gastrointestinal, liver, or kidney cells can be caused by infection, metabolic changes, genetic abnormalities, or toxicity. Direct physical trauma can disrupt tissues and interfere with organ function. Blood cells can also be affected by infection, metabolic changes, or toxicity and can be indirectly affected by trauma to other tissues. Substantial tissue trauma may cause a loss of large amounts of blood from the vascular system, called *hemorrhage*. Hemorrhage has serious and potentially fatal consequences as organs, tissues, and cells become progressively deprived of blood-borne nutrients and oxygen, a process known as *shock*.

The signs of shock reflect the homeostatic effort to maintain blood pressure in the vascular system and blood flow to the internal organs. These signs include pallor (paleness) and cool ("clammy") skin as a result of peripheral vasoconstriction in an effort to preserve blood flow to the internal organs, *hypotension* (low blood pressure) as a result of low blood volume within the vascular system, and *tachycardia* (increased heart rate) in an effort to maintain blood flow to the organs. Shock can also be caused by a response to heart failure (decreasing systemic blood flow)

Table 2-4. Examples of Specialized Cell Types, Location, and Function

CELL TYPE	LOCATION	FUNCTION
Mucosa	Gastrointestinal	Absorb nutrients, secrete mucus for protection and enzymes for digestion
Acinar	Exocrine pancreas	Secrete digestive enzymes
Islet	Endocrine pancreas	Secrete glucagon (alpha cells) Secrete insulin (beta cells)
Hepatic	Liver	Secrete bile, store carbohydrate, form urea, metabolize cholesterol, lipids, and many drugs and toxins
Renal	Kidney	Regulate fluid, form urine
Endocrine	Endocrine glands	Secrete specific hormones

or widespread peripheral vasodilation (in response to autonomic nervous system action, systemic infection, or anaphylaxis).

Endocrine glands are rarely affected by trauma, but physical damage may occur with major injuries and diseases in surrounding organs. More commonly, genetic factors induce abnormal function or tumor development. Environmental factors also potentially affect endocrine function through toxicity. Tumors in the endocrine glands can either reduce or increase secretion of specific hormones, thus upsetting metabolic homeostasis. In addition, because hormones affect multiple organs, signs and symptoms may be produced in several systems.

Response to Injury or Disease

The tissues of the gastrointestinal organs, liver, and kidneys are highly vascularized and display a typical tissue healing response in reaction to cellular damage. The inflammatory response produces clinical signs that are specific to the functions of the affected organ or organs. Many of these cells have a limited ability to regenerate, but if chronic cell damage and inflammation persists, the damage becomes permanent and cells are replaced by scar tissue. With repeated, prolonged, or severe damage, the organs can no longer function properly and may restrict blood flow to surrounding healthy cells, thus propagating cell damage. Examples of this type of pathology include cirrhosis of the liver, chronic renal failure, and inflammatory bowel disease.

Blood Cells

The presence of infection, known as *septicemia*, or a toxin in the blood causes a vigorous inflammatory response throughout the body. The high fever produced in such a condition can destroy other tissues, posing a serious threat to homeostasis and life. The blood can also be affected by genetic diseases, including sickle cell anemia (misshapen red blood cells) and leukemia (proliferation of immature blood cells). These diseases also cause a mild or moderate general inflammatory response.

Summary

Pathophysiology refers to the biological process of disease. The mechanism called homeostasis responds to the changing internal and external environment to maintain chemical, fluid, and energy balances in the body. Many pathological conditions upset this equilibrium. Virtually all pathological processes can be expressed in terms of their effect on individual cells and the cellular effects on organ function. Cells can be damaged by physical, infective, metabolic, genetic, or environmental factors, causing them to either adapt or die. When enough cells die, organ functions are impaired. Inflammation and infection are general responses to cell damage. Each cell and tissue type also produces specific responses to damage. Signs and symptoms are due to these general and specific responses to cell damage.

References

1. National Athletic Trainers' Association. *Athletic Training Education Competencies.* 5th ed. The Commission on Accreditation of Athletic Training Education; 2011.
2. Gould BE, Dyer RM. *Pathophysiology for the Health-Related Professions.* 4th ed. Saunders Elsevier; 2011.
3. McCance KL, Huether SE, Brashers VL, Rote NS, eds. *Pathophysiology: The Biologic Basis for Disease in Adults and Children.* 6th ed. Mosby Elsevier; 2010.
4. Porth CM, Matfin G. *Pathophysiology: Concepts of Altered Health States.* 8th ed. Lippincott Williams and Wilkins; 2010.
5. Hall JE. *Guyton and Hall Textbook of Medical Physiology.* 12th ed. Saunders Elsevier; 2011.

Online Resources

◊ **Medline Plus (U.S. National Library of Medicine, National Institutes of Health)**
  ¤ http://www.nlm.nih.gov/medlineplus/
◊ **MIT Open Courseware, lecture notes for "Principle and Practice of Human Pathology" course by Drs. Gary Tearney and Kamran Badizadegan**
  ¤ http://ocw.mit.edu/courses/health-sciences-and-technology/hst-035-principle-and-practice-of-human-pathology-spring-2003/lecture-notes/

Please visit www.routledge.com/9781630917234 to access additional material.

CHAPTER 3

Pharmacology

CHAPTER OUTLINE AND OBJECTIVES

Introduction

Regulation of Therapeutic Medications

◊ Describe the federal laws and regulations related to the storage and use of medications in an athletic training facility.

¤ Legislative Acts

¤ Food and Drug Administration

¤ Drug Enforcement Agency

Management of Medications

◊ Describe the laws, regulations, and recommended procedures related to the management of medications in an athletic training facility.

¤ Storage and Packaging

¤ Dispensing Versus Administering

¤ Documentation and Inventory Control

¤ Expired Medications

Nomenclature

◊ Use appropriate terminology as it relates to the use, management, and storage of medications in an athletic training facility.

Bhojani RA, O'Connor DP, Fincher AL. *Clinical Pathology for Athletic Trainers: Recognizing Systemic Disease, Fourth Edition* (pp 35-75). © 2022 Taylor & Francis Group.

Classification of Drugs

◊ Describe the classifications of drugs.

   ¤ Over-the-Counter

   ¤ Prescription

   ¤ Controlled Substances

Routes of Administration and Dosage Forms

◊ Describe the common routes of drug administration and dosage forms along with the advantages and disadvantages of each.

   ¤ Oral

   ¤ Injection

   ¤ Inhalation

   ¤ Topical

   ¤ Sublingual and Buccal

   ¤ Rectal

Pharmacokinetics

◊ Explain the processes of pharmacokinetics and the effect of exercise on these processes.

   ¤ Absorption

   ¤ Distribution

   ¤ Metabolism

   ¤ Elimination

Pharmacodynamics

◊ Explain the concepts of bioavailability, half-life, bioequivalence, site of action, onset, and duration of action.

◊ Explain the receptor theory of drug action, dose-response relationship, placebo effect, potency, and drug interactions.

◊ Explain the principles of drug dosing.

◊ Describe the types of drug interactions and adverse reactions.

Therapeutic Medications

◊ Describe the indications, routes of administration, dosage patterns, physiological effects, and side effects associated with common therapeutic medications.

   ¤ Medications for Treating Inflammation

     • Nonsteroidal Anti-Inflammatory Drugs

     • Corticosteroids

   ¤ Medications for Treating Pain

     • Analgesics

     • Acetaminophen (Tylenol)

     • Opioids (Narcotics)

   ¤ Medications for Treating Infections

     • Antibiotics

     • Antifungals

     • Antivirals

- ¤ Medications for Treating Colds and Allergies
  - Antihistamines
  - Decongestants
  - Antitussives
  - Expectorants
  - Multi-Symptom Medications
- ¤ Medications for Treating Asthma
  - Corticosteroids
  - Antileukotrienes
  - Mast Cell Stabilizers
  - Methylxanthines
  - Bronchodilators (short-acting β_2 agonists and long-acting β_2 agonists)
- ¤ Medications for Treating Gastrointestinal Disorders
  - Antiemetics
  - Antidiarrheals
  - Laxatives
  - Antacids
  - Proton Pump Inhibitors
  - H_2 Blockers

Nutritional Supplements and Performance-Enhancing Drugs

- ◊ Describe the routes of administration, dosage patterns, physiological effects, and side effects associated with select nutritional supplements and performance-enhancing drugs.
  - ¤ Creatine
  - ¤ Dehydroepiandrosterone and Androstenedione
  - ¤ Androgenic-Anabolic Steroids
  - ¤ Human Growth Hormone
  - ¤ Erythropoietin
- ◊ Identify supplements and drugs that might be banned by sport or workplace regulations.

Herbal Supplements

- ◊ Describe the intended uses, side effects, and potential drug interactions associated with select herbal supplements.

Drug Resources

- ◊ Use drug resources to access information related to the indications, physiological effects, dosing, and potential side effects associated with common medications.

Summary

Case Study

- ◊ Develop critical-thinking and clinical decision-making skills.

Online Resources

This chapter addresses the following knowledge and skills from the *Athletic Training Education Competencies, Fifth Edition*[1]:

Content Area	Knowledge and Skills
Prevention and Health Promotion (PHP)	48, 49
Therapeutic Interventions (TI)	21-31
Acute Care of Injuries and Illnesses (AC)	31-33

INTRODUCTION

There are hundreds of therapeutic medications used to treat common musculoskeletal and systemic injuries and illnesses. For this reason, it is impossible for athletic trainers to be familiar with every medication that their patients may use. However, athletic trainers should be familiar with the more common types of medications (eg, antihistamines, analgesics, nonsteroidal anti-inflammatory drugs [NSAIDs]) their patients may use and the implications that these medications may have on their patients' ability to participate in sports, work, or rehabilitation. Athletic trainers can also play a role in helping to improve patient compliance with medication usage.

This chapter will review the legal regulations related to the use and management of therapeutic medications in athletic training facilities, introduce the reader to the foundational concepts related to pharmacology, and then discuss the common types of therapeutic drugs, nutritional supplements, performance-enhancing drugs, and herbal medications that athletic trainers might encounter in their clinical practice. Subsequent chapters will also discuss many of the specific drugs used to treat common systemic diseases. A complete and thorough discussion of all concepts and physiological effects of all drugs is beyond the scope of this chapter. We recommend *Principles of Pharmacology for Athletic Trainers, Third Edition*[2] as an additional resource.

REGULATION OF THERAPEUTIC MEDICATIONS

There are multiple federal agencies that regulate the use of medications in the United States. The 2 primary regulatory agencies are the Food and Drug Administration (FDA) and the Drug Enforcement Agency (DEA). There are also several federal legislative acts that relate to the regulation of medications. These acts are summarized in Table 3-1. Athletic trainers should be familiar with the roles of the FDA and DEA in regulating medications, as well as the federal and state laws that apply to this regulation. In most cases, state and federal laws will align with one another. In cases where they differ, the athletic trainer should follow the stricter of the 2 laws.

The Food and Drug Administration

The FDA is housed within the Department of Health and Human Services and is responsible for regulating the safety and effectiveness of over-the-counter (OTC) and prescription drugs. The regulatory efforts of the FDA include the approval of new drugs, as well as the manufacturing and labeling, advertising and marketing, and efficacy and safety of all drugs.

Gaining FDA approval for a new drug can take up to 17.5 years. The multiphase approval process begins with laboratory and animal studies designed to identify the biological activity of the drug. Multiple phases of human clinical trials are then conducted to determine safe dosages, clinical effectiveness, and possible short- and long-term adverse effects. Table 3-2 summarizes the approval process for all new drugs.

The FDA is also responsible for removing unsafe medications from the market. The FDA can learn of unsafe drugs through several different procedures, including:

Table 3-1. Select Federal Acts for Regulating Medications

YEAR	ACT	PURPOSE
1938	Federal Food, Drug and Cosmetic Act	To regulate the safety of drugs
1951	Humphrey Amendment	Established 2 classes of drugs: prescription and nonprescription (OTC)
1962	Kefauver-Harris Amendment	Improve rules for drug safety and require manufacturers to prove drugs' effectiveness
1970	Federal Comprehensive Drug Abuse Prevention and Control Act	To regulate the manufacturing, distribution, and dispensing of drugs that have a potential for abuse
1970	Poison Prevention Act	Required prescription and nonprescription drugs to be packaged in child-resistant containers
1983	Fair Packaging and Labeling Act	Required nonprescription drugs to include their ingredients on their labels
1988	Anti-Drug Abuse Act	Reclassified anabolic steroids as controlled substances
2002	The Best Pharmaceuticals for Children Act	In exchange for studying drug in children, the manufacturer gets 6 months of selling their product without competition
2003	Health Insurance Portability and Accountability Act (HIPAA)	Mandates protection of patient information and confidentiality by all health practitioners involved with protected health information

OTC = over-the-counter.

1. A drug manufacturer may contact the FDA after discovering a problem with one of their drugs.
2. The FDA may identify an unsafe drug while inspecting a manufacturer's facility.
3. The FDA may receive reports of health problems associated with a specific drug.
4. The Centers for Disease Control and Prevention (CDC) may alert the FDA about a specific drug.

FDA drug recalls are categorized into 3 classes based on the seriousness of the threat.[3] Table 3-3 provides a summary of the recall classes for unsafe drugs.

Drug Enforcement Agency

The DEA, which is located within the Department of Justice, is responsible for enforcing the laws and regulations related to the regulation of controlled substances. Federal law requires that all facilities that store, dispense, or administer controlled substances have a DEA certificate. Although not required, it is recommended that athletic training facilities have a DEA certificate for any physician who is responsible for prescription medications stored within the facility.[4]

Table 3-2. FDA New Drug Approval Process

APPROXIMATE YEARS	PHASE	PURPOSE
3 to 6	Preclinical Testing ↓ File Investigational New Drug ↓	Laboratory and animal tests Determine biological activity Obtain FDA approval for clinical trials
1 to 2	Clinical Trials Phase I ↓	20 to 80 healthy volunteers Check pharmacokinetic parameters and safe dosages
2 to 3	Phase II ↓	100 to 300 patients Determine effectiveness and short-term adverse effects
3 to 4	Phase III ↓	1000 to 3000 patients Determine effectiveness and adverse effects compared to other therapy
1.5 to 2.5	FDA review/approval for New Drug Application (NDA) ↓ Postmarketing monitoring Phase IV ↓	Obtain FDA approval for physicians to prescribe General population of patients Monitor for adverse effects; long-term effects Compare with other therapy

FDA = Food and Drug Administration.

Reproduced with permission from Houglam JE, Harrelson GL. *Principles of Pharmacology for Athletic Trainers*. SLACK Incorporated; 2016.

MANAGEMENT OF MEDICATIONS

All athletic training facilities are recommended to have a written policy and procedure document specific to the use of medications.[4,5] This document should address all aspects related to the use and management of medications within the facility. The use of emergency medications (eg, epinephrine auto-injector, β_2 agonist inhaler, insulin) should be documented both within the policy and procedures for medication use and within the emergency action plan. These policies should be reviewed by all members of the sports medicine staff and reviewed against federal and state regulations on the management of medications.

Storage and Packaging

State and federal laws require that medications be kept in a locked cabinet or closet. Controlled substances must be kept separately from prescription medications, which should also be kept separate from OTC medications. If medications are kept within athletic training bags, these bags should be stored within a locked cabinet or closet. Furthermore, all medications (prescription and OTC) must remain in their original containers with their original labels. Repackaging bulk medications into smaller containers for storage in an athletic training kit violates federal law. When possible, medications should be purchased in individual dose packs. Inappropriate use or mismanagement of

Table 3-3. FDA Drug Recall Classes

LEVEL OF THREAT	CLASS	DESCRIPTION OF THREAT
Most serious	I	Potential for serious health problem or death. *Example: Contaminated steroid injections linked to meningitis outbreak (New England Compounding Center, Framingham, MA; 2012)*
	II	Potential for temporary or slight health problem. *Example: Two lots of hydrocodone bitartrate and APAP tablets, USP 10 mg/500 mg found to include tablets that were thicker and darker shade than the other tablets. It is possible that some tablets from lots 519406A and 521759A exceed the weight specification and may contain higher-than-indicated amounts of the ingredients hydrocodone bitartrate and/or acetaminophen.*
Least serious	III	Not likely to cause a health problem. *Example: Ten lots of oral contraceptive Introvale found to have packaging flaw (Sandoz, 2012)*

FDA: Food and Drug Administration; APAP: acetaminophen. (Examples obtained from 2012 Recalls, Market Withdrawals & Safety Alerts. Available at: http://www.fda.gov/Safety/Recalls/ArchiveRecalls/2012/. Accessed February 15, 2013).

medications can have very serious legal ramifications. Athletic trainers should be familiar with their scope of practice as well as state and federal laws related to therapeutic medications. They should also be familiar with all institution and program policies and procedures regarding the use of medications in the athletic training facility.

Dispensing Versus Administering

Dispensing and administering medications are 2 entirely different functions. Dispensing refers to the act of providing multiple doses of a medication to a patient, whereas administering a drug refers to the direct application of a single dose.[4] Unless specifically prohibited by their state practice act, athletic trainers are able to administer OTC medications to their patients. However, it is important to understand that athletic trainers are not legally able to dispense medications to their patients.

Documentation and Inventory Control

A written log should be used to record all medications administered or dispensed in the athletic training facility. This medication log should include the patient's name, date of service, reason for medication, prescription number (if prescription medication is given), physician's name, medication name, strength, dosage form, quantity, expiration date, lot number, initials of the athletic trainer, and initials of the physician. An inventory audit of all medications should be performed at least once every year. The quantity of medications on hand should match the quantity purchased and the quantity administered and/or dispensed. This documentation may be kept in a log and/or in the electronic medical record.

Expired Medications

All expired OTC and prescription medications should be removed from the current inventory, recorded in the medication log, and disposed of properly. Contrary to popular belief, expired medications should not be flushed down the toilet. Expired OTC medications can be placed in a biohazard waste bag and disposed of through the facility's biohazard waste removal procedures.[2] A written log should be attached to the bag or container and should include the drug name, strength, dosage form, quantity, lot number, expiration date, and the initials of the person who completed the log. Athletic trainers can often dispose of expired prescription medications through a local pharmacy. Also, the DEA works with state and local law enforcement agencies to sponsor National Prescription Drug Take Back Days. More information on this program can be found at http://www.deadiversion.usdoj.gov/.

NOMENCLATURE

Drugs are identified by 1 of 3 names: chemical, generic, or trade. The chemical name is rather long and refers to the chemical structure of the drug. The generic name is shorter, nonproprietary, and is derived from the chemical name. The trade name is the recognized brand name that is assigned to a drug by the manufacturer. The trade name is proprietary and therefore cannot be used by other manufacturers. There is only one generic name for each drug, but there may be multiple trade names if more than one company markets the drug. For example, ibuprofen is the generic name both for Motrin (McNeil Consumer Healthcare) and Advil (Wyeth Pharmaceuticals). Any manufacturer can use the name ibuprofen to describe their particular NSAID, whereas the names Motrin and Advil can be used only by McNeil and Wyeth, respectively.

Generic names should not be confused with generic drugs. Every drug has a generic name; however, not every drug is available in a generic form. Generic drugs are copies of brand-name drugs whose patents have expired. They are generally cheaper, with brand-name drugs sometimes costing as much as 4 times that of their generic counterparts. During the patent period of a drug (approximately 20 years), only the original manufacturer may legally market that drug. A large portion of the cost associated with brand-name drugs is related to the original expense of testing and retesting the drug prior to its submittal to the FDA for approval. Once a drug's patent expires, other drug manufacturers can formulate and market their version (generic) of the original drug. Generic drugs must be *therapeutically equivalent*, meaning they must have the same chemical makeup and active ingredients as the original drug and produce the same medical effect. Because manufacturers of generic drugs do not have to pay for additional research and testing of their drugs, they can market their versions of the drugs at a much cheaper cost. Generic drugs are usually marketed using the generic name. Currently, about half of the drugs on the market are available in a generic form.

CLASSIFICATION OF DRUGS

There are 3 major classifications of drugs: OTC, prescription, and controlled substances. Each of these classifications is discussed next.

Over-the-Counter

OTC medications do not require a prescription and are therefore also referred to as nonprescription drugs. Many OTC drugs were originally prescription drugs that have now been approved by the FDA as nonprescription drugs. These medications will typically contain less drug per dose as compared to the corresponding prescription drug. For example, naproxen sodium (Aleve) is a commonly used OTC NSAID and is available in 220-mg tablets. Naproxen is also available by prescription, with a single tablet containing either 250 or 500 mg. OTC medications are typically less expensive than prescription medications and are convenient, allowing consumers to self-medicate for minor conditions rather than going to see their physician.

Table 3-4. Controlled Substances

SCHEDULE	ABUSE POTENTIAL	COMMENTS	EXAMPLE DRUGS
I	Greatest	High potential for abuse, no accepted medical use	Heroin, marijuana, lysergic acid diethylaminde (LSD), tetrahydroxannabiol (THC)
II		May lead to severe psychological or physical dependence	Amphetamines, cocaine, codeine, Demerol, methamphetamine, morphine, oxycodone plus acetaminophen (Percocet), methylphenidate (Ritalin)
III		May lead to moderate or low physical dependence or high psychological dependence	Anabolic steroids, codeine with acetaminophen, hydrocodone with acetaminophen, propoxyphene (Darvon)
IV		May lead to limited physical dependence or psychological dependence	Alprazolam (Xanax), diazepam (Valium), lorazepam (Ativan), phenobarbital (Luminal)
V	Least	Lowest potential for abuse	Cough suppressants containing codeine (Robitussin A-C)
			Antidiarrheal medication containing opium (Kapectolin PG)

Prescription

The purchase of prescription medications requires a written prescription from a physician or nurse practitioner and, by law, must be filled by a pharmacist. These medications are typically associated with a greater potential for adverse reactions and are generally prescribed for a restricted time period. Patients can refill a prescription only when authorized by their physician.

Controlled Substances

Drugs classified as controlled substances have a greater potential for abuse than prescription drugs. The Comprehensive Drug Abuse Prevention and Control Act of 1970, also referred to as the Controlled Substances Act, established the current categories of controlled substances, which are divided into 5 areas or schedules. Schedule I drugs have the highest potential for abuse whereas Schedule V drugs have the least potential for abuse. Table 3-4 provides examples of common drugs within each schedule category. Most narcotic pain medications are classified as Schedule III drugs. Anabolic steroids are also classified as Schedule III drugs. The DEA is responsible for overseeing the manufacturing, distribution, storage, and dispensing of all controlled substances.

ROUTES OF ADMINISTRATION AND DOSAGE FORMS

Therapeutic medications can be administered through a variety of routes and dosage forms, depending on the condition to be treated, the specific drug, and whether the drug is meant to

Table 3-5. Routes of Administration and Dosage Forms

CLASSIFICATION	ROUTES	PRIMARY EFFECT	DOSAGE FORMS (DEVICES)
Enteral	Oral	Systemic	Tablet, capsule, syrup, elixir, softgel, suspension, emulsion
	Buccal	Systemic	Lollipop, film, lozenge, spray
	Sublingual	Systemic	Orally disintegrating tablet
	Rectal	Systemic	Suppository, ointment
Parenteral	Intravenous injection	Systemic	Aqueous solutions, suspensions
	Intramuscular injection	Systemic	Aqueous solutions, suspensions
	Subcutaneous injection	Systemic	Solution (insulin pump, EpiPen®)
	Intra-articular injection	Local	Solution
Inhalation	Inhalation	Local[a]	Crushable tablet (dry powder inhaler), aerosol (metered dose inhaler), liquid (nebulizer)
Topical	Dermal	Local	Ointment, cream, spray
	Transdermal	Systemic	Patch
	Otic	Local[a]	Drops
	Ophthalmic	Local	Drops, ointment

[a] May also produce some systemic effect.

provide a systemic or local effect. The administration route refers to how the drug enters the body (eg, by mouth, injection, inhalation), whereas the dosage form refers to the actual physical form of the drug (eg, tablet, capsule, syrup). Table 3-5 provides a list of the most common routes of administration, the dosage forms that are typically associated with these routes, and the intended effect (systemic or local). Routes of administration that provide entry to the body by way of the alimentary canal or digestive system (ie, oral, sublingual, buccal, and rectal) are referred to as enteral routes. Other route classifications include parenteral, topical, and inhalation. Parenteral routes provide entry into the body through injections (intravenous [IV], intramuscular [IM], and subcutaneous [SC]), whereas topical routes are administered via the skin, eye, ear, and nose. The inhalation route enables drugs to be delivered directly to the lungs, which makes it the ideal route choice for many medications used to treat asthma.

Oral

The oral route is the most commonly used route for administering medication. One disadvantage of the oral route is that stomach acid may completely or partially inactivate some drugs, reducing their therapeutic effectiveness. Also, medications administered orally will take longer to provide a therapeutic effect because they must first be absorbed from the stomach or intestines before they can be distributed. Tablets, caplets, and capsules may take up to 30 minutes to provide their intended therapeutic effect because they must first be broken down or dissolved in the stomach before moving to the small intestine for absorption.[6] It is recommended that oral medications be taken with a full glass of water to help move them into the small intestines for quicker absorption. Also, some foods can interact with certain medications when ingested at the same time; therefore, it is important to read and follow all instructions printed on the medication label.

Some drugs will contain an *enteric coating* that is designed to delay the release of a medication until it reaches the small intestine. This coating is often used to protect an acid-sensitive medication or to protect the gastric mucosa by delaying the breakdown of the drug until after it has passed through the stomach. Extended-release medications may contain an enteric coating or layers of a coating designed to allow a gradual release of medication. Because the medication is released over a prolonged period of time, extended-release medications will typically contain more drug than their normal-release counterparts. Enteric-coated and extended-release medications should never be cut or crushed prior to administration.

Injection

Injections are parenteral routes for drug administration and can be administered directly into the veins (IV drugs) or through IM, intra-articular (IA), or SC tissues. IV drug administration provides an immediate systemic effect, whereas IM and SC injection provides a slower (but still faster than oral) systemic or local effect. IA injections primarily provide a local effect.

Inhalation

Inhalation is a common route of delivery for most asthma medications because it enables the medication to be delivered directly to the bronchial and lung tissues for quicker relief of symptoms (in some cases < 5 minutes). Aerosol mists and dry powders are 2 common dosage forms of inhaled medications and are administered using metered dose inhalers (MDI) and dry powder inhalers (DPI).

Topical

Topical medications are administered through creams, gels, lotions, ointments, sprays, drops, and transdermal patches. Creams, gels, ointments, and lotions are applied to the skin to produce a local effect and are commonly used to treat skin conditions (see Chapter 12). Intranasal sprays enable medications to be administered directly to the mucous membranes within the nose. Drops are used to treat ear and eye conditions.

Unlike most topical dose forms, transdermal patches can produce a systemic effect. Transdermal patches should be applied to clean, dry skin with little or no hair. For prolonged use, the patch should be rotated to a different skin area periodically to avoid skin irritation. Transdermal patches should never be cut in an attempt to adjust dosage or to fit a particular area unless directed by the packaging.

Sublingual and Buccal

Sublingual and buccal medications are administered under the tongue and between the cheek and gum, respectively. Drugs administered through these routes are absorbed quickly because of the rich vascular supply of these mucosal tissues.

Rectal

The suppository is a common dosage form used to administer medication via the rectum. This route of administration is often used to administer antiemetics for treating individuals with severe vomiting when they are unable to keep down oral medications. Some pain medications and laxatives are also administered using suppositories.

PHARMACOKINETICS

Pharmacokinetics describes the physiological processes of how the body acts on a drug and can be divided into 4 distinct phases: absorption, distribution, metabolism, and elimination. Each of these phases is described next.

Absorption

For a drug to produce a therapeutic effect, it must be absorbed into the bloodstream and distributed throughout the circulation to reach its site of action. Absorption of orally administered drugs occurs in the stomach and small intestine, with the majority occurring in the latter structure. The amount of drug that is actually available in the body's tissues is referred to as its *bioavailability*. The bioavailability is usually only a fraction of the original dosage amount. If a drug's bioavailability is 50%, then the body will absorb only 250 mg of a 500-mg dose of medication. Bioavailability varies among drugs. For example, when comparing 2 commonly prescribed NSAIDs, naproxen has a bioavailability of 95% while Voltaren has a 50% bioavailability.

A specific drug's bioavailability is affected both by the amount of drug absorbed and the rate at which it is absorbed. Gastric enzymes can affect whether a drug dissolves completely in the stomach before moving into the intestines or can inactivate a portion of a drug before it leaves the stomach. The "first-pass effect" also influences the bioavailability of a drug and occurs if the drug is absorbed from the intestine into the liver before entering the systemic circulation. The liver serves as the main site for drug metabolism and may cause further inactivation of a portion of the drug. To compensate for the first-pass effect, manufacturers will increase the amount of drug contained within a single oral dose. The first-pass effect is a factor only when drugs are taken orally.

For absorption to occur, a drug molecule must move across one or more membranes through simple diffusion, active transport, or passive diffusion. *Passive diffusion* is the most common mechanism for moving medications across membranes.[2] The lipid solubility of a drug will affect its ability to diffuse across these membranes. With passive diffusion, lipid-soluble drugs will diffuse more quickly and easily and can pass through the blood-brain barrier to affect the central nervous system (CNS). Movement of drug molecules across membranes will typically occur from the side with the greatest concentration to the side with the lowest concentration. When the concentration of molecules becomes equal on both sides, diffusion is stopped.

The *active transport* mechanism requires a protein to move the drug across a membrane. The protein binds to the drug molecule and transports it through the membrane. This mechanism allows selective diffusion of drug molecules in a specific direction, regardless of the concentrations on either side of the membrane. Active transport requires energy to occur. The mechanism of *facilitated diffusion* combines the processes of passive diffusion and active transport. It allows for drug selectivity through the binding of a protein; however, the drug molecule will move only from areas of high concentration to low concentration.

Exercise can delay or reduce the absorption of oral medications because blood is diverted away from the gastrointestinal (GI) tract to the working skeletal muscles. When the body absorbs less of a drug, its therapeutic effectiveness is decreased. For optimum absorption, oral medications should be taken at least 30 minutes prior to beginning exercise. Exercise can increase the absorption of medications delivered via transdermal patches.[7] This increased absorption is due to an increase in subcutaneous blood flow during exercise. Injected medications, particularly intramuscular, also may be absorbed more rapidly during exercise and should be given at least 30 minutes before performing vigorous activity.

Distribution

Once absorption is complete, the drug is transported to its site of action via the circulatory system. Like absorption, a drug's distribution is also affected by its lipid solubility. Drugs with

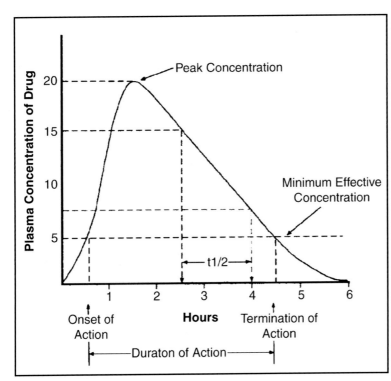

Figure 3-1. Concentration-time curve following a single oral dose of a drug. The onset of action occurs when the concentration is above the level needed to produce an effect (minimal effective concentration). Duration of action (4 hours in this example) is the time between onset and termination of action. The half-life (t½) is the time it takes for the concentration of the drug to be reduced by one-half after it has reached peak concentration. In this example, t½ = 1½ hours; the time it takes for the concentration of drug to decrease from 15 to 7.5. (Reproduced with permission from Houglum JE, Harrelson GL. *Principles of Pharmacology for Athletic Trainers.* 2nd ed. SLACK Incorporated; 2011.)

higher lipid solubility will be able to pass through more membranes providing a wider distribution, particularly with respect to the blood-brain barrier and fat cells. Lipid-soluble drugs are also capable of being stored in the body, producing a longer lasting effect, water-soluble drugs are more easily eliminated or excreted from the body. Blood flow to an area affects the distribution of a drug to that area. For example, the vascular nature of the liver, kidney, and brain enables drug molecules to reach these structures quickly. Structures that are less vascular (bone and fat cells) will typically require more time for drug distribution.

A drug's *onset of action* is the time it takes for drug molecules to reach their site of action in sufficient quantities to produce a therapeutic effect (Figure 3-1). As the drug molecules are metabolized and excreted, their concentration at the site of action is reduced until they are no longer able to exert a therapeutic effect. A drug's *duration of action* is that period of time when concentration levels are sufficient enough to produce a therapeutic effect (see Figure 3-1). Individual drugs differ in their onset and duration of action.

Exercise increases blood flow and therefore may increase the drug distribution rate, depending on the intended site of action. It is important to remember that blood is shunted away from some areas (stomach and intestines) to supply adequate blood to the working skeletal muscles.

Metabolism

Metabolism is the process by which drugs are inactivated and broken down into more water-soluble metabolites in preparation for excretion. The mechanism of metabolism is initiated by enzymes that react with the drug. The liver serves as the primary site for most drug metabolism; however, the kidneys, intestines, lungs, and brain also participate in this process.

Exercise can reduce the metabolism of some drugs, because blood is routed away from the liver and GI tract to the working skeletal muscles. However, in most instances the time necessary for completing the metabolic breakdown of drugs is longer than the duration of exercise, thus negating any overall decrease in drug metabolism.

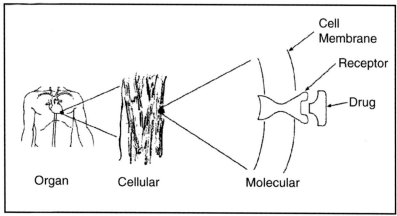

Figure 3-2. Site of action. The site of action is in specific tissues at the cellular and molecular level, often at a receptor on the cell membrane to which the drug chemically fits. (Reproduced with permission from Houglum JE, Harrelson GL. *Principles of Pharmacology for Athletic Trainers.* 2nd ed. SLACK Incorporated; 2011.)

Elimination

Elimination, or excretion, is the process by which the body rids itself of a drug. The kidneys serve as the primary site for drug excretion; however, the intestines (feces), sweat glands (perspiration), and lungs (respiration) also assist in this process. Exercise can decrease the rate of renal excretion because blood flow is directed away from the kidneys to the working skeletal muscles.

The rate at which a drug is excreted from the body is influenced by the drug's half-life. The *half-life* of a drug is the time it takes to reduce the peak blood concentration of the drug by 50% (see Figure 3-1). For example, if a drug has a peak blood concentration of 50 mg and a half-life of 2 hours, then after 2 hours, the blood concentration will be reduced to 25 mg. After 4 hours, it would be 12.5 mg, and after 8 hours it would be 6.25 mg. Drugs with greater half-lives will have greater durations of action and require less frequent dosing. Generally, lipid-soluble drugs have longer half-lives than water-soluble drugs and will therefore stay in the body longer.

PHARMACODYNAMICS

Pharmacodynamics describes the process of how a drug acts on the body. For a drug to produce a therapeutic effect, it must bind with a receptor, which can be a molecule on the cell membrane or within the cell, at the site of action (Figure 3-2). The relationship between a drug and a receptor is very specific, much like that between a lock and key. Any chemical change in the drug or the receptor will change this relationship. These receptors are site specific and exist within the body to regulate certain physiological mechanisms by matching with certain endogenous compounds. A drug that fits the receptor and initiates a mechanism similar to the endogenous compound is referred to as an *agonist*. A drug that fits the receptor but fails to initiate or blocks this mechanism is referred to as an *antagonist*. This process is collectively referred to as the *receptor theory of drug action*.[2]

Drug Dosing

The recommended dose of a drug is based on the potency of the drug, the therapeutic range of the drug, the patient's age, and the patient's condition. *Potency* refers to the strength of the drug. The greater the potency, the smaller the dose needed to produce a therapeutic effect. The therapeutic effectiveness of a drug is greatest when its blood concentration levels consistently stay within a certain range (therapeutic range). Greater blood concentration levels lead to more drug molecules occupying receptor sites. The more receptor sites occupied, the greater the drug's response will be. Once all the receptor sites are occupied, any additional dosing will have no added effect on the drug's response. This concept is referred to as the *dose response relationship*. Maintaining blood levels within the therapeutic range is referred to as *steady state* and is achieved once the blood levels from continued dosing matches the levels of excretion of a drug. In some cases, a physician may prescribe a *loading dose* of a drug, which is usually greater than the *maintenance dose* (dose needed to maintain steady state), to increase the rate at which the drug reaches its therapeutic range.

Drug Interactions and Adverse Reactions

Drug interactions can occur between 2 or more drugs, altering the intended effect of one or all the drugs. Drug interactions can change how the body handles a drug or how a drug acts on the body. For example, antacids can reduce the body's ability to absorb acetaminophen from the intestine but the same is not true for some NSAIDs.

Drug interactions can be additive (agonistic) or inhibitive (antagonistic). *Agonistic interactions* occur when 2 drugs of the same type are taken together (2 stimulants or 2 depressants). The effects of the 2 drugs "add" together, causing an increase in the overall effect. For example, alcohol combined with an antihistamine can cause excessive drowsiness and loss of muscle coordination. *Antagonistic effects* can occur between 2 unrelated drugs. A common example of an antagonistic effect is how antibiotics inhibit or reduce the effectiveness of oral contraceptives.

Adverse drug reactions can range from mild side effects to severe hypersensitivity. Examples of drug side effects include the drowsiness caused by first-generation antihistamines or the loss of appetite or nausea associated with some antibiotics. Also, certain foods or herbal preparations can interact with prescription and OTC medications. Dairy products are known to decrease the absorption of tetracycline antibiotics. When herbs, such as garlic, ginkgo biloba, ginseng, green tea, or grape seed, are taken along with warfarin (Coumadin), aspirin, or other NSAIDs, patients may experience increased bleeding or bruising.[2] Cases of drug hypersensitivity can range from a mild rash to anaphylactic shock. Side effects and hypersensitivity reactions can occur immediately or be delayed.

Most allergic drug reactions are associated with NSAIDs, β-lactam (penicillins and cephalosporins) antibiotics, and sulfonamide antibiotics. People who are allergic to aspirin may experience similar reactions to other NSAIDs. Aspirin and other NSAIDs are also known to cause asthma attacks in 3% to 39% of individuals with chronic asthma.[2] Allergic reactions that produce a rash can often be treated with topical corticosteroids to reduce the acute inflammatory reaction and an antihistamine to reduce the itching. Allergic reactions that progress to anaphylaxis are life-threatening situations requiring activation of the emergency action plan. Epinephrine is commonly used to treat an anaphylactic reaction. The epinephrine is administered subcutaneously using an auto-injectable syringe such as an EpiPen. Chapter 4 provides step-by-step instructions for the use of an epinephrine auto-injectable syringe (see Table 4-10).

Placebo Effect

The *placebo effect* is a phenomenon that results in a patient experiencing a relief of symptoms or an adverse effect that cannot be attributed to the medication taken. For example, if a patient expects pain relief after taking an analgesic, she may experience relief sooner or more significantly than the medication alone provided.[2] It is believed that the patient's anticipation of an effect causes the release of hormones or neuropeptides that in turn contribute to the relief in symptoms.

THERAPEUTIC MEDICATIONS

A large variety of prescription and nonprescription medications are used to treat musculoskeletal injuries and systemic disorders. It is impossible to discuss in detail all the possible medications that athletic trainers may encounter in their clinical practice. This chapter does include a lengthy discussion of NSAIDs because of their widespread use (and abuse) within sport medicine. Analgesics, corticosteroids, antibiotics, antihistamines, decongestants, GI medications, antifungals, and bronchial dilators are discussed in this and subsequent chapters in conjunction with specific systemic disorders. Discussion of each medication will include the drug's mechanism of action,

Figure 3-3. Arachidonic acid pathways.

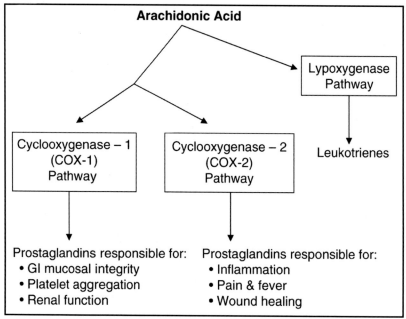

therapeutic indications, common routes for administration, recommended doses, availability (OTC or prescription only), and potential side effects.

Medications for Treating Inflammation

Nonsteroidal Anti-Inflammatory Drugs

NSAIDs are used to treat acute and chronic inflammatory conditions such as sprains, strains, tendonitis, and bursitis. Chapter 2 provided a brief overview of the acute and chronic inflammatory responses and the role of chemical mediators such as prostaglandins, histamine, and bradykinin. Prostaglandins, which are potent vasodilators, are produced by arachidonic acid. They work to sensitize pain receptors to bradykinin and histamine, thereby lowering the threshold of pain and causing increased sensitivity to pain.

During the inflammatory response, arachidonic acid follows 1 of 2 pathways depending on the enzymes that are active in the damaged cells. Figure 3-3 illustrates the cyclooxygenase (COX) and lipoxygenase pathways. The lipoxygenase pathway leads to the production of leukotrienes, which are often involved in the underlying inflammation associated with chronic asthma. Antileukotrienes are also discussed in Chapter 7. The COX pathway involves 2 separate COX enzymes (COX-1 and COX-2), with each enzyme forming a separate pathway. As shown in Figure 3-3, the COX-1 enzyme (housekeeping gene) leads to the production of prostaglandins responsible for protecting the GI mucosa, aiding in platelet aggregation, and maintaining normal renal function. The COX-2 enzyme (inflammatory gene) leads to the production of prostaglandins responsible for inflammation, pain, fever, and wound healing.

NSAIDs work by inhibiting the COX enzyme and reducing the production of prostaglandins. Traditional NSAIDs are referred to as nonselective COX inhibitors since they block the actions along both the COX-1 and COX-2 pathways. By blocking the COX-2 enzyme, nonselective NSAIDs reduce the pain and swelling associated with inflammation along with reducing body temperature. Unfortunately, they also block the COX-1 enzyme, preventing the production of "good" prostaglandins that protect the stomach. As a result, gastric upset and ulcers are 2 side effects commonly associated with extended use of NSAIDs. In addition, by inhibiting platelet aggregation and reducing renal blood flow, other side effects include increased bleeding and impaired kidney function.

Table 3-6. Sample Nonsteroidal Anti-Inflammatory Drugs

CLASS	GENERIC (TRADE) NAME	TYPICAL ANTI-INFLAMMATORY DOSE (ORAL)	AVAILABILITY
Salicylates	Aspirin	500 to 1000 mg qid	OTC
Acetic acid derivatives	Diclofenac (Voltaren)	50 mg tid to qid	Rx
	Etodolac (Lodine)	200 to 400 mg bid to tid	Rx
	Indomethacin (Indocin)	50 mg bid to qid	Rx
	Ketorolac (Toradol)	10 mg qid (do not use more than 5 days)	Rx
Proprionic acid derivatives	Ibuprofen (Advil, Motrin, Nuprin)	400 to 800 mg tid to qid	Rx, OTC
	Ketoprofen (Orudis)	50 to 75 mg tid to qid	Rx, OTC
	Naproxen sodium (Aleve, Naprosyn)	220 to 550 mg bid	Rx, OTC
Oxicam derivatives	Piroxicam (Feldene)	20 mg od	Rx
	Meloxicam (Mobic)	7.5 to 15 mg od	Rx
COX-2 inhibitor	Celecoxib (Celebrex)	200 mg od	Rx

bid = twice a day; COX = cyclooxygenase; od = once daily; OTC = over-the-counter; qid = four times a day; Rx = prescription; tid = three times a day.

Selective COX-2 inhibitors are capable of blocking the COX-2 pathway without affecting the COX-1 pathway. Celecoxib (Celebrex) is an example of a selective COX-2 inhibitor. There were originally 2 additional COX-2 inhibitors on the market: valdecoxib (Bextra) and rofecoxib (Vioxx). These 2 drugs have been recalled by the FDA because of their suspected role in increasing the risk of myocardial infarctions (heart attacks) and strokes.

In addition to their role as an anti-inflammatory agent, NSAIDs are also used as an analgesic (pain reducer) and an antipyretic (fever reducer). Generally, the dosage necessary for reducing inflammation is greater than the dosage necessary for reducing pain or fever. Table 3-6 provides the recommended dosing for anti-inflammatory effects. Also, when the therapeutic goal is to treat inflammation, it is important that dosing be consistent to maintain a steady state within the therapeutic range.

NSAIDs are lipid soluble and are easily absorbed out of the stomach and intestines. Aspirin and diclofenac (Voltaren) are the only NSAIDs that are significantly affected by the first-pass effect in the liver. Most NSAIDs will begin producing an effect within 15 to 30 minutes.[7] In most cases, 7 to 10 days is sufficient time to evaluate the effectiveness of a particular NSAID. If one NSAID is ineffective for a particular patient, another one should be tried. Generally, trying an NSAID from a different class will be more effective than trying another one from within the same class (salicylates, acetic acid derivative). Table 3-6 provides examples of NSAIDs from within each class.

NSAIDs are associated with adverse effects involving several different organ systems. In the GI system, NSAIDs have been reported to cause heartburn, nausea, diarrhea, constipation, GI bleeding, and ulcers.[8] Gastric irritation can be avoided by taking NSAIDs with food, milk, or antacids. Recently, there have been new NSAIDs that are combined with antacids that have been shown to reduce GI side effects. Two examples of this include Vimovo (Naproxen-Esomeprazole) and Duexis

(Ibuprofen-Famotidine). The most common side effects associated with the renal system include sodium retention and edema.[8] In small studies, it has been shown that NSAIDs can alter kidney function leading to nephritis or even acute renal failure. NSAID use has also been linked to adverse effects within the hematological system. Because nonselective COX inhibitors lead to decreased platelet aggregation, these medications may cause increased bleeding in an acute injury, leading to increased swelling and delayed healing.[9] Studies have shown that rheumatoid arthritis patients taking COX-2-selective inhibitors may have an increased risk for heart attacks and strokes. As mentioned earlier, these studies have resulted in 2 of the 3 COX-2 inhibitors being recalled. Side effects involving the CNS include tinnitus, sedation, and dizziness. Although not as common, allergic reactions can also occur when taking NSAIDs. Symptoms will usually present within 3 hours of taking the medication. NSAIDs should not be used by individuals with a history of sensitivity to aspirin or any other NSAIDs. They should be used with caution in patients with bleeding abnormalities, or impaired renal function, and during pregnancy (especially the last trimester) or breast feeding.

Corticosteroids

Corticosteroids are used to treat asthma (Chapter 7), inflammatory bowel disease (Chapter 8), dermatological conditions (Chapter 12), tendonitis, bursitis, and allergic reactions (Chapter 4). They reduce inflammation by inhibiting the synthesis of arachidonic acid and its metabolites along both the cyclooxygenase and lipoxygenase pathways. These actions inhibit the production of prostaglandins and leukotrienes. Corticosteroids are administered through oral, inhalation, injection, and topical routes. Table 3-7 provides a list of sample corticosteroids based on their route of administration. Dosages for corticosteroids vary depending on the route of administration and the specific disorder being treated. Prolonged use of corticosteroids can lead to adrenal insufficiency. For this reason, dosing of corticosteroids is often tapered down to allow time for a return in normal adrenal function.

Side effects associated with using corticosteroids can be categorized as either general or specific to the route of administration. Common general side effects include restlessness, dizziness, sleeplessness, changes in skin color, and unusual hair growth on the face or body. Other general side effects include eye pain; nausea; vomiting; black, tarry stools; fluid retention; skin reactions; menstrual irregularities; and prolonged sore throat, fever, cold, or other signs of infection. Coughing, hoarseness, and oral candidiasis (yeast infection) are side effects specific to the oral inhalation route of administration. Local irritation can occur with nasal inhalation, and joint pain and chondromalacia can result from intra-articular injections of corticosteroids.[5]

Medications for Treating Pain

Analgesics

Analgesics are used to treat pain and are available both in OTC and prescription forms. NSAIDs, discussed above, are also effective in treating pain because of their effect on the COX-2 enzyme. The analgesic dosage for NSAIDs will typically be slightly less than that used for treating inflammation. Acetaminophen, one of the most widely used OTC analgesics, and narcotic analgesics are discussed next.

Acetaminophen (Tylenol)

Tylenol is used effectively to reduce mild to moderate pain and fever. Acetaminophen is known to block the COX enzyme in the brain; however, the exact mechanism that leads to its analgesic effect is not clear. It is available in many different dosage forms, including tablets, capsules, caplets, chewable tablets, suppositories, elixirs, and drops. A single analgesic dose will range from 325 to 1000 mg taken every 4 to 6 hours with a maximum recommended adult dose of 4000 mg a day. The half-life of acetaminophen is approximately 2 hours. It does not inhibit platelet aggregation like

Table 3-7. Sample Corticosteroids

GENERIC (TRADE) NAME	ROUTE OF ADMINISTRATION
Betamethasone (Celestone)	Oral
	Injection
Budesonide (Rhinocort)	Nasal inhalation
Dexamethasone (Decadron)	Oral
	Oral inhalation
	Nasal inhalation
	Injection
Fluticasone (Flonase)	Nasal inhalation
Hydrocortisone (Cortef)	Oral
Hydrocortisone (Solu-Cortef)	Injection
Hydrocortisone cream	Topical cream
Methylpredisolone (Depo-Medrol)	Oral
	Injection
Triamcinolone (Azmacort, Kenalog, Nasacort)	Oral inhalation
	Nasal inhalation
	Injection
Prednisolone (Delta-Cortef)	Oral
	Injection
Prednisone (Orasone, Meticorten, Deltasone, Cortan, Sterapred)	Oral
Cortisone (Cortisone)	Oral
	Injection

aspirin and other NSAIDs. Acetaminophen is often combined with certain opioid analgesics to treat more severe pain.

Acetaminophen is safe to give to children with colds and flus because it does not have the same risk for *Reye syndrome* that aspirin does. The only 2 consistently reported adverse reactions associated with acetaminophen are increased potential for liver toxicity, particularly when combined with alcohol or with overdose. The high rate of overdose is thought to occur because of the number of combination OTC products (antihistamine, decongestant, and analgesic) on the market containing acetaminophen, causing patients to unknowingly self-medicate with multiple doses of acetaminophen.

Opioids (Narcotics)

Opioids are considered controlled substances and are, therefore, available by prescription only. These medications are typically used to treat moderate to severe pain such as postoperative pain, pain associated with significant musculoskeletal injury, and pain associated with some cancers. They are known to cause drowsiness and euphoria and have a potential for abuse and addiction. Constipation is a common side effect reported with most narcotic analgesics. Serious adverse reactions are possible when these drugs are combined with alcohol, benzodiazepines, and/or muscle relaxants.

Table 3-8. Select Opioid Analgesics

GENERIC NAME	TRADE NAME	DOSAGE FORMS	TYPICAL DOSE
Codeine	Codeine	po/im/iv/sc	15 to 60 mg q4h prn
Hydrocodone w/ acetaminophen	Lortab, Norco	po	5 to 10 mg q4 to 6h prn
Meperidine	Demerol	po/im/sc	50 to 150 mg q3 to 4h prn
Oxycodone	OxyContin	po	10 to 80 mg q8 to 12h prn

h = hour; im = intramuscular injection; iv = intravenous injection; po = by mouth; prn = as needed; q = every; sc = subcutaneous injection.

Opioid drugs bind to the opioid receptors in the CNS to decrease the excitability of neurons and thus reduce pain. Although there are 3 opioid receptors in the CNS (mu, delta, and kappa), the mu receptor is believed to be most active with opioid medications. These same receptor sites interact with endogenous opioids (endorphins) released in the brain to produce natural pain relief.

Oxycodone (OxyContin) and meperidine (Demerol) are just 2 examples of opioids. Other examples include morphine and codeine. Opioid analgesics can be administered through oral, rectal, or injectable routes. Doses may vary between routes of administration because of adjustments made to account for first-pass effects in the liver. These drugs are often combined with NSAIDs or acetaminophen to enhance the analgesic effect. Morphine is available in oral and injectable forms. The oral dose of morphine is much larger than any other form because of its excessive first-pass effect. Table 3-8 provides examples of common opioids and their typical doses. Of note, the use of opioids is becoming increasing regulated and will be limited to short duration use for acute pain. Athletic trainers should monitor the use of opioids in post-operative pain management as well as for other acute pain management.

Medications for Treating Infections

Antibiotics

Antibiotics are used to treat bacterial infections; they are ineffective in treating viral infections. Most antibiotics are available for oral, intramuscular, or intravenous administration. A few are also available for topical administration via ointment or drops.

There are several different methods used to classify antibiotics; this chapter will classify them according to their mechanism of action. Eight major classes of antibiotics will be discussed. These classes are grouped according to their mechanism for treating the invading bacteria.

The penicillins, cephalosporins, and carbapenems all have a β-lactam chemical structure and work to inhibit the synthesis of the bacteria's cell wall. These 3 classes are said to be *bactericidal* antibiotics because they work to kill the invading bacteria. The tetracyclines, macrolides, and aminoglycosides disrupt the normal protein synthesis within the bacteria, whereas the sulfonamides inhibit an enzyme used to synthesize tetrahydrofolic acid within the bacteria. Finally, the fluoroquinolones disrupt DNA synthesis within the bacteria. The latter 5 classes of antibiotics are referred to primarily as *bacteriostatic* because they keep the bacteria from reproducing, allowing the immune system time to kill the bacteria. At high doses, or when used in combination with other antibiotics, these drugs can act as bactericidals.

Table 3-9 provides examples of these antibiotic classes, their therapeutic indications, and possible adverse reactions. Several general side effects associated with antibiotics are worth mentioning separately. Many antibiotics interact with oral contraceptives, decreasing their effectiveness; therefore, women taking antibiotics should be warned to use alternate methods of birth control or abstain from sexual intercourse. Also, women who take antibiotics may experience vaginal yeast infections as a result of a change in the normal vaginal flora.

Physicians select antibiotics based on the mechanism of action, the specific bacteria being treated, the site of infection, and individual patient factors (age, allergies). To accurately determine the bacteria involved in an infection, a culture of the infected tissue would need to be performed. However, often antibiotic treatment is often started prior to culture results or without performing a culture. This is possible because there are many infections that are known to be caused by specific bacteria. Athletic trainers should educate their patients regarding the proper use of antibiotics and the importance of finishing their prescribed course of medication. Misuse of antibiotics has led to an increased incidence of antibiotic-resistant *Staphylococcus aureus* infections (eg, methicillin-resistant Staphylococcus aureus, *S. aureus*, [MRSA]). The use of antibiotics is further discussed in subsequent chapters in relation to specific local and systemic infections.

Antifungals

Antifungal medications are used to treat superficial and systemic fungal infections. Athletic trainers are most likely to encounter superficial fungal infections involving the mucous membranes, skin, hair, or nails. These conditions are discussed in Chapter 12 along with the specific antifungal medications recommended for treating each disorder.

Antifungal medications generally work as either fungicidals or fungistatics, depending on the concentration of the drug and the site of action. *Fungicidals* disrupt the cell membrane of the fungus, thus killing the fungal cell, whereas *fungistatics* prevent the fungal cells from replicating, allowing the immune system to manage the infection. Most antifungal medications are administered topically for a local effect; however, some fungal infections (onychomycosis) require systemic treatment administered orally. General side effects associated with the use of oral antifungals include nausea, vomiting, abdominal pain, and headache. Topical antifungals commonly cause itching, burning, or skin irritation. Table 3-10 provides a summary of the more common OTC and prescription antifungal medications.

Antivirals

Antiviral medications can be used to treat herpes (Chapters 9 and 12) and influenza infections (Chapter 4). These medications are effective in preventing and reducing the duration and severity of these viruses. Acyclovir (Zovirax), valacyclovir (Valtrex), and famciclovir (Famvir) are 3 common antivirals used to treat herpes infections. These medications are available only in oral and topical forms and require a prescription. Amantadine (Symmetrel) and rimantadine (Flumadine) are effective in treating influenza A, while zanamivir (Relenza) and oseltamivir (Tamiflu) can be used to treat both influenza A and B.

Medications for Treating Colds and Allergies

Antihistamines

As discussed in Chapter 2, histamines are a chemical mediator released during the inflammatory process. There are 3 types of histamine receptors: H_1, which are located in the respiratory tract; H_2, which are found in the stomach; and H_3, which are in cerebrospinal fluid. H_1 antihistamines are used to treat illnesses affecting the respiratory tract (allergic rhinitis, colds, flu [Chapter 4]) and skin (urticaria and pruritis [Chapter 12]). H_2 antihistamines, referred to as H_2 blockers, are used to reduce gastric acid production and are discussed in Chapter 8.

There are 2 generations of H_1 antihistamines (referred to later as just antihistamines without subtext number): first generation and second generation. The first-generation antihistamines are lipid soluble, making them capable of crossing the blood-brain barrier and affecting the CNS. This characteristic is what causes the side effect of drowsiness so commonly associated with these antihistamines. Commonly used OTC first-generation antihistamines include diphenhydramine (Benadryl),

Table 3-9. Classification of Antibiotics

CLASSIFICATION/ EXAMPLES	MECHANISM OF ACTION	INDICATIONS	ADVERSE EFFECTS
Penicillins [β-lactam] Amoxicillin (Amoxil) Amoxicillin plus clavulatate (Augmentin)	Inhibit cell wall synthesis (bactericidal)	Urinary tract infection, respiratory tract infection, heart infection	Allergic reaction in approximately 10% of population
Cephalosporins [β-lactams] Cephalexin (Keflex) Ceftriaxone (Rocephin)	Inhibit cell wall synthesis (bactericidal)	Urinary tract infection; respiratory tract infection; skin and soft tissue infections	Allergic reactions (not as severe as penicillins) Cross-sensitivity with penicillins
Carbapenems [β-lactams] Imipenem (Primaxin) Meropenem (Merrem)	Inhibit cell wall synthesis (bactericidal)	Lower respiratory tract infections, urinary tract infections, skin infections, intraabdominal and pelvic infections	Patients who have allergic reactions to other β-lactams antibiotics may also have a reaction to the carbapenems.
Tetracyclines Doxycycline (Vibramycin) Minocycline (Minocin)	Inhibit protein synthesis (bacteriostatic)	Rocky Mountain Spotted Fever, Lyme disease; use alternatively when patient is allergic to drug of choice	Epigastric discomfort, nausea, vomiting, diarrhea, not recommended for patients < 8 years old
Macrolides Erythromycin (E-Mycin) Azithromycin (Zithromax)	Inhibit protein synthesis (bacteriostatic)	GI, genital, respiratory tract, skin and soft tissue infections; use alternatively when patient is allergic to penicillin	Epigastric discomfort, nausea, vomiting
Aminoglycosides Gentamicin (Garamycin) Tobramycin (Nebcin) Amikacin (Amikin)	Inhibit protein synthesis (both bactericidal and bacteriostatic)	Eye infections, urinary tract infections, pneumonia, upper respiratory infections	Toxicity in the ear and kidneys
Sulfonamides Sulfisoxazole (Gantrisin) Sulfamethozale (Gantanol)	Inhibits the enzyme used to synthesize tetrahydrofolic acid in bacteria (bacteriostatic)	Urinary tract and upper respiratory infections, pneumonia	Crystallization in urine; patients should increase fluid intake
Fluoroquinolones Ciprofloxacin (Cipro)	Inhibit DNA synthesis (bacteriostatic)	Urinary tract, respiratory tract, prostate, GI, bone, joint, and soft tissue infections	Nausea, vomiting, head-ache, increased risk for tendon rupture and articular cartilage lesions

GI = gastrointestinal.

Table 3-10. Topical Antifungal Agents

GENERIC NAME	TRADE NAME	OTC/RX	DOSAGE FORM
Amphotericin B[a]	Fungizone	Rx	Cream, lotion
Butenafine	Mentax	Rx	Cream
Ciclopirox	Loprox	Rx	Cream, lotion
Clioquinol	Clioquinol	OTC	Cream
Clotrimazole	Lotrimin	OTC, Rx	Cream, lotion, solution
Econazole	Spectazole	Rx	Cream
Fluconazole	Diflucan	Rx	Tablet
Haloprogin	Halotex	Rx	Cream, solution
Ketoconazole	Nizoral	Rx	Cream
Miconazole	Micatin	OTC	Cream, powder, spray
Naftifine	Naftin	Rx	Cream, gel
Nystatin	Mycostatin	Rx	Ointment, powder
Oxiconazole	Oxistat	Rx	Cream, lotion
Sulconazole	Exelderm	Rx	Cream
Terbinafine	Lamisil AT	OTC	Cream, tablet
Tolnaftate	Tinactin	OTC	Cream, powder, solution, spray
Triacetin[b]	Fungoid	Rx	Cream, solution, tincture
Undecylenic acid	Desenex	OTC	Cream, foam, ointment, powder, soap, spray

Except where indicated, these products are effective against infections of tinea pedis, tinea cruris, and tinea corporis.

[a] Not for tinea infections.

[b] Also used for onychomycosis although tolnaftate only as adjunct to systemic therapy.

OTC = over the counter; Rx = prescription.

Reproduced with permission from: Houglam JE, Harrelson GL. *Principles of Pharmacology for Athletic Trainers*. 2nd ed. SLACK Incorporated; 2011.

clemastine (Tavist Allergy), and chlorpheniramine (Chlor-Trimeton). Second-generation antihistamines are less lipid soluble and therefore do not cause drowsiness, making them a better choice for daytime dosing, particularly in athletes and other people who perform physical work or need to be alert during working hours (eg, drivers). Common OTC second-generation antihistamines include loratadine (Claritin) and fexofenadine (Allegra).

Antihistamines are also used to counteract nausea and vomiting caused by other drugs (anesthesia or chemotherapy). Promethazine (Phenergan) is commonly used in patients who do not tolerate anesthesia well; however, it produces significant sedation as a side effect. Finally, diphenhydramine (Benadryl) is commonly used in many sleep agents (Tylenol PM, Simply Sleep) because it produces drowsiness.

Decongestants

Decongestants are used to treat nasal congestion associated with allergic rhinitis and the common cold (Chapter 4). These medications cause vasoconstriction of the blood vessels within the nasal passages and help to reduce swelling of the mucous membranes. Pseudoephedrine (Sudafed) is the most commonly used decongestant and is available in oral form as a stand-alone decongestant or as part of a multi-symptom reliever medication. Nasal decongestant sprays are also available and include tetrahydrozoline (Tyzine), desoxyephedrine (Vicks Vapo Inhaler), phenylephrine (Neo-Synephrine 4-Hour), and oxymetazoline (Afrin 12-Hour Original, Neo-Synephrine 12-Hour). The use of nasal decongestant sprays should be limited to 3 to 5 days because they will cause rebound congestion if used longer than this. General side effects associated with decongestants include nervousness, headache, insomnia, and restlessness. Decongestants should not be used in individuals with hypertension or heart disease unless recommended by a physician. Individuals with diabetes mellitus should also check with their physician before using decongestants because of the risk in changing insulin requirements. Athletes should be made aware that certain decongestants may result in a positive drug test.

Antitussives

Antitussive drugs are used to suppress coughs associated with colds and upper respiratory infections. These medications act to inhibit or suppress the cough reflex in the brain. Antitussives are recommended for dry, hacking (nonproductive) coughs and for coughs that interfere with sleep.

Dextromethorphan (-DM) is the most common OTC antitussive and is available in a variety of dosage forms, including capsules, tablets, syrups, lozenges, and oral disintegrating strips. The typical oral dose for adults ranges from 10 to 30 mg every 4 to 8 hours, with a maximum dosage of 120 mg per day. -DM should not be taken with other CNS depressants, such as alcohol or antihistamines, because it could lead to additive depressant effects.

Opioid antitussives are more effective than -DM; however, because they are controlled substances, they are available only by prescription. Codeine and hydrocodone are the most common opioid antitussives; however, hydrocodone is associated with a greater potential for abuse. Codeine antitussives are available in syrup form with the typical adult dose being 10 to 20 mg every 4 to 6 hours.

Expectorants

Expectorants are used to thin mucous secretions so they can be expelled from the respiratory tract through coughing. Guaifenesin is the most common expectorant and is available both in stand-alone products (Mucinex, 600 to 1200 mg every 12 hours) and combination medications designed to treat the multiple symptoms associated with colds and upper respiratory infections. Expectorants are indicated for chest congestion and productive coughs (those that produce phlegm or mucous)

Guaifenesin is available in capsule, tablet, and liquid forms. Side effects include headache, dizziness, rash, and nausea or vomiting. The typical adult dose is 200 to 400 mg every 4 hours, with a maximum daily dosage of 2.4 g. Guaifenesin is also available in an extended-release form, with a standard dose of 600 to 1200 mg every 12 hours.

Multi-Symptom Medications

There are hundreds of multi-symptom or combination medications on the market for treating the multiple symptoms associated with the common cold, allergies, flu, and upper respiratory infections. Table 3-11 provides examples of these combination products, their individual ingredients, and their recommended dosages. While these combination medications are convenient, they also have the potential for adverse effects. If a combination medication contains acetaminophen, then additional doses of acetaminophen should not be added. Also, when selecting a combination medication, it is important to choose one whose ingredients match the symptoms to be treated.

Medications for Treating Asthma

There are 2 main types of medications used to treat patients with asthma. First, anti-inflammatory medications are used to treat the underlying chronic inflammation associated with asthma. Second, bronchodilators are used to prevent and/or treat acute asthma attacks. Both of these asthma medications are described next. These medications are also discussed in Chapter 7.

Anti-Inflammatory Medications for Asthma

Corticosteroids, antileukotrienes, mast cell stabilizers, and methylxanthines are all examples of medications used for the long-term control of asthma (Table 3-12). These drugs treat the underlying chronic inflammation associated with asthma. For this reason, they should not be used to treat acute asthma attacks.

Corticosteroids

As previously described, corticosteroids reduce inflammation by inhibiting enzymatic activity along both the cyclooxygenase and lipoxygenase pathways. Corticosteroids used to treat asthma are usually administered via inhaler. Table 3-13 provides a list of select corticosteroids commonly prescribed to treat asthma.

Antileukotrienes

Antileukotrienes are effective in reducing the chronic inflammation of asthma by blocking the production and effects of leukotrienes, which are produced along the lipoxygenase pathway (see Figure 3-3). Leukotrienes have been reported to produce bronchial spasms, edema, and mucus formation.[10] They are also associated with the release of other proinflammatory mediators.

Antileukotrienes are taken orally and include montelukast (Singulair), zafirlukast (Accolate), and zileuton (Zyflo) (see Table 3-13). Patients with asthma taking antileukotrienes have often been able to reduce their doses of corticosteroids.[10] This is a valuable benefit given the side effects associated with the long-term use of corticosteroids.

Mast Cell Stabilizers

Mast cell stabilizer medications prevent mast cells from releasing histamine and other chemical mediators that lead to inflammation. These drugs also desensitize the airways to triggers that may cause asthma attacks. Cromolyn (Intal) and nedocromil (Tilade) are 2 examples of mast cell stabilizers that are administered by inhalation (see Table 3-13).

Methylxanthines

Theophylline is the only methylxanthine used to treat asthma. However, it is linked with an increased risk for liver toxicity; therefore, it is used less frequently than other anti-inflammatory agents and mainly in the hospital setting. Athletes or anyone working outdoors who use theophylline should be monitored for dehydration because this drug has some diuretic properties. Theophylline is administered orally and may initially cause nausea and/or vomiting, nervousness, and insomnia. Caffeine is also a methylxanthine and has been reported to improve airway function for up to 4 hours in asthmatics (see Table 3-12).[11] Because of its effect on lung function, patients should avoid consuming caffeine at least 2 hours before performing functional assessments such as peak flow spirometry.

Table 3-11. Select Multi-Symptom Products for Treating Colds, Flus, and Allergies

TRADE NAME	ANTIHISTAMINE	DECONGESTANT	ANTITUSSIVE	EXPECTORANT	ANALGESIC	DOSAGE
Tylenol Cold Multi-Symptom Severe (Liquid)		Phenylephrine HCl 5 mg/tbsp	Dextromethorphan HBr 10 mg/tbsp	Guaifenesin 200 mg/tbsp	Acetaminophen 325 mg/ tbsp	2 tbsp q4h
Tylenol Cold Multi-Symptom Nighttime (Liquid)	Doxylamine succinate 6.25 mg/ tbsp	Phenylephrine HCl 5 mg/tbsp	Dextromethorphan HBr 10 mg/tbsp		Acetaminophen 325 mg/ tbsp	2 tbsp q4h
Tylenol Cold Multi-Symptom Daytime (Caplet)		Phenylephrine HCl 5 mg/caplet	Dextromethorphan HBr 10 mg/caplet		Acetaminophen 325 mg/ caplet	2 caplets q4h
Alka-Seltzer Plus Cold & Cough (Liquid Gel Capsules)	Chlorpheniramine maleate 2 mg/ capsule	Phenylephrine hydrochloride 5 mg/ capsule	Dextromethorphan HBr 10 mg/capsule		Acetaminophen 325 mg/ capsule	2 capsules q4h
Benadryl Allergy Plus Sinus Headache (Gelcaps)	Diphenhydramine HCl 12.5 mg/gelcap	Phenylephrine HCl 5 mg/gelcap			Acetaminophen 325 mg/ gelcap	2 gelcaps q4h
Vicks DayQuil Cold and Flu Relief (Liquicaps)		Phenylephrine HCl 5 mg/liquicap	Dextromethorphan HBr 10 mg/liquicap		Acetaminophen 325 mg/ liquicap	2 liquicaps q4h
Sudafed Cold + Cough (Caplets)		Phenylephrine HCl 5 mg/caplet	Dextromethorphan HBr 10 mg/caplet	Guaifenesin 100 mg/caplet	Acetaminophen 325 mg/ caplet	2 caplets q4h

q4h = every 4 hours.

Table 3-12. Adult Dosages of Selected Long-Term Asthma Control Medications

GENERIC NAME	TRADE NAME	OTC/RX	DOSAGE FORM; TYPICAL ADULT DOSAGE
Albuterol	Proventil Repetabs	β_2-agonist, LA	Oral extended release; 4 mg q12h
Beclamethasone	QVAR	Corticosteroid	MDI; 2 puffs (40 to 80 mcg each) bid
Budesonide	Pulmicort	Corticosteroid	DPI; 1 to 2 inhalations (200 mcg each bid)
Budesonide + formoterol	Symbicort	Corticosteroid + β_2-agonist, LA	MDI; 2 puffs (80 to 160/4.5 mcg, respectively) bid
Ciclesonide	Alvesco	Corticosteroid	MDI; 1 puff (80 mcg each) bid
Cromolyn	Intal	Mast cell stabilizer	MDI; 2 to 4 puffs (800 mcg each) qid
Flunisolide	AeroBid	Corticosteroid	MDI; 2 puffs (250 mcg each) bid
Fluticasone	Flovent	Corticosteroid	MDI; 2 puffs (110 mcg each) bid
Fluticasone + salmeterol	Advair	Corticosteroid + β_2-agonist, LA	DPI; 1 inhalation (100, 250, or 500/50 mcg, respectively) bid
Mometasone	Asmanex	Corticosteroid	DPI; 1 inhalation (220 mcg) od
Montelukast	Singulair	Antileukotriene	Oral tablets; 10 mg od
Nedocromil	Tilade	Mast cell stabilizer	MDI; 2 to 4 puffs (1.75 mg each) qid
Theophylline	Theo-Dur	Methylxanthine	Oral extended release; 300 mg bid
Triamcinolone	Azmacort	Corticosteroid	MDI; 2 puffs (100 µg each) bid
Zafirlukast	Accolate	Antileukotriene	Oral tablets; 20 mg twice/day
Zileuton	Zyflo	Antileukotriene	Oral tablets; 600 mg qid

bid = twice per day; DPI = dry-powder inhalers; LA = long-acting; MDI = metered dose inhaler; od = once per day; q12h = every 12 hours; qid = 4 times per day.

Reproduced with permission from: Houglam JE, Harrelson GL. *Principles of Pharmacology for Athletic Trainers*. 2nd ed. SLACK Incorporated; 2011.

Table 3-13. Select Quick-Relief Asthma Medications

GENERIC NAME	TRADE NAME	CATEGORY	DOSAGE FORM; TYPICAL ADULT DOSAGE
Albuterol	Proventil, Ventolin	β_2-agonist, SA	MDI; 2 puffs (90 mcg each) q4h to q6h prn
Ipratropium	Atrovent	Anticholinergic	MDI; 2 to 3 puffs (18 mcg each) q6h
Levalbuterol	Xopenex	β_2-agonist, SA	MDI; 2 puffs (45 mcg each) q4h to q6h prn
Pirbuterol	Maxair	β_2-agonist, SA	MDI; 2 puffs (0.4 mg) q4h to q6h

MDI = metered dose inhaler; prn = as needed; SA = short-acting.

Adapted with permission from Houglam JE, Harrelson GL. *Principles of Pharmacology for Athletic Trainers*. 2nd ed. SLACK Incorporated; 2011.

Bronchodilators

Bronchodilators are used by individuals with asthma to reduce bronchial spasms and expand airways. These medications are typically categorized as either short-acting (onset of action: 2 to 15 minutes; duration: 2 to 4 hours) or long-acting (onset of action: 20 to 30 minutes; duration: 12 hours). Short-acting β_2-agonists and anticholinergics are examples of bronchodilators that provide a quick onset of action and are therefore used for managing an acute asthma attack. Because of their role in treating acute attacks, these short-acting bronchodilators are also commonly referred to as "rescue" inhalers. Table 3-13 provides a listing of common short-acting β_2-agonists. Long-acting β_2-agonists are often used in combination with inhaled corticosteroids for the long-term management of chronic asthma. Because of their delayed onset of action, long-acting β_2-agonists are not effective for treating acute bronchial spasms and should never be confused with the rescue inhalers.

There are 3 main types of inhalers commonly used by people who have asthma: MDI, DPI, and breath-actuated MDIs (Figure 3-4). The standard MDI is the most common type of inhaler used and delivers a metered dose of medication in the form of an aerosol mist. This type of delivery, however, requires good technique in timing the inhalation to coincide with the propelled mist. Poor technique results in a decreased amount of medication actually reaching the lungs. Plastic spacers can be used to extend the distance between the inhaler and the mouth and help reduce the effects of poor technique on medication delivery (Figure 3-5). For optimum dosing, patients should be instructed in the proper techniques for using their inhalers. Step-by-step instructions for using a standard MDI are provided in Table 7-5 in Chapter 7.

Nebulizers are another device that can be used to deliver bronchodilators and corticosteroids for treating asthma and other respiratory diseases (Figure 3-6). There are multiple types of nebulizers ranging in size from large, tabletop models that must be plugged into an electrical outlet to small, hand-held, battery-operated units. Each type of nebulizer converts a small dose of liquid medication into a fine aerosol mist that the patient breathes in through a mouthpiece. Nebulizer treatments are often referred to as "breathing treatments" and typically last 10 to 15 minutes. Table 7-6 in Chapter 7 describes the steps to follow when administering a nebulizer treatment.

General side effects associated with bronchodilators include tachycardia, increased blood pressure, increased blood sugar, nausea, vomiting, nervousness, restlessness, and sleeplessness.

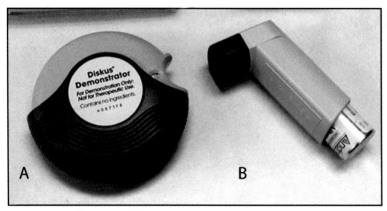

Figure 3-4. Types of inhalers: (A) DPI (B) and MDI.

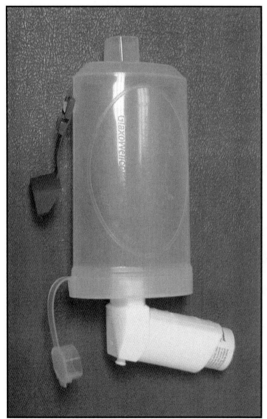

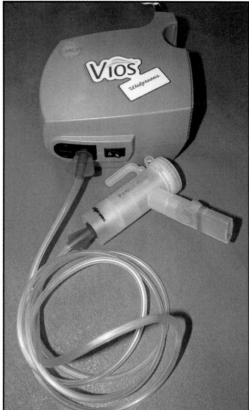

Figure 3-5. Plastic spacer used to improve medication delivery from an inhaler.

Figure 3-6. Nebulizer.

Bronchodilators can be administered both through oral and inhalation routes; however, the inhaled drugs are able to act more quickly and are generally associated with fewer systemic side effects.

Medications for Treating Gastrointestinal Disorders

There are a variety of medications used to treat GI disorders, including antiemetics, antidiarrheals, antacids, laxatives, proton pump inhibitors, and H_2 blockers. Tables 3-14 through 3-16 provide examples of these types of medications and whether they are available OTC. These medications are further discussed in Chapter 8 in conjunction with the specific disorders they treat.

Table 3-14. H₂ Blockers

GENERIC NAME	TRADE NAME	RX/OTC	TYPICAL ADULT DOSAGE			
			Heartburn	Gerd	Peptic Ulcer Disease	Peptic Ulcer Maintenance
Cimetidine	Tagamet	OTC	200 mg prn od to bid	400 mg qid or 800 bid	800 mg hs or 300 mg qid or 400 mg bid	400 mg hs
Famotidine	Pepcid	OTC	10 mg prn od to bid	20 mg bid	40 mg hs or 20 mg bid	20 mg hs
Nizatidine	Axid	OTC	75 mg prn od to bid	150 mg bid	300 mg hs or 150 mg bid	150 mg hs
Ranitidine	Zantac	OTC	75 mg prn od to bid	150 mg bid	300 mg hs or 150 mg bid	150 mg hs

bid = twice a day; GERD = gastroesophageal reflux disease; hs = at bedtime; od = once a day; OTC = over the counter; prn = as needed; Rx = prescription.

Table 3-15. Side Effects Associated With Abuse of Anabolic-Androgenic Steroids

SYSTEM	SIDE EFFECT
Cardiovascular	Increase in cholesterol, high blood pressure, stroke, heart disease
Central nervous	Mood disorders, increased aggression, depression, dependence on AAS and other drugs
Hepatic	Hepatitis, jaundice, liver tumors
Integumentary	Facial and body acne, exacerbation of existing skin condi-tions (ie, psoriasis, rosacea)
Immune	Reduction of antibody synthesis, lymphocyte maturation, natural killer cell activity
Musculoskeletal	Delay in tissue healing, tendon ruptures, premature closing of epiphyseal growth plates leading to limb length discrepancies
Neuroendocrine/reproductive	Female-like breast enlargement in males, masculinization in females, deepening of voice in females, reduction in testicular size, reduction of sperm production, decreased libido, impotence in males, enlargement of the prostate gland, enlargement of the clitoris, increased insulin resistance, decreased glucose tolerance, male patterned baldness in women, premature baldness in men
Renal	Kidney stones, proteinuria, tumors

Antiemetics

Antiemetics are used to treat nausea and vomiting. These symptoms are regulated by the medulla in the brain. Nausea and vomiting occur when the vomiting center in the medulla is stimulated by 1 of 3 pathways. The neurotransmitters (serotonin, histamine, acetylcholine, and dopamine) along these 3 pathways are the targets for prescription antiemetics. OTC antiemetics include bismuth subsalicylate (Pepto-Bismol) and Emetrol (Table 3-17).

Antidiarrheals

Antidiarrheals are used to treat the symptoms of diarrhea; however, they generally do not treat the underlying cause of the diarrhea. There are 3 types of antidiarrheals: opioids, absorbents, and bismuth subsalicylate. The opioids function by decreasing gastrointestinal motility. Examples of opioids include loperamide (Imodium), diphenoxylate (Lomotil), and difenoxin (Motefen). Loperamide is available OTC; however, diphenoxylate and difenoxin are controlled substances because of their potential for abuse. Absorbent antidiarrheal agents function by absorbing water and other compounds to increase the viscosity of the stool. Kapectolin is an example of this type of agent. Bismuth subsalicylate (Pepto-Bismol) can be used to treat nonspecific diarrhea and to prevent traveler's diarrhea. When broken down in the stomach, bismuth subsalicylate is converted to salicylic acid and bismuth oxychloride, which provide both an anti-inflammatory and antibacterial effect. Because it is converted to salicylic acid, individuals with an allergy or sensitivity to aspirin should not take bismuth subsalicylate[2] (see Table 3-14).

Table 3-16. Common Herbal Supplements

HERB	INDICATION OR PURPOSE	SIDE EFFECTS	POSSIBLE DRUG INTERACTIONS
St. John's Wort	Depression, inflammation	GI side effects	Oral contraceptives, anticoagulants, antivirals, cardiac glycosides, immunosuppressants
Gingko	Cardiovascular and peripheral vascular disease, memory, cognitive function	Bleeding, mild GI side effects, headache, allergic skin reactions	Anticoagulants, diuretics, antiplatelet drugs, NSAIDs
Ginseng	Boost immune system, depression, chronic fatigue, GI irritation,	Diarrhea, skin lesions, menopausal bleeding	MAOIs (antidepressants), anticoagulants, corticosteroids, hypoglycemic drugs
Garlic	Hypertension	Heartburn, gas, allergic reactions, dermatitis, GI symptoms	Anticoagulants, antihyperlipidemic drugs, antihypertensive drugs, protease inhibitors
Echinacea	Stimulate immune system, promote wound healing	Liver toxicity if taken longer than 8 weeks	Immunostimulants, corticosteroids, anabolic steroids

GI = gastrointestinal; MAOIs = monoamine oxidase inhibitors; NSAIDs = nonsteroidal anti-inflammatory drugs.

Laxatives

Laxatives are used to treat constipation, and fall into 1 of 4 categories: bulk-forming, osmotic, stimulant, and stool softeners. Common dosage forms for laxatives include tablets, liquids, enemas, and suppositories. *Bulk-forming laxatives* are made of a fiber or cellulose that swells once combined with fluid, producing a thick substance that stimulates peristalsis and pushes the intestinal content forward. To be effective, these laxatives should be taken with a full glass of water. Bulk-forming laxatives may require 12 to 72 hours to produce a result. Psyllium (Metamucil) and methylcellulose (Citrucel) are examples of this type of laxative. *Osmotic laxatives* function to increase peristalsis by drawing water into the intestinal lumen. This type of laxative is effective in providing acute relief of constipation, with onset of action times ranging from 1 hour or less up to 3 hours. Polyethylene glycol (MiraLax) is an example of an osmotic laxative. *Stimulant laxatives* work by increasing motility of the bowels. The onset of action for this class of laxatives is generally 6 to 10 hours. These medications are also known for producing stomach cramps. Senna (Ex-Lax) and basacodyl (Dulcolax) are both examples of stimulant laxatives. *Stool softeners* require 12 to 72 hours to produce a result and are therefore more effective in preventing constipation. Docusate (Colace) is an example of a stool softener (see Table 3-14).

Antacids

Antacids work to neutralize stomach acid and increase gastric pH. They can be used to treat peptic ulcers, heartburn, and mild cases of gastroesophageal reflux disease (GERD), although they are much less effective than proton pump inhibitors and H_2 blockers. All antacids are available as OTC medications in a variety of dosage forms including tablets, caplets, liquids, suspensions, and

Table 3-17. Common Antiemetics, Antidiarrheals, Antacids, and Laxatives

TYPE	GENERIC NAME	TRADE NAME	OTC/RX	TYPICAL ADULT DOSAGE
Antiemetic		Emetrol	OTC	1 to 2 tbsp q15 min until symptoms resolve
	Bismuth subsalicylate	Pepto-Bismol	OTC	2 caplets q0.5 to 1h prn; 2 tbsp q0.5h to q1h prn
	Dimenhydrinate	Dramamine	OTC	1 to 2 tablets q4 to 6 hrs
	Promethazine hydrochloride	Phenergan	Rx	Oral, rectal, IM or IV: 12 to 25 mg q4 to 6 hours prn
Antidiarrheals	Loperamide	Imodium	OTC	2 caplets (4 mg) followed by 1 caplet (2 mg) after each additional unformed stool; not to exceed 16 mg in 24 hours
	Bismuth subsalicylate	Kaopectate	OTC	2 tbsp (30 mL) q0.5 to 1h prn
	Diphenoxylate	Lomotil	Rx	2 tablets qid; 2 tsp qid
	Bismuth subsalicylate	Pepto-Bismol	OTC	2 caplets q0.5 to 1h prn; 2 tbl q0.5 to 1h prn
Antacids	Sodium bicarbonate	Alka-Seltzer	OTC	1 to 2 chewable tablets q2 to 4h
	Aluminum hydroxide and magnesium hydroxide	Maalox tablets	OTC	1 to 2 tablets prn, not to exceed 8 tablets in 24 hours
	Magnesium hydroxide	Milk of Magnesia	OTC	1 tablet q4h, not to exceed 4 tablets in 25 hours
	Calcium carbonate and magnesium carbonate	Mylanta Gelcaps	OTC	2 to 4 tablets or capsules prn, not to exceed 12 tablets/capsules in 24 hours
	Aluminum hydroxide and simethicone	Mylanta Liquid Regular Strength	OTC	2 to 4 tsp prn, not to exceed 24 tsp in 24 hours
	Calcium carbonate	Tums	OTC	2 to 4 chewable tablets, not to exceed 15 tablets in 24 hours

(continued)

Table 3-17 (continued). Common Antiemetics, Antidiarrheals, Antacids, and Laxatives

TYPE	GENERIC NAME	TRADE NAME	OTC/RX	TYPICAL ADULT DOSAGE
Laxatives	Methylcellulose	Citrucel (bulk-forming)		1 scoop powder in 8 ounces water, not to exceed 3 scoops in 24 hours 2 caplets, not to exceed 6 caplets in 24 hours
	Polyethylene glycol solution	Miralax (osmotic)		1 packet of powder daily dissolved in 8 ounces (0.23 kg) liquid
	Senna	Ex-Lax (stimulant)	OTC	Chew 2 pieces od or bid
	Bisacodyl	Dulcolax (stimulant)	OTC	1 to 3 tablets daily

bid = twice per day; IM = intramuscular; IV = intravenous; od = once per day; OTC = over the counter; prn = as needed; q0.5 to 1h = every half to 1 hour; q2 to 4h = every 2 to 4 hours; q4h = every 4 hours; qid = four times per day; Rx = prescription; tbsp = tablespoon; tid = three times per day; tsp = teaspoon.

powders, and include one or more of the following: aluminum hydroxide, magnesium hydroxide, calcium carbonate, and sodium bicarbonate. Typically, antacids are taken after meals and at bedtime and can provide relief within 5 to 15 minutes. Antacids can inhibit or reduce the absorption of other medications; therefore, they should be taken at least 2 hours before or after other medications (see Table 3-14).

Proton Pump Inhibitors

Proton pump inhibitors (PPIs) work to decrease acid production in the stomach. They are available in prescription and generic form and are recommended for the treatment of GERD, as well as gastric and duodenal ulcers. Exact dosage amounts depend on the specific condition being treated. Because stomach acid will inactivate PPIs, they commonly contain an enteric coating. Like other enteric-coated medications, PPIs should not be chewed or crushed. For optimal dosing, the makers of PPIs recommend that they be taken 30 minutes before a meal (Table 3-18). Long term use of PPIs have associated safety concerns, including and not limited to increased risk for C. difficile infections, malabsorption of magnesium/calcium/B12/iron, and kidney damage. Patients using PPIs daily should be referred to physicians to determine if there are other treatment modalities to use.

H₂ Blockers

H_2 blockers work as antagonists to the histamine receptors in the stomach. By blocking these receptors, H_2 blockers are able to decrease acid production in the stomach. H_2 blockers are available OTC and are commonly used to treat mild heartburn, GERD, and peptic ulcers. Like PPIs, dosages vary depending on the condition being treated. For example, higher dosages are used when treating GERD as compared to when treating mild heartburn (see Table 3-14).

Table 3-18. Proton Pump Inhibitors

GENERIC NAME	TRADE NAME	RX/OTC	TYPICAL ADULT DOSAGE[a]			
			Peptic Ulcer Disease	Gerd	Gerd with Erosive Esophagitis	Gerd Maintenance
Esomeprazole	Nexium	Rx/OTC[b]	na	20 mg	20 to 40 mg	20 mg
Lansoprazole	Prevacid (Novartis)	Rx/OTC[c]	15 to 30 mg	15 mg	30 mg	15 mg
Omeprazole	Prilosec	Rx/OTC[d]	20 to 40 mg	20 mg	20 mg	20 mg
Pantoprazole	Protonix	Rx	40 mg	na	40 mg	na

[a] All doses are once a day for 4 to 8 weeks (except maintenance therapy).

[b] Nexium 24-hour available as OTC at 20 mg only.

[c] Prevacid 24-hour available as OTC at 15 mg only.

[d] Prilosec OTC available as OTC at 20.6 mg.

GERD = gastroesophageal reflux disease; na = not approved by Food and Drug Administration (FDA); OTC = over-the-counter; Rx = prescription.

Adapted with permission from Houglam JE, Harrelson GL. *Principles of Pharmacology for Athletic Trainers.* 2nd ed. SLACK Incorporated; 2011.

Nutritional Supplements and Performance-Enhancing Drugs

There are thousands of nutritional supplements and performance-enhancing products currently on the market, which makes it impossible for the athletic trainer to be familiar with them all. In fact, many times athletes become aware of these new types of products long before the athletic trainer does. The 1994 Dietary Supplements and Health Education Act prevents the FDA from having any regulatory control over nutritional supplements. As a result, manufacturers of nutritional supplements are not required to list the ingredients on the labels of their products. This is particularly concerning for athletes who are competing at levels with banned substances and regular drug testing.

There are entire textbooks that focus on nutritional supplements and performance-enhancing substances. This chapter will discuss a few of the more commonly used substances, including creatine, androstenedione, anabolic steroids, human growth hormone, and erythropoietin. Athletic trainers can play a vital role in educating and counseling athletes to help them make informed decisions regarding nutritional supplements and performance-enhancing drugs. Research has shown that scare tactics are not effective in preventing the abuse of these substances. In fact, this approach often pushes young athletes to abuse performance-enhancing drugs rather than avoid them. Athletic trainers should be able to talk honestly and factually with their athletes or patients regarding nutritional supplements and performance-enhancing drugs. There are 3 key questions that must be answered regarding these substances:

1. Are they safe?
2. Are they legal?
3. What do they do physiologically?

Creatine

Endogenous creatine, which is formed by the amino acids arginine, glycine, and methionine, is synthesized in the liver, pancreas, and kidney and then transported to the muscles via the circulatory system. Once in the muscle cell, creatine binds with a phosphate group to form creatine phosphate. Muscles need energy to contract. As energy is produced in a contracting muscle, adenosine triphosphate (ATP) is broken down into adenosine diphosphate (ADP). Stored creatine phosphate can be used to convert ADP back into ATP. After being used for energy production, creatine phosphate is transformed to creatinine and released back into the bloodstream, where it is filtered and excreted by the kidneys.

Synthetic creatine is used therapeutically to increase strength or muscle function in patients with muscular dystrophy or amyotrophic lateral sclerosis. Athletes take creatine in the form of creatine monohydrate (CrM) to improve performance during repeated, brief, high-intensity exercise that requires sudden bursts of energy (sprinting, swinging a baseball bat, jerking a weight bar, starting a new football play every minute or so). This product is ineffective in improving performance in endurance sports.

CrM is available in a variety of dosage forms including capsules, effervescent tablets, effervescent powder, dry powder, and wafers. Two common dosing patterns for CrM include a loading dose or a steady dosing regimen. Loading doses include 20 g/d for 5 to 6 days, followed by a maintenance dose of 2 to 5 g/d.[12] Steady dosing patterns include 3 g/d.[13] It seems to be absorbed quicker when taken with glucose or another sugar source. Most doses are taken just prior to exercise. Individuals taking CrM are advised to drink 6 to 8 glasses of water per day.

There are 2 working theories behind supplementing with CrM. First, an increased amount of creatine phosphate in the muscle helps to increase the rate at which ATP can be regenerated from ADP. Regeneration of the ATP results in decreased fatigue, allowing the muscles to work for longer periods of time. The high levels of ATP also minimize the body's dependency on glycolysis (glucose breakdown) that can lead to lactic acid build-up, muscle pain and burning, and eventual muscle inactivity. The second theory suggests that increased levels of creatine within the muscle draws fluid into the muscle cell, causing an increased muscle cell volume. The increased volume produces a larger cross-sectional area that influences strength development. Following this theory, the increased cross-sectional area will allow the muscle to lift more weight, which in turn builds more muscle mass.

Most reported side effects with taking CrM have been anecdotal and include dehydration, electrolyte imbalance, heat-related illness, muscle cramping, muscle injury, kidney dysfunction, GI upset, weight gain, and skin rash. With the exception of weight gain, research has failed to link these side effects with CrM use.[12,14,15] Of note, upon cessation of CrM use, there is loss of muscle mass changes and slow restoration of baseline muscle prior to use.

Dehydroepiandrosterone and Androstenedione

Dehydroepiandrosterone (DHEA) and androstenedione are steroid hormones produced by the adrenal glands and gonads (ovaries and testicles). Endogenously, DHEA and androstenedione serve as precursors for the production of testosterone and estrogen.[16] The synthetic or exogenous versions of these substances are touted by their manufacturers as being "natural" steroids.

The theory behind using DHEA and androstenedione as performance enhancers is based on the fact that increased levels of testosterone are known to increase protein synthesis, muscle strength, and lean body mass. However, research has failed to show that increased levels of exogenous DHEA and androstenedione, when taken at the recommended doses, actually increase levels of testosterone. In fact, in healthy normal males, DHEA and androstenedione may lead to an increase in the production of estrogen. There are studies that have shown that low levels of DHEA may correlate with chronic fatigue and increase risk of diabetes, anxiety, and cardiovascular disease with greater likelihood of insulin resistance.

Extended use of DHEA and androstenedione can lead to a decrease in high-density lipoprotein cholesterol, which increases the risk of developing cardiovascular disease. Long-term use of these substances, particularly when taken at higher than recommended doses, may lead to serious side effects.[15] Potential side effects for males include enlarged breasts, decreased size of testicles, decreased libido, premature balding, enlarged prostate (may lead to prostate cancer), reduced sperm count, and increased aggression. Females may develop menstrual irregularities, increased masculinization, and increased hair growth.

Androgenic-Anabolic Steroids

Androgenic-anabolic steroids (AAS), a derivative of testosterone, produce both masculinizing (androgenic) and tissue-building (anabolic) effects. Athletes and other individuals who take steroids do so in an effort to gain the physiological effects of increased muscle size and strength, as well as enhancement of physique or body image. These outcomes are achieved through protein synthesis, as well the inhibition of glucocorticoids, which normally produce catabolism. The Anabolic Steroid Control Act of 1990 classifies testosterone and anabolic steroids as Schedule III drugs, making them illegal for possession or distribution without a prescription.

Androgenic-anabolic steroids are lipid-soluble hormones that are available in a variety of dosage forms, including oral, injectable, buccal, transdermal patches, creams, and gels.[16] Although there are FDA approved AAS available for the treatment of specific disorders, these medications require a prescription from a physician. Also, since AAS are controlled substances, athletes and others seeking to purchase these drugs for performance-enhancing purposes must turn to unreliable sources (eg, Internet, teammates, workout partners, gyms). This practice results in the purchase of non-FDA-approved AAS such as "designer steroids," veterinary-grade steroids, and other potentially contaminated or impure formulations.

Abusers of AAS typically take dosages that are significantly greater than the FDA-approved therapeutic doses. Also, they often "stack" or combine multiple AAS with different half-lives in order to maximize sustained blood levels and physiological effects. Athletic trainers should be aware that it is common practice for athletes and others who abuse AAS to alternate between cycles of use and nonuse. Periods of AAS use typically range from 4 to 12 weeks, following by cycles of nonuse. Often the dosage of AAS is varied within the cycle of use following a pyramid pattern, with the maximum dose occurring during the middle of the cycle.[17]

The side effects associated with long-term use of AAS have been well documented and can be categorized into the following areas: cosmetic, hepatic, cardiovascular, reproductive, musculoskeletal, and psychological. These side effects are summarized in Table 3-17. When recognized, these side effects can serve as signs or indicators that an individual may be abusing AAS. Athletic trainers can play a vital role in educating athletes, parents, and coaches about the side effects and health risks associated with steroid use.

As previously mentioned, AAS are classified as controlled substances, making them illegal to purchase or use for performance-enhancing purposes. For this reason, AAS are banned from all competitive sports organizations (ie, high school, university, professional, Olympic).

Human Growth Hormone

Endogenous human growth hormone (hGH) is secreted by the pituitary and is responsible for regulating several metabolic and growth functions in the body. Clinically, hGH, also known as somatotropin, is taken to treat growth deficiencies in children; however, recently this hormone has gained attention for its alleged ability to slow aging and build strength. Research, however, has shown that hGH does increase the size of the muscle, but it does not increase strength. Many athletes and body-builders take hGH for its reported effects in reducing body fat, increasing lean mass, increasing energy levels, and boosting the immune system. These changes in body composition are due in part to hGH's ability to selectively burn fats as fuel rather than carbohydrates.

As an ergogenic aid or performance enhancer, hGH is known to produce the anabolic effects of building muscle through increased amino acid uptake and protein synthesis. Although hGH is not classified as a controlled substance, it is illegal to use this drug for any type of performance enhancement. The hormone is administered via intramuscular or subcutaneous injection. Unfortunately, hGH can also lead to increased growth in bone and cartilage, especially in the jaw and forehead (acromegaly). Other side effects associated with hGH use include water retention, carpal tunnel syndrome, insulin resistance and increased risk for diabetes, increased risk for osteoporosis, sexual dysfunction, enlargement of the liver and spleen, and risk of heart damage. The use of hGH is banned by the National Collegiate Athletic Association (NCAA), the International Olympic Committee, and the World Anti-Doping Agency (WADA).

Erythropoietin

Produced in the kidney, the endogenous hormone erythropoietin (EPO) stimulates the production of red blood cells, which increases hemoglobin levels. This increase in hemoglobin in turn increases the circulating levels of oxygen. Recombinant EPO (r-EPO) was developed to treat bone marrow disorders and certain anemias. Competitive athletes, particularly endurance athletes, are known to use r-EPO to boost the oxygen-carrying capacity of their blood cells and thus gain an advantage over their opponents.

R-EPO is administered through IM or SC injection and is associated with several dangerous side effects. Increasing the number of red blood cells without also increasing plasma volume increases the viscosity of the blood. Use of r-EPO is linked with an increased potential for clotting incidents, heart attacks, and strokes. This substance is banned by the NCAA, the International Olympic Committee, and WADA.

Table 3-19. Drug Resources

PRINT RESOURCES

AHFS Drug Handbook: American Society of Health-System Pharmacists and Lippincott Williams & Wilkins.

Drug Facts and Comparisons: Facts and Comparison.

Physician's Desk Reference: Medical Economics Company Inc.

PDR for Nutritional Supplements: Thomson PDR.

PDR for Herbal Supplements: Thompson PDR.

PDR for Nonprescription Drugs and Dietary Supplements: Thompson PDR.

ONLINE RESOURCES

Drug Information Online: http://www.drugs.com

FDA: www.fda.gov

Medline Plus: http://www.nlm.nih.gov/medlineplus/druginformation.html

RxList: www.rxlist.com

WebMD: http://www.webmd.com/medical_information/drug_and_herb/default.htm

HERBAL SUPPLEMENTS

Many individuals take herbal supplements instead of, or in addition to, therapeutic medications to treat a variety of medical conditions. Like nutritional supplements, herbal supplements are not regulated by the FDA and therefore are not required to undergo testing or a strict drug approval process. Manufacturers of herbal supplements are allowed to make broad claims for the use of their products; however, they cannot claim that their product is effective in treating a specific disease.

Most side effects associated with herbal supplements are relatively minor; however, drug interactions with therapeutic medications could be potentially serious. Athletic trainers, when possible, should be aware of the herbal supplements that their patients are taking. Because many herbal supplements exhibit an antiplatelet effect, athletic trainers should specifically determine whether their patients are taking any herbal supplements before recommending the use of NSAIDs.[18,19]

DRUG RESOURCES

As mentioned at the beginning of this chapter, it would be virtually impossible for athletic trainers to be familiar with every drug that might be used to treat the injuries or illnesses of their patients. However, there are a variety of resources available in print, through computer software, and from the Internet that the athletic trainer can use to quickly obtain information about a medication.[13]

Table 3-19 provides a sample list of resources for drug information. It is also recommended that the athletic trainer seek out a local pharmacist who is willing to serve as a resource for questions regarding medications.

Case Study

During preparticipation physical examinations, you notice that Tim, one of your baseball athletes, has really bulked up over the summer. While visiting with him, he explains to you how he spent most of his summer in the weight room. He wants this year, his senior year, to be his best season ever.

Later in the semester, Tim comes into your athletic training facility complaining of shoulder pain. As he takes his shirt off for you to examine his shoulder, you notice that Tim's back is covered in severe acne. You don't remember Tim having acne before. When you question him about it, he says it started this past summer. He just figured it was due to all of the sweating he did while working out. After evaluating his shoulder, you determine that Tim has some impingement due to rotator cuff weakness, so you start him on a treatment and rehabilitation program. A few days later, while completing his shoulder exercises in the athletic training facility, Tim gets into a fight with another athlete. You've never seen Tim act this way. He has always been a very mild-mannered young man. You start to worry about Tim and what might be going on with him.

Critical Thinking Questions

1. Given his clinical presentation over the course of the semester, what do you think might be influencing Tim's behavior? What signs cause you to suspect this?
2. Following the policies and procedures set forth at your institution, what would you do to follow-up on your suspicions?
3. How would you address your concerns with Tim?

References

1. National Athletic Trainers' Association. *Athletic Training Education Competencies*. 5th ed. The Commission on Accreditation of Athletic Training Education; 2011.
2. Houglam JE, Harrelson GL. *Principles of Pharmacology for Athletic Trainers*. 3rd ed. SLACK Incorporated; 2016.
3. *2012 Recalls, Market Withdrawals & Safety Alerts*. Available at: http://www.fda.gov/Safety/Recalls/ArchiveRecalls/2012/. Accessed February 15, 2013.
4. Chu DA. *Jumping into Plyometrics*. Leisure Press; 1992.
5. Courson R, Patel H, Navitskis L, Reifsteck F, Ward K. Policies and procedures in athletic training for dispensing medication. *Athl Ther Today*. 2005;10(1):10-14.
6. *Therapeutic Medications in Athletic Training*. 2nd ed. Human Kinetics; 2007.
7. Lenz TL, Gillespie N. Transdermal patch drug delivery interactions with exercise. *Sports Med*. 2011;41(3):177-183.
8. Biederman RE. Pharmacology in rehabilitation: nonsteroidal anti-inflammatory agents. *J Orthop Sports Phys Ther*. 2005;35:356-367.
9. Mautner KR. Nonsteroidal anti-inflammatory drugs and sports injuries: helpful or harmful? *Athl Ther Today*. 2004;9:48-49.
10. Gawchik SM, Saccar CL. Role of antileukotrienes for in asthma therapy. *J Am Osteopath Assoc*. 2000;100(1):32,37-43.
11. Welsh EJ, Bara A, Barley E, Cates CJ. Caffeine for asthma. *Cochrane Database Syst Rev*. 2010;1:CD001112.
12. Bemben MG, Lamont HS. Creatine supplementation and exercise performance. *Sports Med*. 2005;35:107-125.
13. Jordan BF. What you need to know about PEDs. *Athl Ther Today*. 2006;11:56-57.
14. Greenwood M, Kreider RB, Greenwood L, Byars A. Cramping and injury incidence in collegiate football players are reduced by creatine supplementation. *J Athl Train*. 2003;38(3):216-219.
15. Powers ME. The safety and efficacy of creatine, ephedra, and anabolic-steroid precursors. *Athl Ther Today*. 2004;9:57-63.
16. Reents S. *Sports and Exercise Pharmacology*. Human Kinetics; 2000.
17. Dandoy C, Gereige RS. Performance-enhancing drugs. *Pediatr Rev*. 2012;33(6):265-272.
18. Martin M, Kishman M. Drug-herb interactions: are your athletes safe? *Athl Ther Today*. 2005;10:15-19.
19. Zhang X, Donnan PT, Guthrie B. Non-steroidal anti-inflammatory drug induced acute kidney injury in the community dwelling general population and people with chronic kidney disease: systematic review and meta-analysis. *BMC Nephrol*. 2017;18(1):256.

ONLINE RESOURCES

◊ **Food and Drug Administration Recalls and Safety Alerts**
  ¤ http://www.fda.gov

◊ **Medline Plus (U.S. National Library of Medicine, National Institutes of Health). Provides information on prescription and over-the-counter medications as well as herbs and supplements.**
  ¤ http://www.nlm.nih.gov/medlineplus/druginformation.html

◊ **NCAA Banned Drug List**
  ¤ http://www.ncaa.org

◊ **United States Antidoping Agency**
  ¤ http://www.usantidoping.org

◊ **World Anti-Doping Agency: Home**
  ¤ http://www.wada-ama.org/

Please visit www.routledge.com/9781630917234
to access additional material.

CHAPTER 4

Immune System

CHAPTER OUTLINE AND OBJECTIVES

Introduction

Review of Anatomy, Physiology, and Pathogenesis

◊ Review the basic physiology of the immune system.

◊ Review pathophysiological mechanisms of the immune system, including contributions to homeostasis.

◊ Describe the effect of exercise on the immune system.

Signs and Symptoms

◊ Identify the general signs and symptoms of pathology involving the immune system.

Pain Patterns

◊ Identify the general pain patterns associated with pathology involving the immune system.

Medical History and Physical Examination Procedures

◊ Discuss medical history findings relevant to pathology involving the immune system.

◊ Describe the physical examination procedures used to assess conditions involving the immune system.

Pathology and Pathogenesis

◊ Discuss the signs, symptoms, management, medical referral guidelines, and, when appropriate, the return to participation criteria for pathology involving the immune system.

  ¤ Infections

   • Infectious Mononucleosis

   • Musculoskeletal Infections

Bhojani RA, O'Connor DP, Fincher AL. *Clinical Pathology for Athletic Trainers: Recognizing Systemic Disease, Fourth Edition* (pp 77-102).
© 2022 Taylor & Francis Group.

- ¤ Autoimmune Disorders
  - • Rheumatoid Arthritis
  - • Systemic Lupus Erythematosus
- ¤ Chronic Fatigue and Overtraining Syndrome
- ¤ Blood-Borne Viral Diseases
  - • Human Immunodeficiency Virus and Acquired Immunodeficiency Syndrome
  - • Hepatitis B Virus
- ¤ Vector-Borne Diseases
  - • Lyme Disease
  - • West Nile Virus
- ¤ Prevention of Infectious Disease
- ¤ Allergic Reactions and Anaphylaxis
  - • Urticaria
  - • Cholinergic Urticaria
  - • Anaphylaxis
  - • Exercise-Induced Anaphylaxis
  - • Insect Stings and Bites

Pediatric Concerns

- ◊ "Childhood" Infectious Diseases
  - ¤ Chicken Pox
  - ¤ Mumps
  - ¤ Measles

Summary

Case Study

- ◊ Develop critical-thinking and clinical decision-making skills.

Online Resources

This chapter addresses the following knowledge and skills from the *Athletic Training Education Competencies, Fifth Edition*[1]:

Content Area	Knowledge and Skills
Prevention and Health Promotion (PHP)	17g
Clinical Examination and Diagnosis (CE)	1-3, 20j, 21p, 22
Acute Care of Injuries and Illnesses (AC)	6, 7, 35, 36j, 36o
Therapeutic Interventions (TI)	30, 31

INTRODUCTION

Infections occur because of the immune system defending the body against foreign microorganisms such as viruses, bacteria, fungi, or parasites (Table 4-1). Physical, behavioral, psychological, environmental, and nutritional factors can all affect immune system function.[2] Contact with infected tissues or body fluids, contact with contaminated objects or substances, or inhaling airborne

Table 4-1. Types of Infectious Organisms

TYPE	STRUCTURE	MODE OF REPLICATION	ENVIRONMENTAL FACTORS
Bacteria	Simple single-celled organisms	Replicate independent of host	Do not depend on host for survival
Viruses	Non-cellular genetic strands	Use host's cellular mechanisms to replicate	Cannot exist outside the biological environment of the host(s)
Parasites (protozoa)	Complex single-celled organisms with multiple or undifferentiated cells	Replicate independent of host	Exist in the environment of the host
Fungi (mycoses)	Primitive single-celled plants, commonly yeasts and molds	Replicate by spores	Dependent on host for growth (but not necessarily for reproduction)

microbes are methods of person-to-person exposure to infectious organisms.[3] Athletes may be at an increased risk for infection because of frequent travel, close and frequent physical contact with other individuals, sharing of facilities and equipment, and altered sleep patterns, all of which affect the immune system.[2,4]

In general, infectious organisms perpetuate themselves by passing from host to host. A *host* is a person (or animal) that harbors an infectious organism. Life cycles of some infectious organisms include a *vector*, often an insect, which transmits the disease-causing organism between 2 individual hosts. The vector is usually not affected itself but can pass the infectious organism to many hosts. Infectious diseases that can pass from person-to-person without vectors are called *contagious*. *Communicable* diseases can be passed from any animal to any other, and thus include vector-mediated diseases.

Failure of the immune system to fully protect the human body can lead to several types of pathology including (1) *immunodeficiency disorders*, which occur when the body is unable to mount the appropriate immune responses to foreign microorganisms; (2) *autoimmune disorders*, which occur when the body mounts an immune response against itself; and (3) *allergic reactions*, which occur when a normal immune response damages normal tissues. This chapter will discuss infections, blood-borne viral diseases (which include immunodeficiency disorders), autoimmune disorders, chronic fatigue and overtraining syndrome, and allergic reactions. System-specific infections (ie, urinary tract infections, upper respiratory tract infections, skin infections) are addressed in the corresponding system chapters.

REVIEW OF ANATOMY, PHYSIOLOGY, AND PATHOGENESIS

Key components of the immune system include the thymus, spleen, lymph system, bone marrow, white blood cells, antibodies, and complement system. The thymus is located in the chest between the sternum and the heart and is responsible for producing T cells. The thymus is active from infancy through adolescence; however, it becomes less active in adults. The thymus functions to help

Figure 4-1. Lymphatic system.

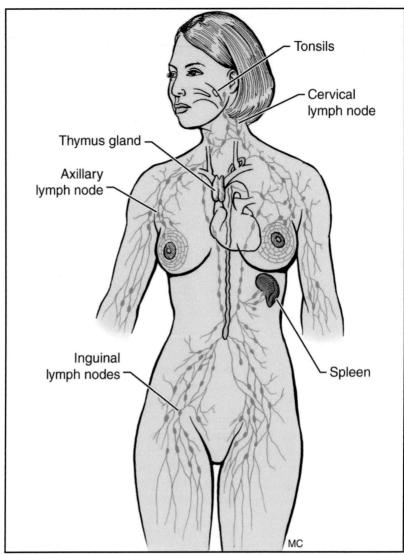

T lymphocytes mature and become immunocompetent (able to recognize and bind to antigens). The spleen, which is about the size of a fist, is located in the left upper quadrant of the abdomen, just under the diaphragm. It functions to filter blood and lymph to remove abnormal red blood cells and platelets and to initiate an immune response against antigens through the actions of T and B cells. Macrophages located in the spleen work to remove cellular debris, bacteria, viruses, and toxins from the blood. Illness and injury to the spleen are discussed in Chapter 8.

The lymph system includes the lymph fluid, lymphatic vessels, and lymph nodes (Figure 4-1). Lymph is a clear fluid, rich in white blood cells, that circulates throughout the interstitial tissues. The lymph collects plasma and debris from the interstitial tissues and is then reabsorbed into the lymphatic vessels, which are located throughout the body alongside blood vessels. Lymphatic vessels range in size from small lymphatic capillaries to large lymphatic ducts. Like veins, lymphatic vessel walls are very thin and contain one-way valves to help move the lymph unidirectionally toward the lymph nodes and then onto the lymphatic and thoracic ducts where it is dumped back into the circulatory system. The lymphatic duct receives lymph drained from the right arm and the right side of the thorax, neck, and head. The thoracic duct is much larger and receives lymph from all remaining areas of the body. Lymph nodes are located throughout the body in clusters and function

Table 4-2. Components of the Immune Response

COMPONENT	INNATE (NONSPECIFIC) RESPONSE	ADAPTIVE (SPECIFIC) RESPONSE
Humoral (blood borne)	Protein complement	Immunoglobulins (antibodies)
Cell-mediated	Phagocytosis (macrophages, monocytes)	B cells, T cells (lymphocytes)

to filter the lymph fluid, as well as to monitor for antigens. The largest collections of lymph nodes occur in the axillary, neck, groin, popliteal, supraclavicular, popliteal, abdominal, pelvic, and chest areas. Only the first 3 of these areas are easily palpated and are often found to be swollen and tender when someone is "fighting" an infection.

The bone marrow is the site for the production of red and white blood cells. The red blood cells mature in the bone marrow, whereas the white blood cells enter the blood stream and are transported to other sites for maturation. There are many different types of white blood cells including *granulocytes* (neutrophils, eosinophils, and basophils), *lymphocytes* (T and B cells), and *monocytes* (macrophages). All of these white blood cells are collectively referred to as *leukocytes*. Regardless of the type, all leukocytes are produced in the bone marrow from stem cells.

Antibodies, also called immunoglobulins, or Ig, are proteins that bind to antigens to deactivate them, prevent them from moving through cell walls, or to mark them for the complement system to destroy. There are 5 classes of Ig: IgM, IgA, IgD, IgG, and IgE. The Ig within each of these classes play different roles within the immune response. An *antigen* is any substance that triggers an immune response. Each antibody is capable of binding with a specific antigen. The *complement system*, also made up of proteins, produces a cascade of chemical mediators that amplify the inflammatory or immune response. This process helps or "complements" the work of antibodies in destroying antigens.

Immune Response Systems

The body's immune system is made up of 2 types of response systems: the innate (or nonspecific) and the adapted (also referred to as acquired or specific) (Table 4-2).[5] Both of these response systems also include humoral (blood-borne) and cell-mediated components.[6] The *humoral response* involves activated proteins and Ig (B cell antibodies) that circulate in the bloodstream. These B cell antibodies work to neutralize microorganisms, toxins, and cancer cells or mark these antigens for destruction by the T cells. The *cell-mediated* component involves the activation of specific immune system cells (T cells, phagocytes, neutrophils, and macrophages), which start a chemical cascade of events to eliminate the microorganism or other tissue debris.[6] Table 4-3 lists the immune responses to the various types of invading organism.

The *innate immune response* system provides the body's first and second lines of defense against foreign invaders (eg, microorganisms, bacteria, viruses).[7] The first line of defense is provided by the physical barriers of the skin and the mucus membranes lining the mouth, nose, digestive tract, respiratory tract, urinary tract, and reproductive tract. Any opening in the skin or mucus membranes allows an invading microorganism to enter the body. The second line of defense is provided by a combination of cellular and chemical defenders. As part of the innate immune response, chemical mediators (eg, histamine, complement, kinins, prostaglandins) are released, which in turn attract phagocytes and natural killer cells to the area. The innate response is further enhanced by the work of antimicrobial proteins (interferon and complement). The interferon proteins protect the uninfected cells in the area, while the complement proteins kill invading microorganisms and enhance phagocytosis.[7]

Table 4-3. Response of Immune System to Various Invading Organisms

MICROBE	IMMUNE RESPONSE
Bacteria or fungi	Macrophages stimulate T cells to stimulate neutrophils (general, cell-mediated) Some B cell and antibody action
Parasites	Macrophages stimulate T cells to stimulate eosinophils (general, cell-mediated) B cells, particularly if toxins produced by parasite Some humoral mechanisms
Viruses	Macrophages stimulate T cells to stimulate "killer" cells and cytotoxic T cells B cells and some humoral proteins that are effective against some viruses

The innate immune response increases overall metabolism to mobilize energy sources and nutrients to meet the increased demands caused by the infection.[5] This generalized immune response can cause muscle catabolism, which releases proteins into the blood to provide extra energy (through gluconeogenesis) and supplies amino acids for white blood cells to combat infection.[5] Fast-twitch muscle fibers, followed by slow-twitch and ultimately cardiac muscle, are affected. Inhibition of muscle energy through both the oxidative and glycolytic pathways impedes aerobic and strength performance. Insulin increases to enhance glucose uptake, and fat metabolism is inhibited.[5] In individuals with diabetes mellitus, the lack of insulin prevents the uptake of glucose; therefore, blood sugar levels increase. This is an important point to remember when dealing with patients with diabetes who are ill or recovering from surgery.

Substances released from macrophages, monocytes, and T cells in the cell-mediated innate response activate protein complement in the blood, which binds foreign particles as part of the humoral general response.[6,8] This sequence of events occurs during the fever phase in proportion to the *virulence* (aggressiveness) of the infection.[5,6]

During recovery from infection, strength remains limited until the metabolized muscle protein is replaced, usually in 2 to 4 weeks. Aerobic function is affected by decreases in blood volume (dehydration), hemoglobin, cardiac efficiency, and muscle mass and may not recover for up to 3 months.[5]

The *adaptive immune response* system provides the body's third line of defense and includes both cell-mediated and humoral components (see Table 4-2). The cell-mediated adaptive response involves activated T and B cells (lymphocytes). This response is stimulated by antigens, which are proteins on the outer cell wall of the invading microbes.[6] The B cells then produce antibodies specific to the invading antigen, thus providing the humoral specific response. These antibodies cue phagocytes to recognize and destroy a foreign microbe. Vaccinations are an example of this adaptive immune response. The B cells "remember" antigens and secrete the appropriate antibodies when subsequently stimulated by those specific antigens.[6,8] The T cells are critical to immune function because they regulate B cell activity and stimulate the general immune responses.[6]

Effect of Exercise on Immune Function

Acute bouts of moderate exercise have been shown to produce transient decreases in the normal functioning of both the innate and acquired immune systems.[9] These transient effects, which include decreases in the circulating blood levels of lymphocytes, including T and B cells, typically

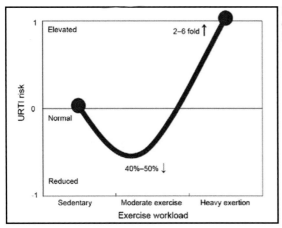

Figure 4-2. J Curve Model on the relationship between exercise workload and risk of upper respiratory tract infections.

return to normal (pre-exercise levels) within 24 hours. However, prolonged, high-intensity exercise, such as marathon or triathlon training, can lead to sustained depression of the immune system. This chronic reduction in immune system functioning is more prevalent when individuals follow intense training schedules that fail to incorporate adequate recovery time between training sessions.[9] In contrast, following a consistent program of moderate exercise with adequate recovery time seems to have a small beneficial effect on the immune system.[10,11] Multiple studies have shown a correlation between exercise training with immune responses, specifically upper respiratory infections. In Figure 4-2, there is a J curve distribution of the risk of upper respiratory infections with regards to training intensity.

Exercise in the presence of an active infection may be contraindicated.[5] Most bacterial infections do not worsen with exercise, but viral and parasitic infections nearly always increase.[6] In addition, viruses may migrate through the bloodstream to additional organs and tissues, such as the myocardium. Myocarditis, a viral infection of the heart, is discussed in Chapter 6. In determining if an athlete may exercise in the presence of infection, the "neck check" rule may provide a general guide to symptom management. If the athlete does not have symptoms below the neck, they may attempt to exercise to tolerance. Any symptoms below the neck warrant cessation of exercise until resolved.

Regardless of the invading organism, athletic performance nearly always decreases when an infection is present because body temperature is increased.[6] Chest pain, tightness, or palpitations during exercise with an infection requires rest from athletics until fever and other symptoms resolve.[5] Classifying an infection as bacterial or viral is impossible to determine without medical tests, so the athletic trainer should recommend rest from physical activity during fever.

SIGNS AND SYMPTOMS

Most systemic infections produce pain and edema in the affected organ or system, resulting in signs and symptoms specific to that system (see Chapters 6 through 13). The signs and symptoms described next are common to infections regardless of the system involved.

Fever

Fever is the most common sign of infection and defined as a temperature of greater than 100.4°F. Fever can generally be classified as low-grade (less than 102°F) and high-grade (102°F and above). While both indicate pathology, high-grade fever suggests more serious pathology. Sustained body temperature over 104°F kills brain cells and may cause irreversible cell necrosis in other organs. Fever causes other symptoms, such as arthralgia, myalgia, anorexia, fatigue, and diaphoresis. See Algorithm 4-1 for clinical decision making related to fever.

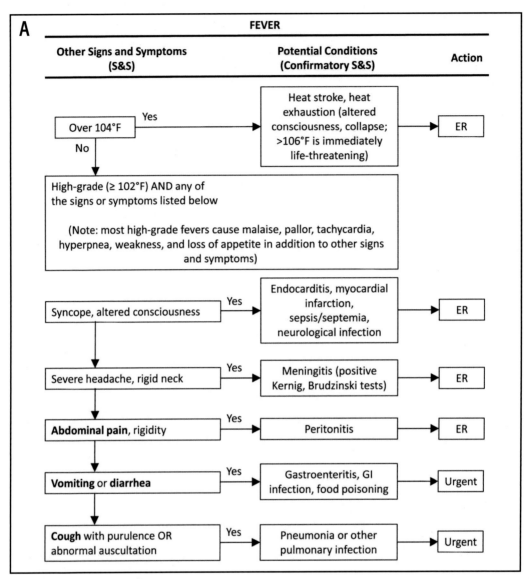

Algorithm 4-1. (A) *(continued)*

Fatigue

Metabolic rate increases with infection. Increased energy demand from the immune response causes catabolism of muscle and other tissues for fuel, resulting in a progressive and persistent fatigue. A chronic infection that continually stimulates the immune response results in chronic fatigue.

Lymphadenitis

Swelling of the lymph nodes (lymphadenitis) may indicate the presence of infection; reaction to mediators from injured tissues and antigens causes the swelling. In general, the infection is usually located distal to the swollen lymph nodes. See Algorithm 4-2 for clinical decision making related to lymphadenitis.

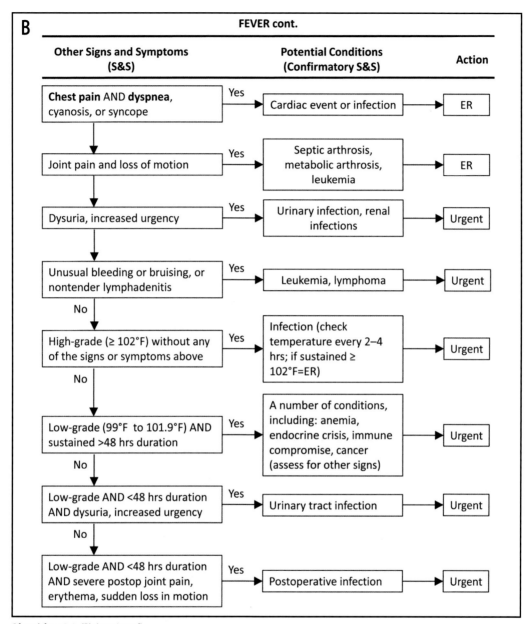

Algorithm 4-1. (B) *(continued)*

Localized Pain, Redness, Heat, and Swelling

These signs occur with inflammation caused by local infection and are easily observed when superficial tissues are affected. Distinctive red streaks or bands that run longitudinally may appear in limbs that have a distal infection, proximal to the infected site.

Unusual Muscle and Joint Pain

Infection may cause muscle or joint pain as a result of the inflammatory response to the invading organism. This type of muscle or joint pain does not change with movement and becomes progressively worse over time.

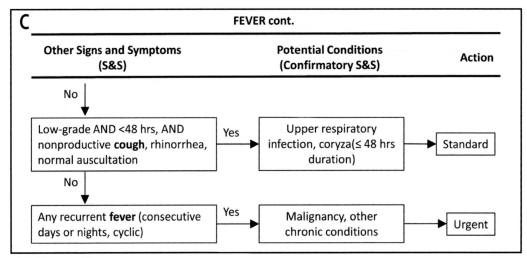

Algorithm 4-1. (C)

PAIN PATTERNS

An infection produces signs and symptoms related to the involved system. Signs and symptoms may also arise in other systems that become secondarily infected.

MEDICAL HISTORY AND PHYSICAL EXAMINATION PROCEDURES

Family and Personal History

Family history may reveal that a family member is experiencing or has experienced symptoms in the recent past similar to those reported by the patient, suggesting an infection spreading within the family. Personal history may identify symptoms consistent with infection, such as fever, fatigue, arthralgia, or myalgia. The course of the symptoms is important, including origin, intensity, and duration of symptoms.

Inspection and Physical Examination

Fever is the primary sign of a systemic infection. Body temperature can be evaluated using a glass, digital, or electronic oral thermometer, a tympanic thermometer, or a rectal thermometer. Normal body temperature is 37°C (98.6°F), although it may range 1 or 2 degrees either way in individuals. Rectal and tympanic temperatures are approximately 0.5°C to 0.9°C (0.9°F to 1.4°F) higher than oral temperatures.[12] Oral temperature fluctuates to a greater extent because it is influenced by hot or cold food and drink, ambient temperature, smoking, and anything that affects mouth temperature. Body temperature also varies throughout the day. It is highest in the evening, low in the morning, and lowest while asleep. Women have a higher body temperature during ovulation. Exercise also increases body temperature, as do emotionally stressful states.

Assessing Oral Temperature

Glass thermometers contain a liquid and must be read manually. Before using a glass thermometer, it should be "shaken down" until the liquid drops below 35.5°C (96°F). To do this, hold the end opposite the bulb tightly between your thumb and fingers and flick your wrist sharply several times. The thermometer is then inserted into the patient's mouth and placed under the tongue with the

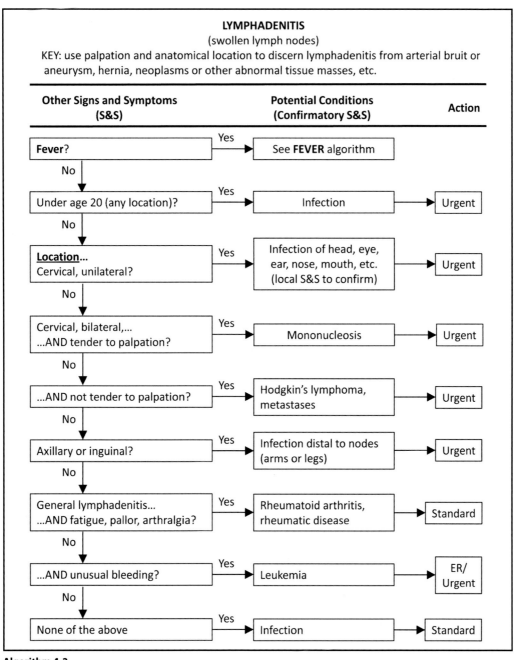

Algorithm 4-2.

mouth closed for 3 minutes. If a high temperature is suspected, read the thermometer, reinsert it for 1 minute, and read it again. If the second temperature is higher than the first, repeat the process until the temperature reading stabilizes. To read the glass thermometer, hold the end opposite the bulb between the thumb and index finger. Roll the thermometer back and forth between the thumb and index finger until the liquid column becomes visible. The number at the end of the column is the temperature. Glass thermometers should be disinfected after each use. Digital and electronic thermometers supply a reading within 10 to 15 seconds. These thermometers should be covered with a disposable latex or vinyl cover and placed under the tongue with the mouth closed.

Figure 4-3. Tympanic thermometer.

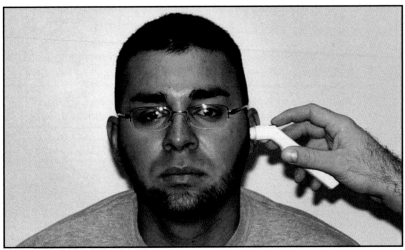

Assessing Tympanic Temperature

Tympanic thermometers assess body temperature via the external auditory canal. These thermometers are battery operated and provide an easy-to-read digital display. Each model may have slightly different operational instructions; however, in general, the following steps can be followed:

1. Place a disposable, protective tip on the end of the tympanic thermometer.
2. Turn on the thermometer.
3. Insert the tip of the thermometer fully into the external auditory canal and aimed at the tympanic membrane (Figure 4-3).
4. Press the button to obtain a temperature reading.
5. Remove the thermometer after the beep.
6. Remove the disposable cover.

Assessing Rectal Temperature

Rectal temperature can be assessed using a glass thermometer with a stubby end or using a flexible probe attached to an electronic temperature device. Instruct the patient to lie on their side with the hips flexed. Lubricate the thermometer or probe and then insert it approximately 3 to 4 cm (1.5 inches) into the anal canal in a direction pointing toward the umbilicus.[12] The glass thermometer should be left in place for 3 minutes. The examiner should wear gloves and the thermometer should be disinfected after each use. As previously mentioned, rectal temperatures are a more accurate reflection of core temperature and will be higher than oral temperatures (0.4°C to 0.5°C or 0.7°F to 0.9°F).[12]

Assessing Other Forms of Temperature

Of note, due to technological advances, there are now cutaneous thermometers that have been used in pediatrics as well in the hospital. These newer forms may not readily be available to the athletic trainer and have not been tested reliably in athletes.

Inspection

Purulent (containing pus) drainage from a wound or body part is a sign of local infection. Likewise, erythema and edema in joints and deep body tissues indicate the presence of an inflammatory response, possibly caused by an infection.

Swollen lymph nodes (lymphadenopathy), particularly if tender, are highly suggestive of infection. As mentioned previously, the lymph node clusters in the anterior neck, axilla, and inguinal areas are most easily palpated. Swelling in the anterior neck nodes is associated with infections involving the mouth, throat, and ear. The axillary nodes drain the arm, lateral chest, and abdominal walls, while the inguinal nodes filter the lower extremities, genitalia, lower abdomen, and buttocks.

PATHOLOGY AND PATHOGENESIS

Infections

Infectious Mononucleosis

Caused by the Epstein-Barr virus (EBV), a variant of herpes virus carried in saliva, *mononucleosis* ("Mono") is most common among persons age 15 to 25 years.[8,11,13] Repeated and prolonged exposure is required to induce an active infection, although an estimated 90% of Americans over age 30 show antibodies to EBV.[11]

Mononucleosis follows a typical course. The incubation period lasts over 1 month and is then followed by a 3- to 5-day prodromal period in which the patient presents with headache, fatigue, loss of appetite, and myalgia.[8,13] The following 1 to 2 weeks are characterized by a severe sore throat, enlargement of the tonsils, moderate fever, bilateral cervical lymphadenopathy, small red spots on the soft palate, splenomegaly in more than half of all cases, and hepatomegaly in about one third of all cases.[8,11,13,14]

A maculopapular rash (flat red areas with small raised bumps) is common in 10% of patients and 90% of patients who are treated with the antibiotic ampicillin.[13] This is important as mononucleosis can mimic "strep throat" or pharyngitis/tonsillitis and can be misdiagnosed. Patients with these symptoms should be referred to a physician for assessment and treatment.

The diagnosis of mononucleosis is made based on clinical symptoms and findings from blood tests. The Monospot blood test screens for the presence of heterophil antibodies, which are common in patients infected with mononucleosis. Blood tests for patients with "mono" will also typically show increased white cell counts (with atypical lymphocytes on the differential) and abnormal liver enzymes.[13] In addition, the new gold standard for confirmation of diagnosis in athletes is the EBV antibody panel.

Treatment for mononucleosis consists of rest, hydration, and acetaminophen or a nonsteroidal anti-inflammatory drug (NSAID) for sore throat pain and fever.[4,11] Occasionally, corticosteroids are prescribed for symptomatic relief of sore throat and swollen tonsils; however, this practice is controversial because of concern for immune suppression.[13] Antibiotics are not indicated unless a bacterial infection occurs concurrently. Patients with mononucleosis do not need to be quarantined.[13] Standard procedures for preventing the spread of infections are sufficient to prevent the transmission of this disease.

Although the signs and symptoms rarely persist more than 1 month, athletic performance may be impaired for up to 3 months.[11] Mononucleosis causes splenomegaly, which predisposes the spleen to rupture. Although spleen rupture in patients with mononucleosis is rare, it will typically occur during the first 3 weeks of symptoms.[4,8,11] Thus, to protect the spleen, a minimum of 3 weeks after onset of clinical symptoms should pass before allowing return to athletics[11] or other strenuous activity. A physician should make all return-to-participation decisions in patients with mononucleosis. These decisions should be individualized, but will typically require the resolution of symptoms.[13,15] There is disagreement in the literature as to whether the determination of spleen size, through physical examination or diagnostic ultrasound, or liver function laboratory tests should be included in return to participation decisions.[13,15] When the return-to-participation criteria have been met, athletes may begin light, noncontact activities.[15] Return to full participation should be gradual and may take an additional 1 to 2 weeks because of continued fatigue.[11] Weightlifting may require extended activity restrictions because the associated sudden increases in intra-abdominal pressure may increase risk of splenic rupture.[15]

Musculoskeletal Infections

Osteomyelitis describes an infection of bone. Usually an infection in the surrounding tissue is transmitted to a bone. Open fractures, recent orthopedic surgery, and prosthetic joints also increase the risk of osteomyelitis because of exposure of bone to the environment. Once a bone is infected, the blood supply becomes compromised, increasing necrosis and infection in the surrounding bone. Signs and symptoms of osteomyelitis include fever, weight loss, fatigue, and inflammation in the affected area. Definitive diagnosis usually requires x-rays or other imaging studies, with biopsy (surgical tissue harvesting) used to identify the organism. Antibiotic therapy, surgical debridement, and/or bone grafting may be necessary to halt progression of the infection.

Septic arthrosis is an infection of a joint, which may result in destruction of synovium and cartilage, called *septic arthritis*. Immunocompromise or malnutrition increases the risk of septic arthrosis. Infectious organisms may invade a joint through wounds, the bloodstream, or surrounding tissues. The athletic trainer may encounter this condition among individuals who have had a recent orthopedic surgery, a penetrating wound into a joint, or a deep subcutaneous wound. Rapid inflammation of the joint occurs, well beyond the normal postoperative inflammatory response, and extreme pain and intolerance for joint movement may be present. Fever may or may not occur if the infection is contained in only one joint. Orthopedic referral for the appropriate antibiotic treatment is necessary.

Autoimmune Disorders

As previously discussed, the immune system is designed to protect the body from invading microorganisms such as bacteria, viruses, and fungi. In some cases, the immune system mistakenly attacks healthy tissues in the body, which can lead to tissue damage and altered functioning within one or more bodily systems. These conditions are referred to as *autoimmune disorders*.

Athletic trainers may encounter a number of autoimmune disorders throughout their clinical practice, including Type I diabetes (Chapter 10), Crohn's disease (Chapter 8), ulcerative colitis (Chapter 8), multiple sclerosis (Chapter 13), eczema (Chapter 12), celiac disease (Chapter 8), rheumatoid arthritis, and lupus. The latter 2 of these disorders are discussed in this chapter. The remaining autoimmune disorders identified above are addressed with the corresponding system chapter as noted above.

Rheumatoid Arthritis

Rheumatoid arthritis (RA), a chronic condition characterized by progressive degeneration of multiple joints, occurs when the immune system mistakenly perceives the synovial lining of a joint as a foreign tissue and attacks it. Morning stiffness in the joints lasting greater than 1 hour before maximal improvement, greater than 3 joints affected with symmetry (small joints of the hands, wrist, elbow, knee, ankle, and MTP joint), with radiographical findings and/or nodules are part of the diagnostic criteria for RA. As RA progresses, joint deformities, ruptured tendons, and disability develop. Persons with RA require lifetime medications and may undergo multiple reconstructive surgeries. Precautions, such as avoiding high loads and extremes of range of motion, are required.

Systemic juvenile idiopathic arthritis (formerly known as Still's disease or systemic juvenile RA) occurs among adolescents with a clinical presentation similar to standard RA in addition to fevers and rash, although the prognosis is considerably better. NSAIDs and occasionally corticosteroids are prescribed to limit synovial inflammation. Participation in athletics should be under the guidance of the treating physician and depends on the severity of the disease.

Table 4-4. Types of Lupus

TYPE	DESCRIPTION
Systemic lupus erythematosus	Most common form; affects major organ systems (kidneys, brain, heart)
Cutaneous lupus erythematosus	Primarily affects the skin; can present with a malar rash or discoid rash (raised, disc shaped, red, and scaly lesions)
Drug-induced lupus erythematosus	Caused by certain prescription drugs used to treat hypertension, arrhythmias, and tuberculosis; rarely affects organs
Neonatal lupus	Passed from mother to child; infant is born with rash; signs and symptoms resolve within several months

Systemic Lupus Erythematosus

Systemic lupus erythematosus (SLE) is an autoimmune disease that usually affects multiple organs or systems including the skin, joints, kidneys, heart, lungs, and brain. There are 4 types of lupus; however, SLE is the most prevalent. Table 4-4 provides a description of the other types of lupus.

SLE occurs most commonly between the ages of 15 and 44 years and affects women more often than men. Two to 3 times as many Black women develop lupus compared to women of other races. Signs and symptoms differ, depending on the systems involved. The most common signs and symptoms include fatigue; butterfly rash across the nose and cheeks (malar rash) (Figure 4-4); swollen, painful joints; fever; sensitivity to light (photosensitivity); abnormal blood clotting; and ulcers in the mouth or nose. SLE is often referred to as the "great imitator" because its signs and symptoms mimic those of other conditions, such as Lyme disease, RA, fibromyalgia, diabetes, thyroid disorders, chronic fatigue syndrome, and a number of musculoskeletal disorders. Individuals with SLE typically experience periods of active signs and symptoms followed by periods of remission.

Athletic trainers should refer patients who present with fatigue and unexplained joint pain or swelling, particularly when accompanied by a malar rash. As previously described, SLE is difficult to diagnose since it can mimic so many other conditions. Table 4-5 summarizes the diagnostic criteria established by the American College of Rheumatology and used by physicians to identify SLE. A diagnosis of SLE requires the presence of at least 4 of the criteria listed in Table 4-5.

Treatments for SLE are structured around the following 5 goals:[16]

1. Decrease overall inflammation
2. Suppress the immune system
3. Prevent flare-ups, and treat them when they are present
4. Control symptoms (ie, joint pain and fatigue)
5. Decrease organ damage

Athletic trainers should be aware that patients with SLE typically have decreased levels of physical fitness and functional capacity[17]

Chronic Fatigue and Overtraining Syndrome

Overtraining is excessive athletic conditioning without allowing for adequate recovery. Overtraining may result in behavioral and physical changes. Increases in cortisol in response to chronic physical stress impairs the ability to respond to hypoglycemia during and after exercise and suppresses the immune system.[18] This produces irritability, apathy, unusual fatigue, declining performance, loss of appetite, excessive thirst, and insomnia.[18,19] In addition, certain physical signs,

Figure 4-4. Malar (butterfly) rash associated with lupus.

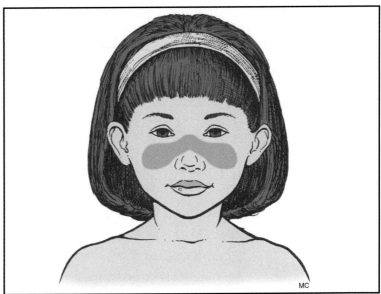

such as increases in resting heart rate, blood pressure, body temperature, or changes in body weight or bowel habits, may occur.[19] Prolonged rest until resolution of signs and symptoms following by a change in training routine to allow recovery between intense exercise sessions is the definitive treatment.

Blood-Borne Viral Diseases

Human Immunodeficiency Virus and Acquired Immunodeficiency Syndrome

Although no confirmed cases of *human immunodeficiency virus* (HIV) transmission have occurred in sports (2 unconfirmed cases have been reported)[6], it is hypothetically possible to contract the virus through fist-fighting or other violent physical contact.[3] Hence, standard precautions (using latex gloves, avoiding contact with body fluids) should be followed to avoid exposure to blood or other body fluids. HIV has been documented among health care workers after exposure to body fluids of infected individuals. Most cases among the general population are contracted through sexual contact or sharing of intravenous needles.

HIV primarily impairs T cells, but also affects B cells, phagocytes, and other immune system cells, thus impairing both the adapted and innate responses of the cell-mediated component of the immune system. In addition, the responses of the humoral aspect of immunity are also impaired because the B cells, which mediate protein complement and Ig (antibody) function, are affected. This results in suppression of the immune system, which increases the risk of multiple opportunistic infections.

Initial signs and symptoms, which appear within 1 month of HIV infection, include fever, arthralgia, skin rash, and lymphadenitis throughout the body. These signs and symptoms, which may be mistaken for influenza or other viral infection, persist for 1 to 3 weeks and then subside. The person can communicate HIV to others in this asymptomatic stage. Without treatment, neurological, hematological, gastrointestinal, dermatological, and pulmonary infections appear within 3 to 10 years. The presence of certain infections that are otherwise rare (eg, cytomegalovirus retinitis mycobacteriosis, Kaposi's sarcoma, pneumocystis carinii pneumonia) as a result of HIV infection are called *Acquired Immunodeficiency Syndrome* (AIDS). About half of people infected with HIV develop AIDS within 10 years.

Table 4-5. Diagnostic Criteria for Systemic Lupus Erythematosus[a]

Malar rash (butterfly-shaped fixed erythema rash across the cheeks and nose sparing the nasolabial folds)

Discoid rash (raised, round-shaped, red patches with scaling and follicular plugging)

Photosensitivity (development of a rash following sun exposure)

Mouth or nose ulcers (usually painless)

Arthritis that is not erosive in two or more peripheral joints (typically presents with joint pain and swelling)

Serositis (pericarditis and/or pleuritis)

Neurological disorder (seizures and/or psychosis without a medication/metabolic cause)

Renal disorder (persistent proteinuria >500mg/24hrs or cellular casts)

Hematologic disorder (hemolytic anemia, low white blood cell count, low platelet count)

Elevated antinuclear antibodies (ANA)

Presence of anti-double stranded DNA antibodies and/or anti-Smith antibodies

[a] Diagnosis requires 4 or more of these criteria.

Treatment of initial HIV infection includes a complex regimen of antiviral agents, which inhibits HIV replication and delays onset of AIDS. AIDS, once developed, is also treated with antiviral medications. Other treatments are provided depending on comorbid infections. Exercise can provide HIV-infected individuals with both immunological and psychological benefits.[6] Athletes with HIV should be under the care of a physician. Healthy asymptomatic athletes can continue to participate in competitive athletics; however, they should avoid overtraining.[20]

Currently, no cure exists for HIV or AIDS. HIV remains contagious for life regardless of antiviral therapy. Strict avoidance of contact with body fluids prevents communication of HIV. Of note, the United States Preventative Services Task Force and the Centers for Disease Control and Prevention recommends that individuals between the ages of 15 and 65 get tested for HIV at least once as part of their routine health care and higher risk individuals get checked more frequently.

Hepatitis B Virus

Hepatitis B virus (HBV) is more common, present in more body tissues and fluids, more durable outside the body, and more easily communicated than HIV. Fortunately, standard precautions prevent exposure to HBV.[21] To date, the United States has no reported cases of HBV transmission during sports, although it has occurred in other countries.[3] Vaccination against HBV is available. Health care workers should undergo the 8-month series of 3 injections to decrease their risk of contracting HBV.[21] Of note, there are new guidelines for screening for HBV in the pregnant and nonpregnant population. Chapter 8 reviews the signs, symptoms, and treatment of hepatitis.

Vector-Borne Diseases

Vector-borne diseases are bacterial and viral diseases that are transmitted to humans through the bite of infected insects and arachnids.

Lyme Disease

Lyme disease, which is the most common vector-borne disease in the United States, is caused by the bacterium Borrelia burgdorferi and is transmitted to humans by the blacklegged tick. The immature blacklegged tick (nymph) is responsible for the majority of Lyme disease cases. During

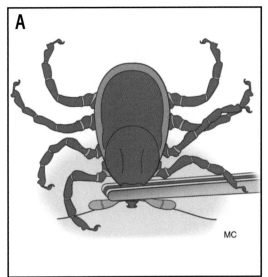
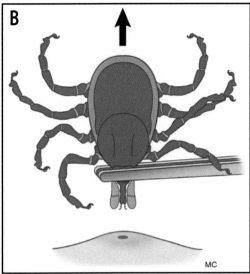

Figure 4-5. Correct technique for removing a tick. (A) Using tweezers, grasp the tick very close to the skin. (B) Remove by pulling straight away from the skin in a slow, smooth motion.

the nymph stage of development these ticks are about the size of a poppy seed and are most active in the spring and summer months. The adult blacklegged tick, which is also capable of transmitting Lyme disease, is about the size of a sesame seed and is more active during the fall and winter months.

Infected ticks must remain attached for 36 to 48 hours before the Borrelia burgdorferi bacterium is transmitted. Removing the tick prior to this time may prevent the transmission of Lyme disease. Figure 4-5 illustrates the proper procedures for removing a tick. Contrary to popular belief, it is not recommended to "smother" the tick with petroleum jelly or to apply a previously lit match to the tick.

The clinical sequelae of Lyme disease can progress through multiple stages, which, in some cases, can last for years after the initial tick bite. Table 4-6 describes the stages of disease progression and the signs and symptoms associated with each stage. The diagnosis of Lyme disease is made on the basis of clinical presentation and laboratory tests. Early stages of Lyme disease typically respond well to oral antibiotics, whereas more advanced cases may require intravenous administration of antibiotics. Physically active patients can typically return to participation following antibiotic treatment and the resolution of symptoms.

Early recognition and treatment can prevent Lyme disease from progressing to the point of central nervous system involvement. Any patient who presents with flu-like symptoms and a bullseye rash (Figure 4-6) should be referred to their physician, even when there is no known history of a tick bite. Similarly, any patient with a history of a tick bite who presents with early or late signs and symptoms of Lyme disease should also be referred to their physician.

Prevention of tick bites is the best strategy for preventing Lyme disease. Table 4-7 outlines strategies for avoiding ticks and preventing tick bites. Ticks are most prevalent in wooded or bushy areas with tall grass or leaf debris. Although cases of Lyme disease are reported throughout the United States annually, most cases occur in the northeast, upper Midwest, and West Coast areas of the country. In 2015, 95% of the reported cases of Lyme disease were from 14 states (Table 4-8).

West Nile Virus

West Nile virus (WNV) is a vector-borne disease that is spread to humans by infected mosquitos. WNV is considered a seasonal epidemic in North America with most cases reported during the summer and early fall.[22] Symptoms, when present, will typically begin 3 to 14 days following a bite from an infected mosquito. About 80% of the people infected with WNV will not develop any

Table 4-6. Stages of Lyme Disease

STAGE	DISEASE PROGRESSION	TIME PERIOD (POST TICK BITE)	SIGNS AND SYMPTOMS
Stage 1: Early, localized	Bacteria is localized; has not spread throughout body	3 to 30 days	Erythema migrans (EM) or "bullseye" rash • Flu-like symptoms • Fever • Fatigue • Chills • Muscle and joint pain • Headache • Swollen lymph nodes
Stage 2: Early disseminated	Bacteria begins to spread throughout body	Weeks to months	Additional EM rashes Facial paralysis (Bell's Palsy) Palpitations Chest pain Shortness of breath
Stage 3: Late disseminated	Bacteria has spread throughout body	Months to years	Muscle pain and weakness Joint pain and swelling (arthritis) of knees and other large joints Numbness and tingling Speech disorder

clinical symptoms. The majority of those who become symptomatic will display flu-like symptoms (eg, headache, fever, malaise, fatigue, body aches, nausea, and vomiting) that can last from several days to several weeks. This mild form of WNV is also referred to as West Nile fever. Approximately 1 in 150 persons infected with WNV will develop severe neurological symptoms similar to meningitis or encephalitis (eg, severe headache, fever, stiff neck, disorientation, coma, muscle weakness, vision loss, numbness, and paralysis). There is no treatment for WNV; however, patients with neuroinvasive symptoms may require hospitalization for supportive treatment (eg, intravenous fluids, respiratory care).

The CDC provides recommendations for preventing exposure to mosquitos that might be infected with WNV. Mosquitos are most active between dusk and dawn; however, they can still be present during other times of the day. People who work or play outdoors should use insect repellent that contains DEET (N, N-diethyl-m-toluamide) or Picaridin. When possible, wearing long-sleeve shirts and pants can provide some degree of protection from mosquito bites. Permethrin can also

Figure 4-6. Bullseye rash associated with Lyme disease.

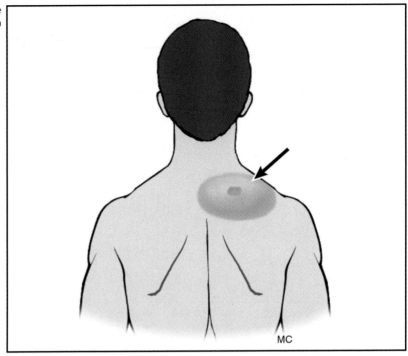

be applied to clothing to repel mosquitos. Standing water should be emptied or changed regularly, because these areas can become breeding sites for mosquitos. Also, practice and playing field should be treated with outdoor mosquito sprays.

Prevention of Infectious Disease

Table 4-9 provides general guidelines for the prevention of infectious diseases in athletic and health care environments.[3,6,11,21,23] Position statements of various medical associations and regulations for health care facilities regarding control of infectious disease are available.[23-25]

Allergic Reactions and Anaphylaxis

An allergy is an exaggerated, cell-mediated immune response that is caused by an exposure to an antigen. Allergic reactions can occur immediately after exposure (eg, anaphylaxis, allergic rhinitis) or be delayed for hours or days (eg, contact dermatitis). Potential antigens associated with allergic reactions include certain foods (eg, peanuts, shellfish), drugs (eg, antibiotics, aspirin or other NSAIDs), pollens, molds, animal dander, insect bites, and latex rubber. Immune reactions can also occur locally or systemically and are associated with the release of histamine, antileukotrienes, and other vasodilatory and inflammatory chemical mediators.

Urticaria

Urticaria is a generalized, allergic skin reaction that produces *wheals* (hives) in response to an antigen. The skin rash associated with urticaria may start out with itching and progress to red welts. Mechanical, psychogenic, or physical agents can also produce urticaria. Urticaria is typically treated with antihistamines.

Table 4-7. Preventing Tick Bites

Avoid wooded or bushy areas with tall grass or leaf debris.

Use insect repellent that contains at least 20% DEET on all areas of exposed skin.

Treat all clothing (shirts, pants, socks, shoes, hats) with permethrin.

Bathe or shower within 2 hours of returning from possible tick-infested area.

Conduct full-body inspection for ticks after returning from possible tick-infested area.

Properly remove any tick found (see Figure 4-5).

Table 4-8. Prevalence of Lyme Disease Cases (2015)[a]

Connecticut	Minnesota	Rhode Island
Delaware	New Hampshire	Vermont
Maine	New Jersey	Virginia
Maryland	New York	Wisconsin
Massachusetts	Pennsylvania	

[a] Centers for Disease Control and Prevention (http://www.cdc.gov/lyme/stats/index.html).

Cholinergic Urticaria

Cholinergic urticaria results in a systemic reaction to a rapid increase in core temperature of 1.8°F or greater, such as may occur during physical exercise. Other causative factors may include hot showers or baths, fever, or anxiety. Although the pathophysiology is not completely understood, cholinergic urticaria is believed to be caused by a cascade of events that starts with the release of acetylcholine, which leads to mast cell degranulation (the release of cytotoxic molecules such as histamine from granules within the mast cell).

In some cases, this inflammatory reaction may present as itching on the extremities without a specific rash. Other individuals will develop either diffuse hives or distinct wheals ranging in size from small (2 to 4 mm) to large (5 to 10 mm), with itching still a common complaint. In most cases, these symptoms will resolve within 3 to 4 minutes.

In moderate to severe cases, cholinergic urticaria may produce systemic symptoms such as labored breathing or tightness of the throat. These more advanced cases are often difficult to distinguish from exercise-induced anaphylaxis, which can be life threatening. Active individuals with a known history of systemic symptoms associated with cholinergic urticaria should see a physician to discuss the need for an EpiPen prescription.

Implementing a more gradual warm-up program may help to prevent cholinergic urticaria reactions. Taking a non-sedating antihistamine, such as loratadine (Claritin) or cetirizine (Zyrtec), 1 hour before exercise can also be helpful in preventing cholinergic urticaria during exercise.[26,27]

Anaphylaxis

Anaphylaxis is a potentially life-threatening, systemic allergic response. The response leads to widespread vasodilation, which in turn produces shock. Anaphylaxis is caused by exposure to specific antigens, most commonly insect bites and certain foods and drugs. Although rare, anaphylaxis can also be caused by physical activity (exercise-induced anaphylaxis [EIA]). Signs and symptoms of anaphylaxis can include a rash that may or may not itch, difficulty swallowing, shortness of breath, wheezing, stridor, hypotension, and swelling of the face, mouth, or tongue.[28] Avoidance of known physical triggers or allergens constitutes primary prevention. Emergency treatment to counter the

Table 4-9. Preventing Infectious Diseases

Appropriate diet, recovery time between workouts, and sleep

Individual water bottles, towels, uniform, and personal equipment

Individual-dose packaging for ointments and topical medications

Immediate showering after participation

Frequent laundering of uniforms

Recognition, proper care, and protection of infectious skin lesions

Vaccination of athletes and health care workers against preventable diseases (eg, measles, mumps, rubella, DPT, influenza, HBV)

Prompt cleaning and covering of open wounds and body-fluid saturated uniforms

Disinfecting soiled surfaces or equipment promptly

Personal protective equipment and strict enforcement of hand washing and standard precautions protocols for medical and laundry personnel

Immunization, particularly tetanus, measles, and childhood vaccinations should be current; may need to update immunizations when traveling to specific regions or countries

Avoid exertion and contact with teammates during active infection

Avoid possibly contaminated water (lakes, rivers)

Meticulous environmental control of public areas (showers, swimming pools, weight rooms, etc)

DPT = diptheriadiphtheria, pertussis, and tetanus toxoids; HBV = hepatitis B virus.

histamine response, such as injectable epinephrine, may be necessary in extreme reactions (Table 4-10 provides step-by-step instruction on the use of an EpiPen). History of known allergens and reactions should be obtained during the preparticipation examination and a plan of care should be developed to manage accidental exposures. Athletes with known anaphylactic reactions should have epinephrine available while participating in activities where exposure to the triggering antigen is possible.

Exercise-Induced Anaphylaxis

A history of breathing problems during exercise combined with a chronic use of NSAIDs increases the risk of EIA, an abnormal immune response to vigorous physical activity.[29] In some individuals, eating certain foods (seafood, celery, wheat, cheese) or taking certain medications (aspirin, NSAIDs) prior to exercise appears to be a predisposing factor for EIA.[30] The anaphylactic reaction causes a widespread release of histamine, an inflammatory chemical that causes vasodilation throughout the body. This reaction also causes acute bronchospasm. Recognition of EIA is important; in contrast to exercise-induced bronchospasm, which is not typically an emergency, EIA is always life threatening.

EIA causes a "flush" sensation in the head and neck during exercise that is rapidly followed by coughing, wheezing, stridor, and shock.[31] Multiple skin lesions (*urticaria* or hives) 1 to 1.5 inches in size may appear.[29] Hypotension and tachycardia herald the onset of shock.

Treatment for EIA includes injecting epinephrine, maintaining an airway, administering supplemental oxygen, and emergency transport to a hospital for monitoring and/or further interventions. Intravenous medications, such as adrenaline, are required to reverse the vasodilation and open the airway.[29] Modifying behavior, such as avoiding known irritants or exercising several hours after exposure to an irritant, and use of antihistamines may be preventive.[32]

Table 4-10. Use of an Epinephrine Auto-Injectable Syringe

1. Remove the epinephrine auto-injectable syringe from its case.
2. Form fist around the syringe, black tip pointing downward.
3. Using your other hand, pull off the gray safety release.
4. Hold black tip to outer thigh.
5. Swing (at 90-degree angle) and jab firmly into outer thigh until pen clicks.
6. Continue to hold epinephrine auto-injectable syringe firmly against outer thigh for approximately 10 seconds.
7. Remove the syringe from thigh and massage injection area for 10 seconds.
8. Carefully place the used epinephrine auto-injectable syringe (without bending the needle), needle end first, into the storage tube.

Insect Stings and Bites

Insect stings and bites have the potential to cause serious systemic allergic reactions. Approximately 1% of children and 3% of adults are allergic to some type of insect sting or bite. Bees, wasps, hornets, yellow-jackets, and fire ants are the insects most commonly linked to allergic reactions. Allergic reactions to insect stings in children tend to be localized and subcutaneous, whereas reactions in adults tend to be more systemic in nature. These systemic symptoms may range from generalized urticaria, dizziness, throat tightness, and shortness of breath to anaphylactic shock. Adults who have experienced a previous localized reaction have a 10% to 15% chance of experiencing a systemic reaction in the future. Also, adults who have had at least one systemic reaction to an insect sting have up to a 70% chance of experiencing future systemic reactions. Therefore, athletic trainers should be aware of those patients who have a history of an allergy to insect stings, particularly those who work or exercise outdoors.

Local reactions to insect stings can be treated with antihistamines to reduce the itching and oral corticosteroids to reduce the inflammation and swelling. Anaphylactic reactions, however, require immediate emergency care. It is essential to have an epinephrine auto-injector on hand for the treatment of these individuals. Although guidelines state that the standard adult dose of epinephrine (0.2 to 0.5 mg) can be administered a second or third time (waiting 10 to 15 minutes between doses) for individuals who do not respond to the first dose,[33] epinephrine auto-injectors are single-dose devices. Individuals with a history of severe anaphylactic reactions should have multiple epinephrine auto-injectors on hand. If multiple doses of epinephrine are required, the individual must be closely monitored, because the epinephrine may cause cardiac arrythmias. Anaphylactic reactions can be recurrent; therefore, all individuals suffering from anaphylaxis, regardless of the dose of epinephrine administered, should be monitored closely for 3 to 6 hours following an attack.[33]

At least 50 deaths are attributed to allergic reactions from insect stings each year.[33] Individuals with a known allergy to insect stings should avoid contact with these insects whenever possible. Individuals who are stung or bitten by an insect during athletic or recreational participation should be monitored closely. Return-to-participation decisions should be made on a case-by-case basis; however, anyone demonstrating a systemic allergic reaction should be removed from activity.

PEDIATRIC CONCERNS

"Childhood" Infectious Diseases

Chicken pox (varicella virus), mumps (paramyxovirus), and measles (rubeola) are common among children but can be contracted at any age. These conditions spread rapidly in day care centers and schools. Close physical proximity and contact, insulated environments, and sharing of food utensils and toys between children contribute to such outbreaks. While relatively harmless in otherwise healthy children, these diseases can cause severe complications among children with immunosuppression and susceptible (ie, not previously infected) adults. Thus, controlling spread of these diseases is important.

Chicken Pox

Chicken pox incubates for approximately 2 weeks and then causes general systemic symptoms (low-grade fever, fatigue, headache) and widespread skin vesicles that erupt, itch, and drain. The virus is most contagious immediately preceding and during vesicle formation. Chicken pox often causes epidemics in schools or other children's peer groups (eg, sports teams). Once all vesicles burst, drain, and crust, the virus is no longer contagious. The lesions should not be scratched; itching may be controlled by topical antipruritic. Acetaminophen may be used to control fever, but aspirin should be avoided completely because of the risk of Reye syndrome. Infection ensures lifetime immunity; adults who have not been exposed to varicella are at risk of several severe medical problems if they acquire chicken pox. A vaccine is available for children and adults to prevent chicken pox and has become a required immunization for all children enrolled in public schools.

Mumps

Mumps incubates for 2 to 4 weeks and then causes general systemic signs and symptoms shortly before salivary and parotid glands begin to swell. This bilateral swelling causes a characteristic swollen ("chipmunk") face. Additional signs and symptoms include dysphagia (difficulty swallowing), high-grade fever, and tenderness in the swollen glands. The virus is contagious (less so than chicken pox or measles) from about 1 week before glandular swelling through resolution. As a result of immunization programs, including use of a 2-dose protocol, mumps has become relatively rare in the US, with fewer than 500 cases reported per year, although larger outbreaks occasionally occur.

Measles

Measles (rubella or German measles; Morbillivirus or 7-day measles) incubates for approximately 2 weeks, then initiates a "flu-like" syndrome (fever, myalgia, malaise) followed within 1 week by numerous, characteristic red skin eruptions. A high-grade fever (over 102°F) develops and lasts several days, after which the condition resolves. Measles is contagious from the time of infection until the rash subsides. Similar to mumps, immunization programs have reduced reported measles cases to fewer than 200 cases per year in the United States.

SUMMARY

Infection is the invasion of a tissue or organ by colonies of organisms, such as bacteria, viruses, parasites, or fungi. The immune system combats infection by using both innate and adapted mechanisms. Infection produces signs and symptoms that are both general, including fever, myalgia, malaise, and fatigue, and specific to the affected organ or system. Contagious diseases are extremely common and affect physical performance. The majority of these conditions can be treated with rest and support of the immune system, although some require antibiotic medications or other medical care. Following relatively simple procedures can significantly reduce the risk of spreading most infectious diseases.

CASE STUDY

During the preparticipation examination, you discover that Mark, an 18-year-old college freshman baseball player, is allergic to bee stings. He has known this since he was 10 years old.

Critical Thinking Questions

1. Based on Mark's history, what other questions might you ask during the preparticipation examination? What else do you need to know about Mark's history with respect to his allergy?
2. What steps will you take to prepare for Mark's participation on the college's baseball team? What specific equipment and supplies might you need? What kind of education and training might you have to provide and to whom might you provide it? Is there anything you could potentially do to the baseball field to help prevent a bee sting?

REFERENCES

1. National Athletic Trainers' Association. *Athletic Training Education Competencies*. 5th ed. The Commission on Accreditation of Athletic Training Education; 2011.
2. Pyne DB, Gleeson M. Effects of intensive exercise training on immunity in athletes. *Int J Sports Med*. 1998;19(Suppl 3):S183-S194.
3. Mast EE, Goodman RA. Prevention of infectious disease transmission in sports. *Sports Med*. 1997;24:1-7.
4. Hosey RG, Rodenberg RE. Training room management of medical conditions: infectious diseases. *Clin Sports Med*. 2005;24:477-506.
5. Friman G, Ilbäck NG. Acute infection: metabolic responses, effects on performance, interaction with exercise, and myocarditis. *Int J Sports Med*. 1998;19(Suppl 3):S172-S182.
6. Brenner IKM, Shek PN, Shepard RJ. Infection in athletes. *Sports Med*. 1994;17:86-107.
7. Marieb EN. *Anatomy and Physiology*. Benjamin Cummings; 2002.
8. Roberts JA. Viral illnesses and sports performance. *Sports Med*. 1986;3:296-303.
9. Walsh NP, Gleeson M, Shephard RJ, et al. Position statement. Part one: immune function and exercise. *Exerc Immunol Rev*. 2011;17:6-63.
10. Peters EM. Exercise, immunology and upper respiratory tract infections. *Int J Sports Med*. 1997;18(Suppl 1):S69-S77.
11. Sevier TL. Infectious disease in athletes. *Med Clin North Am*. 1994;78(2):389-412.
12. Bickley LS, Szilagyi PG. *Bates' Pocket Guide to Physical Examination and History Taking*. 4th ed. Lippincott Williams & Wilkins; 2004.
13. Howe WB. Infectious mononucleosis in athletes. In: Garrett WE Jr, Kirkendall DT, Squire DL, eds. *Primary Care Sports Medicine*. Lippincott Williams & Wilkins; 2001:239-246.
14. Nichols AW. Nonorthopedic problems in the aquatic athletic. *Clin Sports Med*. 1999;18:395-411.
15. Krafczyk MA, Vikram M. Infectious mononucleosis in the athlete. *Int J Athl Ther Train*. 2012;17(6):10-13.
16. Tucker LR. Some mathematical notes on three-mode factor analysis. *Psychometrika*. 1966;31:279-311.
17. Balsamo S, Santos-Neto LD. Fatigue in systemic lupus erythematosus: an association with reduced physical fitness. *Autoimmun Rev*. 2011;10:514-518.
18. Allen DB. Effects of fitness training on endocrine systems in children and adolescents. *Adv Pediatr*. 1999;46:41-66.
19. Johnson MB, Thiese SM. A review of overtraining syndrome: recognizing the signs and symptoms. *J Athl Train*. 1992;27:352-354.
20. McGrew CA. Blood-borne pathogens in sports. In: Garrett WE Jr, Kirkendall DT, Squire DL, eds. *Principles and Practice of Primary Care Sports Medicine*. Lippincott Williams & Wilkins; 2001:247-250.
21. Buxton BP, Daniell JE, Buxton BH, Okasaki EM, Ho KW. Prevention of hepatitis B virus in athletic training. *J Athl Train*. 1994;29:107-112.
22. West Nile Virus (WNV) Fact Sheet, Centers for Disease Control and Prevention, 2013.
23. Arnold BL. A review of selected blood-borne pathogen position statements and Federal regulations. *J Athl Train*. 1995;30:171-176.
24. Brkich M. Infectious waste disposal plan of the high school athletic trainer. *J Athl Train*. 1995;30(3):208-209.
25. National Athletic Trainers Association. Blood-borne pathogens guidelines for athletic trainers. *J Athl Train*. 1995;1995:3.
26. Fisher AA. Sports-related cutaneous reactions: part II. Allergic contact dermatitis to sports equipment. *Cutis*. 1999;63:202-204.
27. Sweeney TM, Dexter WW. Cholinergic urticaria in a jogger. *Phys Sportsmed*. 2003;31(6):32-36.

28. Delves PJ. Anaphylaxis. The Merck Manual. Merck & Co. Inc. Available at: http://www.merckmanuals.com/professional/immunology_allergic_disorders/allergic_autoimmune_and_other_hypersensitivity_disorders/anaphylaxis.html. Accessed June 10, 2013.
29. Kyle JM. Exercise-induced pulmonary syndromes. *Sports Med.* 1994;78:413-421.
30. Hosey RG, Carek PJ, Goo A. Exercise-induced anaphylaxis and urticaria. *Am Fam Physician.* 2001;64(8):1367-1372.
31. Mellman MF, Podesta L. Common medical problems in sports. *Clin Sports Med.* 1997;16:635-662.
32. Truwit J. Pulmonary disorders and exercise. *Clin Sports Med.* 2003;22:161-180.
33. Golden DB. Stinging insect allergy. *Am Fam Physician.* 2003;67:2541-2546.

ONLINE RESOURCES

◊ **American College of Rheumatology**
  ¤ http://www.rheumatology.org/practice/clinical/patients/diseases_and_conditions/lupus.asp

◊ **Asthma and Allergy Foundation of America:**
  ¤ http://www.aafa.org/index.cfm

◊ **CDC Division of Vector-Borne Diseases**
  ¤ http://www.cdc.gov/ncezid/dvbd/

◊ **Healthcare Associated Infections**
  ¤ http://www.cdc.gov/hai/

◊ **Lupus Foundation of America**
  ¤ www.lupus.org/

CHAPTER 5

Oncology

CHAPTER OUTLINE AND OBJECTIVES

Introduction

Review of Anatomy, Physiology, and Pathogenesis

◊ Describe the etiology and pathophysiological mechanisms of cancer.
◊ Explain the process of metastasis.

Risk Factors

◊ Identify the modifiable and nonmodifiable risk factors associated with cancer.

Signs and Symptoms

◊ Identify the signs and symptoms of cancer.
◊ Identify potential early warning signs of cancer.

Medical History and Physical Examination Procedures

◊ Identify medical history findings that are suggestive of cancer.
◊ Identify conditions that would warrant inclusion in a differential diagnosis.
◊ Identify physical examination techniques that may be useful when cancer is suspected.
◊ Determine when the findings of an examination warrant referral of the patient.

Diagnosis and Staging

◊ Describe the TNM System for staging cancer.
◊ Explain the concept of survival rates and its relation to cancer staging.

Bhojani RA, O'Connor DP, Fincher AL. *Clinical Pathology for Athletic Trainers: Recognizing Systemic Disease, Fourth Edition* (pp 103-115).

Cancer Treatment Options

◊ Describe the types of treatment used for cancer, including surgery, radiation, chemotherapy, and other methods.

◊ Explain the process of recovery from cancer.

Return to Activity

◊ Describe the factors that may affect a cancer patient's ability to return to participation during or following adjuvant treatment.

Pathology and Pathogenesis

◊ Discuss the clinical presentation, treatment options, prognosis, and survival rates for common types of cancers.
  ¤ Leukemia
  ¤ Hodgkin's lymphoma
  ¤ Non-Hodgkin's lymphoma
  ¤ Skeletal tumors and bone cancers

Pediatric Concerns

◊ Acute lymphocytic leukemia
◊ Ewing's sarcoma

Summary

Case Study

◊ Develop critical-thinking and clinical decision-making skills.

Online Resources

This chapter addresses the following knowledge and skills from the *Athletic Training Education Competencies, Fifth Edition*[1]:

Content Area	Knowledge and Skills
Prevention and Health Promotion (PHP)	3, 5, 25
Clinical Examination and Diagnosis (CE)	6, 13, 17, 18, 20a-c, 22
Psychosocial Strategies and Referral (PS)	6

INTRODUCTION

Cancer is not just one disease, but rather a group of more than 100 diseases. Cancer begins at the cellular level and occurs when cells become damaged or changed, causing the growth and proliferation of abnormal cells. The American Cancer Society estimates the lifetime risk for people in the United States to develop cancer during their lifetime to be approximately 1 in 2 males and 1 in 3 females.[2] Fortunately, many cancers are now curable thanks to advances in cancer detection and treatment protocols. As of January 1, 2016, it was estimated that more than 15.5 million Americans were living as cancer survivors (either cancer free or in treatment).[2] Because of the increasing number of cancer survivors, it is very likely that athletic trainers will encounter patients in their clinical practice who are at some stage of cancer survivorship. By educating their patients about risk factors, early warning signs, and the importance of self-examination techniques, athletic trainers can play a role both in cancer prevention and early detection. Athletic trainers may also play a role in helping cancer patients and survivors to restore function and return to physical activity. For these reasons, athletic trainers should be aware of the common cancer treatments, their side effects, and the precautions and contraindications relative to physical activity and rehabilitation.

This chapter will provide an overview of cancer, including the general signs and symptoms, common diagnostic procedures, staging methods, and treatment options. Additionally, this chapter will discuss several specific cancers including leukemia, Hodgkin's lymphoma, non-Hodgkin's lymphoma, and skeletal tumors. Other common system-specific cancers are discussed in their associated system chapters including lung (Chapter 7); colorectal (Chapter 8); breast, testicular, ovarian, and prostate (Chapter 9); and skin (Chapter 12).

REVIEW OF PHYSIOLOGY AND PATHOGENESIS

Cancer is a disease of the cell and can occur in virtually any system of the body. Damaged DNA within the cell leads to rapid proliferation of abnormal cells, which causes tumors to develop. Cancers form tumors in affected organs, although not all tumors are cancerous. *Benign* tumors are often only abnormal accumulations of normal cells and are not usually harmful.[3,4] Benign tumors typically grow slowly and act like the cells in the tissue of origin. *Malignant* (cancerous) tumors, however, consist of undifferentiated, or nonspecific, cells.[4] These cells do not function like cells of the original tissue, but rather divide very rapidly because of abnormal chromosomal composition. Malignant tumors are progressive and invasive, interfering with the function of normal cells in the affected organ or system.[3,4]

The chromosomal defects associated with cancer can be inherited or acquired through exposure to environmental *carcinogens* (substances known to cause genetic mutation).[3,4] The abnormal cells do not function properly and replicate at a very high rate. Eventually, healthy, functional cells are either completely replaced by cancerous cells or the resulting tumor grows large enough to impair the organ or surrounding structures such as blood vessels or nerves.

Cancer cells may also migrate to other tissues in adjacent or associated systems through a process called *metastasis*.[3,4] Cancer metastases spread to multiple sites, most commonly the spine, lungs, and brain, subsequently causing tumors and impairment of function in those organs. This migration or spreading of the disease occurs when cancer cells enter the bloodstream or lymph system, allowing them to be transported throughout the body. Once cancer has metastasized, the *prognosis*, the most likely recovery or outcome, becomes significantly worse.

Cancers are typically named according to the organ or tissue of their origin. When cancer cells metastasize to another organ or tissue, they still look and behave like the original tumor cells. For example, when bone cancer cells metastasize to the lung and form a new tumor, this condition is referred to as metastatic bone cancer rather than lung cancer. If examined under a microscope, the new cancer cells found in the lung would be identified as bone cancer cells.

RISK FACTORS

Certain risk factors increase the potential for cancer to develop, including a positive family history, smoking, high-fat low-fiber diet, increased body fat, alcohol abuse, prolonged exposure to sunlight, psychoemotional stress, occupation, and gender (for certain cancers). Although people have no control over nonmodifiable risk factors such as a positive family history or gender, they can limit or modify other risk factors simply by choosing to follow a healthy diet and lifestyle.

Table 5-1. CAUTION: American Cancer Society's Warning Signs for Potential Cancer

• Change in bowel or bladder habits	• Indigestion or difficulty swallowing	• White patches inside the mouth or white spots on the tongue
• A non-healing wound(s)	• Obvious change in wart or mole	• Unexplained weight loss
• Unusual bleeding or discharge	• Nagging, persistent cough or hoarseness	• Fever
• Thickening of tissue or lump (particularly breast)		• Fatigue
		• Pain

SIGNS AND SYMPTOMS

Many cancers may initially present with general signs and symptoms (listed later); however, the disease eventually interferes with organ function, leading to system-specific signs and symptoms, which are discussed in Chapters 6 through 13. To aid in early detection, the American Cancer Society has identified several early warning signs of cancer (Table 5-1).

Fever

Cancer can produce a low-grade fever as part of the immune system's response to the disease as well as to the increased metabolic activity in cancer cells.

Fatigue

Increased demand for energy on the part of cancer cells can lead to fatigue. Meeting these energy demands can lead to the catabolism of muscle and other tissues, which in turn causes a persistent and progressive fatigue and decreased tolerance for activity.

Lymphadenopathy

Lymphomas are cancers that originate and proliferate in the lymph nodes and lymphatic system, producing swelling in multiple lymph nodes. In addition, the lymph nodes are common sites of metastases for many types of cancer.

Night Symptoms

Night sweats, pain that worsens at night, or other symptoms that wake a person during the night may be an early sign of cancer. Organ systems dominated by parasympathetic control, such as gastrointestinal, hepatic-biliary, and renal-urogenital, are more active at night and may therefore become more symptomatic when affected by cancer.

Cyclical Pain Pattern

The regular occurrence of intermittent pain cycles may reflect pathology of organ-systems that function in such a manner (eg, gastrointestinal, hepatic-biliary, and renal-urogenital). In addition, symptoms associated with certain body functions, such as digestion (following a meal), urination, or breathing, may be associated with underlying cancer in that system.

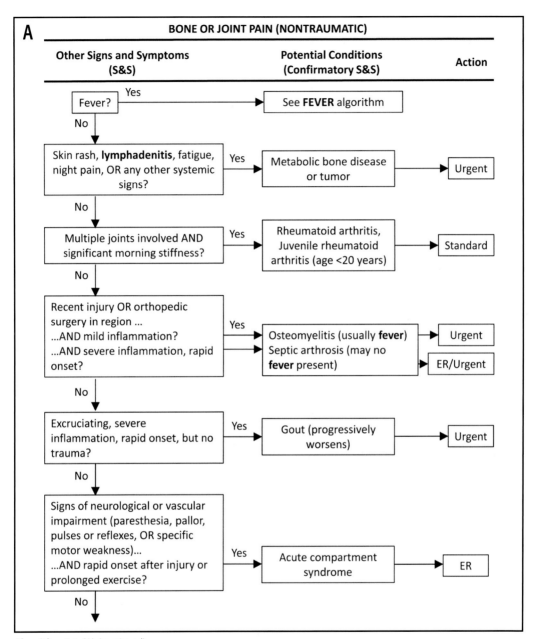

Algorithm 5-1. (A) *(continued)*

Unusual Muscle and Joint Pain

Muscle or joint pain that does not change with posture or movement and becomes progressively worse over time suggests serious underlying pathology, potentially including cancer. See Algorithm 5-1 for clinical decision making related to nontraumatic muscle and joint pain.

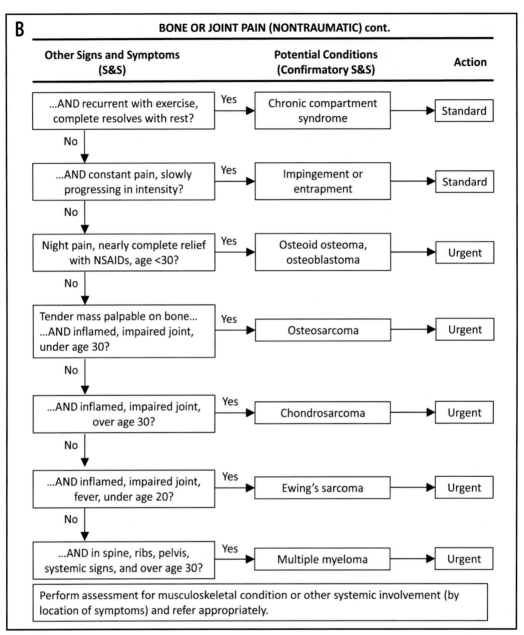

Algorithm 5-1. (B)

Pain Patterns

An organ system that develops cancer may produce signs and symptoms related to that system. Secondary signs and symptoms, however, commonly arise in other systems, including the lungs, bone, brain, and central nervous system once metastasis has occurred. Sometimes signs and symptoms at the sites of metastases are noticed before those of the primary system. Pain patterns associated with specific cancers are dependent on the system(s) involved and are discussed in Chapters 6 through 13.

MEDICAL HISTORY AND PHYSICAL EXAMINATION PROCEDURES

Family and Personal History

Family history can be a significant risk factor for certain cancers, particularly those of the breast, ovary, and colon. Personal history may reveal presence of the early warning signs (see Table 5-1) or general signs and symptoms associated with cancer. The symptomatic course is important, including cycle (rhythm), intensity, and duration of symptoms, as well as how much time has passed since the symptoms began.

Inspection/Palpation

Changes in the appearance or size of moles and mucous membranes can indicate cancerous changes. New, growing, or tender masses; lymphadenopathy; and nonhealing wounds occur with certain types of cancer. Tumors (neoplasms) of bone or connective tissue often become large enough to palpate. Tumors in the abdomen may also be palpable, although considerable practice and skill is necessary to discern normal abdominal anatomy from pathology (see Chapter 8).

Physical Examination

As mentioned previously, the signs of cancer are usually associated with the tissue, organ, or system of origin or tumor site. Many of the examination procedures presented in Chapters 6 through 13 may be used to identify functional changes in the systems as a result of cancer.

DIAGNOSIS AND STAGING

Many cancers are initially identified when tumors are found during self-examination or medical imaging tests (eg, mammogram, computed tomography [CT], magnetic resonance imaging [MRI], ultrasound). However, the accurate diagnosis of cancer requires pathological testing of sample tissue taken either during surgery or through biopsy. In most cases, once a cancer diagnosis is made, the disease is staged using the TNM System to determine treatment options and prognosis.[3,5] The TNM System is based on tumor size (T), involvement of lymph nodes (N), and metastasis to other organs (M).[4,5] In cancers that involve a tumor, the size of the mass can be estimated through diagnostic imaging and confirmed during surgical removal. The degree of lymph node involvement can be determined through a sentinel node biopsy. During this procedure, radioactive dye is injected into the soft tissue around the tumor. The dye is picked up by the lymphatic system, allowing surgeons to identify the sentinel lymph node, or the first node that cancer cells would affect should they enter the blood stream to travel to other parts of the body. This sentinel node is removed by the surgeon, along with several other area nodes, for subsequent microscopic examination. Identification of cancer cells within any of these nodes determines to what extent, if any, the nodes are involved. Medical imaging studies, such as a chest x-ray, bone scan, CT scan, MRI scan, or positron emission tomography scan, are used to determine whether the cancer has metastasized to any other organ(s). Laboratory blood work may also be performed since many cancers have specific serum tumor markers associated with them.

Once the cancer has been described by the TNM System, it is classified into 1 of 4 stages, ranging from stage I, indicating limited cellular changes that remain self-contained within the organ, to stage IV, indicating widespread cellular changes and metastasis.[3,4] Prognosis for cancer is described in terms of 5-year survival rates, or the proportion of patients who remain alive 5 years after diagnosis. If all patients were still alive 5 years after diagnosis, the 5-year survival rate would be 100%. If only half of the patients are still alive 5 years after diagnosis, the 5-year survival rate would be 50%. Many patients live much longer than 5 years after diagnosis for many cancers, but the 5-year survival rate is the standard measure of prognosis.

CANCER TREATMENT OPTIONS

Treatment options are driven somewhat by the stage of the disease and the philosophy of the *oncologist* (a physician who specializes in the treatment of cancer). The most common treatment options for most cancers include surgery, radiation, and chemotherapy; however, hormonal therapy and other biological treatments are also used.[3] Many cancer treatments are used in sequence or combination.

When indicated, surgery can be used to remove the tumor from the diseased tissue.[3] Even when the entire tumor can be effectively removed, radiation and chemotherapy are often still used to kill any cancer cells that might be left in the body. Depending on the type of cancer and the surgeon's and oncologist's philosophy, radiation or chemotherapy may be used first in an effort to shrink the tumor prior to surgery. Radiation and chemotherapy treatments that are given after surgery to increase the chances of a cure are referred to as *adjuvant therapy*.

Radiation can be focused on the particular tumor or tissue area, whereas chemotherapy has a more systemic effect. Each treatment has advantages and disadvantages. Surgery, when indicated, can provide a sure way to limit the spread of cancer, but may be disfiguring or disabling. Radiation uses high-energy x-rays or other forms of radiation to attack cancer cells and prevent them from proliferating.[3] Radiation is most often delivered externally through a high-powered x-ray machine that sends radiation through the tissues, but it can also be administered internally using radioactive needles, seeds, or wires implanted in and around the target tissue. Although radiation provides a fairly localized treatment field, nearby healthy tissues can also be affected, and their function impaired. Most patients experience some degree of fatigue during the course of their radiation treatments.

Chemotherapy can be used to target specific cell types, particularly those that divide rapidly; unfortunately, the chemotherapy drugs cannot distinguish normal, rapidly dividing cells from cancer cells. Therefore, chemotherapy drugs also damage healthy tissues, such as bone marrow, and produce many unpleasant and disabling side effects, such as nausea, fatigue, memory problems, neuropathy, and impairment of blood cell production leading to anemia, clotting delays, and immune system suppression. Because the hair, nails, and mucous membranes are made up of rapidly dividing cells, most patients undergoing chemotherapy will also typically lose their hair, experience discoloration or loss of nails, and inflammation of mucous membranes within the mouth, esophagus, and stomach.

Chemotherapy is most often administered through injection into a vein, although some forms of cancer respond well to oral doses. High-dose chemotherapy is also being used but usually requires a bone marrow transplant afterward. Because the high-dose chemotherapy destroys the blood-forming cells, stems cells are harvested prior to the treatment, frozen, and then thawed again after treatment completion. The stem cells are then transplanted through infusion to help produce new blood cells.

Cancer treatment is specific to the type, extent, and severity of the disease. Research has led to other treatment options, usually used in concert with surgery, radiation, and chemotherapy. Immunotherapy attempts to stimulate the body's immune system to attack cancerous cells. Blood product transfusions may be necessary to replace blood cells lost from impairment of bone marrow. Similarly, bone marrow transplantation may be needed to restore immune function. Antiangiogenesis treatments prevent tumors from becoming vascularized; with no blood supply, the tumor cannot grow. The manipulation of a person's genes (gene therapy) to stop cancer cell division, repair faulty genes, or label cancer cells to make them more vulnerable to radiation, chemotherapy, or immune response is currently being investigated. In addition, there are cancer treatment programs that use a holistic approach to treatment, including nutritional and lifestyle modifications in addition to medical treatments.

RETURN TO ACTIVITY

Return to activity during or after recovery from cancer depends on several factors, including the extent and duration of the disease, patient's age, type of cancer, presence of metastases and related complications, and overall health and fitness prior to disease onset. With nearly all types of cancer, deconditioning occurs from relative inactivity during the illness, from metabolic muscle wasting that accompanies severe illness, and as a side effect of chemotherapy, radiation, and surgery. Although many people survive cancer and return to very active lives, the recovery process is extremely individualized.

Many cancer survivors continue to experience fatigue long after their cancer treatments have ended. Exercise interventions have been shown to reduce cancer-related fatigue during and after adjuvant cancer treatment[6] as well as improve health-related quality of life.[7] Athletic trainers should consult the attending oncologist or primary care physician to obtain specific precautions or contraindications relative to rehabilitation or return of a patient to a desired level of physical activity.

PATHOLOGY AND PATHOGENESIS

Leukemia

Leukemia describes cancers of the white blood cells (WBCs) and involves the bone marrow, circulating WBCs, lymph nodes cells, and spleen.[8] Abnormal WBCs do not respond to infection normally, so immune system function is compromised.[9] In addition, the high rate of proliferation of undeveloped WBCs in the bone marrow inhibits formation of red blood cells and platelets, causing anemia and clotting disorders (see Chapter 6).[9]

About 35,000 people are diagnosed with leukemia each year. Leukemia, unlike most cancers, is not staged using the TNM System because the disease is known to involve the bone marrow and, in most cases, has spread to other sites at the time of diagnosis. Leukemia is classified according to the type (acute or chronic) and subtype (lymphocytic or myeloid) of the disease, with the most common forms including acute lymphocytic leukemia (ALL), acute myelocytic leukemia, chronic lymphocytic leukemia, and chronic myelocytic leukemia.[8] The acute forms of leukemia are associated with rapid deterioration, while the chronic forms typically progress more slowly. Survival rates vary by the type of leukemia and phase of disease (eg, chronic, accelerated, blast). Acute types of leukemia have a worse prognosis, with 5-year survival rates between 24% to 35%.[2] By contrast, treatment of some types of chronic leukemia leads to complete remission in most patients.[10]

The most common signs and symptoms of acute leukemia include anemia, chronic recurrent infections, easy bruising, and abnormal bleeding from the gums or nose or in mid-menstrual cycle.[8,11] Additional signs and symptoms depend on the other organs that are affected, but may include fatigue, weight loss, fever, lymphadenopathy, hepatomegaly, splenomegaly, deep bone pain, headache, cranial nerve effects, and vomiting.[3,8,9] ALL is the most common cancer diagnosed in children; however, it also affects adults. Acute myelocytic leukemia can occur at any age.[8]

The clinical presentation of chronic leukemia typically occurs gradually over time. Signs and symptoms include fatigue, weight loss, shortness of breath with exertion, lymphadenopathy, splenomegaly, and hepatomegaly.[8] Chronic myelocytic leukemia is most commonly diagnosed in young adults, whereas chronic lymphocytic leukemia typically presents in individuals who are middle age or older.[8]

Unless treated, all leukemias are fatal. Chemotherapy and bone marrow transplant are the main methods of treatment.[10] Leukemia may go into remission for many years, then recur and cause death within weeks or months. Early diagnosis techniques and advances in treatment have been able to cure leukemia in many patients.

Hodgkin's Lymphoma

Hodgkin's lymphoma is a cancer that develops in one or more lymph nodes and occurs most commonly between the ages of 15 and 40 years.[12] Approximately 8000 cases of Hodgkin's lymphoma are diagnosed each year, with almost 1000 deaths each year attributed to the disease.[2] Hodgkin's lymphoma metastasizes to many lymph nodes and organs, including the spleen, liver, lungs, and bone.[9,13] Most commonly, the first sign is painless, swollen lymph nodes that are palpated as firm, movable masses in the unilateral groin or neck.[10-12] Other signs and symptoms may include fever, night sweats, weight loss, fatigue, loss of appetite, and itching of the skin. General systemic signs and symptoms may also be present if the cancer has spread to other systems. In untreated advanced stages, chronic recurrent infections, and multiple symptomatic metastases occur.[9] With early recognition, Hodgkin's lymphoma is treated with radiation and chemotherapy and has a good prognosis; the 5-year survival rate is 80% to 90% and the 15-year survival rate is 68%.

Non-Hodgkin's Lymphoma

Non-Hodgkin's lymphoma is several types of lymphatic cancer that present clinical signs and symptoms similar to Hodgkin's lymphoma. Non-Hodgkin's lymphoma is diagnosed in 74,000 people annually and causes approximately 19,000 deaths annually.[2] Non-Hodgkin's lymphoma is usually more widespread, aggressive, and has a worse prognosis in comparison to Hodgkin's disease. Hence, lymph node swelling, particularly if reported as persisting more than a couple of weeks, requires medical referral.

Non-Hodgkin's lymphomas can form in B and T cells, which have immune system functions, as well as the lymph nodes and organs with lymphatic tissue (spleen, bone marrow). If the cancer obstructs the flow of lymph, localized swelling occurs; this is most common in the abdomen, neck, and brain. Lymphoma growth may encroach on the superior vena cava, causing swelling in both arms and legs. The 5-year survival rate for all types of non-Hodgkin's lymphoma is 70%; 10-year survival is 42%.

Skeletal Tumors and Bone Cancers

Bone cancers are relatively rare, with approximately 3000 cases per year diagnosed and 1400 deaths annually[14]; primary bone cancer accounts for 0.2% of all cancers. There are many types of bone cancer, and some are more severe than others. Five-year survival for all types of bone cancer is approximately 64% if detected in early stages, but decreases to less than 10% for advanced disease.

Benign Bone Tumors

Osteoid Osteoma/Osteoblastoma

These benign but painful bone tumors may impair joint motion or impinge nerves or blood vessels as they grow. Most prevalent before the age of 30 years, a recurrent, dull, aching pain that increases at night and nearly completely disappears with anti-inflammatory use suggests *osteoid osteoma* (< 2 cm) or *osteoblastoma* (> 2 cm). Soft tissue swelling and deformity may also be visible depending on the location. These benign tumors have been reported to occur more frequently in men than women and most commonly involve the femur or tibia. Treatment is by surgical excision and bony stabilization, if needed.[15] After postoperative healing and rehabilitation, return to full unlimited activity can be anticipated.

Osteochondroma and Chondroblastoma

Osteochondroma and chondroblastoma are 2 additional types of benign bone tumors, both of which present similarly to osteoid osteoma and osteoblastoma. An *osteochondroma* is made up of cartilage and bone and is most commonly seen near the epiphyseal plates in the shoulder or knee. These tumors present as hard, immobile masses that may or may not be symptomatic; however, the adjacent soft tissue may become sore. *Chondroblastomas* occur within the epiphysis and are most commonly seen in the shoulder, hip, or knee. Symptoms are similar to those of osteochondromas. The diagnoses for both chondroblastomas and osteochondromas are made through x-rays, CT scans, or MRIs. Treatment for both types of tumors involves surgical excision and bone grafting, when necessary. Generally, recovery is complete, although lengthy, if large sections of bone are involved.

Malignant Bone Tumors

These malignant tumors occur in the metaphysis of long bones and articular cartilage, respectively.[16] *Osteosarcoma* is most common among adolescent and young adult males, whereas *chondrosarcoma* presents more often among middle-aged adults.[15,16] Osteosarcoma has an affinity for the rapidly growing epiphysis, often in the distal femur, and causes pain, swelling, and joint impairment without a history of injury. Pathological fracture may also occur if the bone is sufficiently weakened. Metastases to the lungs and brain occur early in osteosarcoma and are associated with a worse prognosis.

In contrast, chondrosarcoma progresses more slowly and is less likely to metastasize. Clinical signs are few, with a gradually increasing tender bone mass as the most frequent sign. Surgery is an integral part of the treatment for bone tumors; however, chemotherapy is commonly used prior to surgery in an effort to shrink the tumor. Prognosis is considerably better than that of osteosarcoma. Recent advances in diagnosis and treatment continue to increase the survival rates for both tumors.

PEDIATRIC CONCERNS

Acute Lymphocytic Leukemia

As previously mentioned, ALL is the most common cancer in children, appearing most often in early childhood (under 5 years of age).[8,9] Signs and symptoms follow those outlined for acute leukemia above. Bone pain in the chest or tibia is also common. Clinical presentation of ALL is initially suggestive of acute infection, with high-grade fever and rapid physical collapse. ALL is a medical emergency, but timely treatment leads to a 5-year survival rate of 89%.

Ewing's Sarcoma

Ewing's sarcoma can affect any part of the bone, usually appearing in the lower extremity. Nontraumatic pain of the affected region is the main symptom, accompanied by limb swelling and a low-grade fever.[15] A tender mass may be palpable over the bone in more advanced stages. Neurologic signs and symptoms occur if the tumor impinges a nerve. Like other bone cancers, treatment consists of radiation, chemotherapy, and surgery, including wide-scale tissue resection or amputation as necessary to remove all cancerous cells. Between 50% to 70% of children with Ewing's sarcoma survive at least 5 years, with better prognosis for earlier diagnosis and lack of metastases. Ewing's sarcoma is detectable by routine x-ray. Any child or adolescent with unexplained, vague limb or joint pain should be promptly referred for appropriate diagnostic testing.

SUMMARY

Cancer can affect any organ system and at any age. These diseases can produce signs and symptoms of both general illness and specific illness to a particular system, presenting a clinical picture of chronic or acute severe illness. Athletic trainers should be aware of risk factors and early warning signs for cancer. In addition, they should be aware of potential precautions for physical activity for persons recovering from cancer. Education of students, athletes, and patients with respect to warning signs and self-examination techniques may help them detect cancer in earlier stages, thereby increasing probability and duration of survival.

CASE STUDY

Casey is a 15-year-old male soccer athlete who plays on the varsity soccer team at your school and on an elite soccer team outside of school. He is complaining of medial knee pain (5/10) in his left leg. He doesn't remember any particular injury, but rather remembers that his knee just started aching about 2 or 3 weeks ago and has been hurting ever since. He explains that his knee aches all the time, but the pain is worse at night. Initially he didn't think anything of the knee pain since he had played in 2 tournaments that weekend, one with his high school team and another one with his elite team. He just thought that maybe he had overdone it.

As you begin your physical examination, you notice some mild swelling along the medial aspect of the knee. On palpation, you find him to be tender over the distal medial femoral condyle; however, all other palpation findings are negative. Range of motion is slightly limited in the left knee with the following measurements: right knee flexion = 130 degrees, left knee flexion = 118 degrees. Although his history does not indicate ligamentous injury, you decide to perform a thorough physical examination that includes valgus, varus, lachman, and McMurray tests. All of these tests are also negative. Your evaluation fails to yield any clues as to the cause of Casey's knee pain, and you are concerned that he reports his pain worsens at night. You decide to refer Casey to Dr. Smith, a local orthopedist, to see what he might find.

A few hours after his doctor's appointment, Casey and his mother show up at your office. After looking at his x-rays, Dr. Smith is concerned that Casey might have a bone tumor. He has ordered an MRI and would like for Casey to see Dr. Jones, a local oncologist for consultation and further tests.

Critical Thinking Questions

1. Casey and his mother have many questions for you. First, what causes bone tumors and are there different kinds of bone tumors? If he does have a bone tumor, does that mean he has cancer? Also, what does this mean for Casey's soccer career?

2. Casey's mother also asks what kinds of tests that you think Dr. Jones is likely to conduct. What will these tests be looking for?

REFERENCES

1. National Athletic Trainers' Association. *Athletic Training Education Competencies*. 5th ed. The Commission on Accreditation of Athletic Training Education; 2011.
2. *Cancer Facts and Figures*. American Cancer Society; 2019.
3. Caudell KA. Alterations in cell growth and replication: neoplasia. In: Porth CM, ed. *Essentials of Pathophysiology: Concepts of Altered Health States*. 6th ed. Lippincott Williams & Wilkins; 2002:64-83.
4. Damjanov I. Neoplasia. In: Damjanov I, ed. *Pathology for the Health-Related Professions*. WB Saunders Co.; 2000:71-98.
5. Unger P, Goodman CC. The integumentary system. In: Goodman CC, Boissonnault WG, eds. *Pathology: Implications for the Physical Therapist*. W.B. Saunders Company; 1998:173-215.

6. Puetz TW, Herring MP. Differential effects of exercise on cancer-related fatigue during and following treatment: a meta-analysis. *Am J Prev Med.* 2012;43:e1-e24.

7. Knobf MT, Musanti R, Dorward J. Exercise and quality of life outcomes in patients with cancer. *Semin Oncol Nurs.* 2007;23:285-296.

8. Rytting ME. Overview of leukemia. The Merck Manual. Merck & Co., Inc. Available at: http://www.merckmanuals.com/professional/hematology_and_oncology/leukemias/overview_of_leukemia.html. Accessed June 7, 2013.

9. Gould BE. Cardiovascular and lymphatic disorders. In: *Pathophysiology for the Health Care Professions.* W.B. Saunders Co; 1997:159-212.

10. Caudell KA, Gaspard KJ. Alterations in white blood cells. In: Porth CM, ed. *Essentials of Pathophysiology: Concepts of Altered Health States.* Lippincott Williams & Wilkins; 2002:191-205.

11. Damjanov I. The hematopoietic and lymphoid systems. In: Damjanov I, ed. *Pathology for the Health Related Professions.* 2nd ed. W.B. Saunders Co.; 2000:209-240.

12. Portlock CS. Hodgkin's Lymphoma. The Merck Manual. Merck & Co, Inc. Available at: http://www.merckmanuals.com/professional/hematology_and_oncology/lymphomas/hodgkin_lymphoma.html. Accessed June 7, 2013.

13. Goodman CC. The hepatic, pancreatic, and biliary systems. In: Goodman CC, Boissonnault WG, eds. *Pathology: Implications for the Physical Therapist.* W.B. Saunders Co; 1998:496-531.

14. Boissonnault WG. Urinary tract disorders. In: Goodman CC, Boissonnault WG, eds. *Pathology: Implications for the Physical Therapist.* W.B. Saunders Co; 1998:532-546.

15. Gunta KE. Alterations in the skeletal system: trauma, infection, and developmental disorders. In: Porth CM, ed. *Essentials of Pathophysiology: Concepts of Altered Health States.* Lippincott Williams & Wilkins; 2002:789-813.

16. Damjanov I. Bones and joints. In: Damjanov I, ed. *Pathology for the Health-Related Professions.* W.B. Saunders Co; 2000:439-462.

ONLINE RESOURCES

◊ **The American Cancer Society**

¤ www.cancer.org

◊ **The Leukemia and Lymphoma Society**

¤ www.lls.org

◊ **National Cancer Institute**

¤ www.cancer.gov

CHAPTER 6

Cardiovascular and Hematological Systems

CHAPTER OUTLINE AND OBJECTIVES

Introduction

Review of Anatomy, Physiology, and Pathogenesis

◊ Describe basic cardiovascular and hematological anatomy and function.

◊ Explain the pathophysiological mechanisms of the cardiovascular and hematological systems.

◊ Describe the response of the cardiovascular and hematological systems to exercise.

◊ Explain the role of the preparticipation physical examination in identifying potential cardiovascular or hematological conditions that might predispose an athlete to sudden cardiac death.

◊ Identify the minimum cardiovascular screening components that should be included in a preparticipation physical examination, as recommended by current guidelines.

◊ Identify the risk factors and mechanisms for illnesses involving the cardiovascular and hematological systems.

Signs and Symptoms

◊ Identify signs and symptoms of common cardiovascular and hematological pathology.

Pain Patterns

Medical History and Physical Examination Procedures

◊ Discuss medical history results that are relevant to cardiovascular and hematological pathology.

◊ Perform physical examination tasks and interpret findings relevant to the cardiovascular and hematological systems.

  ¤ Heart Rate

  ¤ Respiration Rate

  ¤ Blood Pressure

Bhojani RA, O'Connor DP, Fincher AL. *Clinical Pathology for Athletic Trainers: Recognizing Systemic Disease, Fourth Edition* (pp 117-159).
© 2022 Taylor & Francis Group.

¤ Auscultation

¤ Palpation

Pathology and Pathogenesis

◊ Explain the precautions and risk factors associated with physical activity in individuals with common congenital and acquired abnormalities and diseases involving the cardiovascular and hematological systems.

◊ Explain the prevention guidelines associated with the common causes of sudden death in physically active individuals.

◊ Describe etiology, signs, symptoms, interventions, and, when appropriate, return-to-participation criteria for cardiac conditions.

¤ Sudden (Cardiac) Death

¤ Hypertrophic Cardiomyopathy

¤ Coronary Artery Anomalies

¤ Disorders of the Myocardium and Coronary Artery Disease

¤ Valve Disorders

¤ Cardiac Conduction Disorders

¤ Marfan Syndrome

¤ Commotio Cordis

◊ Describe etiology, signs, symptoms, interventions, and, when appropriate, return-to-participation criteria for hypertension.

◊ Describe etiology, signs, symptoms, interventions, and, when appropriate, return-to-participation criteria for disorders of the blood.

¤ Anemia

¤ Sickle Cell Disease and Sickle Cell Trait

¤ Hemophilia

◊ Describe etiology, signs, symptoms, interventions, and, when appropriate, return-to-participation criteria for vascular disorders.

¤ Trauma

¤ Occlusion Syndromes

¤ Thoracic Outlet Syndrome

¤ Deep Vein Thrombosis and Pulmonary Embolism

¤ Aneurysm

¤ Headaches

Pediatric Concerns

◊ Describe etiology, signs, symptoms, interventions and, when appropriate, return-to-participation criteria for pediatric cardiovascular conditions.

¤ Chest Pain

¤ Congenital Heart Conditions

Summary

Case Study

◊ Develop critical-thinking and clinical decision-making skills.

Online Resources

This chapter addresses the following competencies from the *Athletic Training Education Competencies, Fifth Edition*[1]:

Content Area	Competency #
Prevention and Health Promotion (PHP)	3, 5, 8, 9, 17a
Clinical Examination and Diagnosis (CE)	13, 16, 17, 18, 20b, 20h, 21i, 22
Acute Care of Injury and Illness (AC)	6, 7, 36a, 36e, 41
Therapeutic Interventions (TI)	30
Healthcare Administration (HA)	22, 23
Clinical Integration Proficiencies (CIP)	3, 5, 6

INTRODUCTION

The incidence of cardiovascular disease has declined in the United States over the past 20 years, but heart disease and stroke remain among the leading causes of death.[2] The American College of Sports Medicine and the American Heart Association (AHA) recommend that all people who exercise regularly be routinely evaluated for signs of potential cardiovascular disease.[3] Coronary artery disease (CAD) is the leading cause of exercise-associated death for physically active people older than age 35 years.[3,4] Unfortunately, the first sign of a cardiovascular abnormality in children, adolescents, and young adults is often sudden cardiac death (SCD). Cardiovascular events are a leading cause of on-the-field sudden deaths among athletes. For this reason, one of the primary purposes of the preparticipation physical examination is to identify athletes who may be at risk for a cardiac incident.[5,6]

Athletic trainers work with clients and patients from across the lifespan. Consequently, athletic trainers should be familiar with the signs and symptoms of cardiovascular disease and the common cardiovascular and hematological abnormalities in all age groups. Additionally, it is essential that athletic trainers be able to perform a basic cardiovascular assessment.

REVIEW OF PHYSIOLOGY AND PATHOGENESIS

The cardiovascular system consists of the heart, blood, and blood vessels, including arteries, veins, and capillaries. The heart (Figure 6-1), a 4-chambered organ made of a type of muscle called *myocardium*, pumps blood throughout the entire body. Muscular septa, or walls, separate the left and right atria in the superior part of the heart and separate the left and right ventricles, which lie inferior to the respective atrium. A sac of connective tissue, called the *epicardium*, surrounds the entire heart. Tissue called *pericardium* attaches the epicardium (and therefore, the heart) to the thorax. Potential pathology affecting the myocardium includes heart failure, cardiomyopathy, congenital defects, trauma, and ischemia (a loss of blood supply). The epicardium and pericardium are subject to infection, and edema can form in between these tissues.

Arteries, veins, and capillaries circulate blood to and from the heart (Figure 6-2). The walls of arteries and veins have 3 layers: an inner layer (tunica intima) of endothelium, a middle layer (tunica media) of elastic fibers and smooth muscle, and an outer layer (tunica adventitia) of connective tissue. The relative thickness of these layers, as well as the proportion of elastic fibers or smooth muscle, depends on the vessel type and location in the body. Capillary walls are very thin and contain only a single layer of cells, the tunica interna.

Arteries carry oxygenated blood (except for the pulmonary artery which carries deoxygenated blood) from the heart and are classified as either muscular or elastic. Muscular arteries contain

Figure 6-1. Structure of the heart. IVC = inferior vena cava; LA = left atrium; LV = left ventricle; P trunk = pulmonary trunk; PA = pulmonary artery; PV = pulmonary vein; RA = right atrium; RV = right ventricle; SVC = superior vena cava.

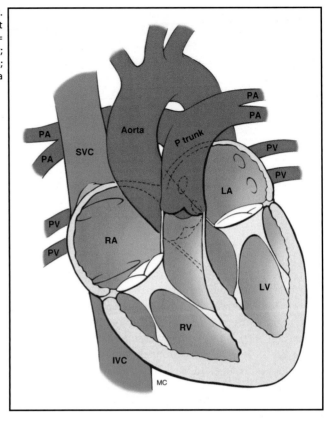

Figure 6-2. Cross-section of typical artery, vein, and lymphatic vessels.

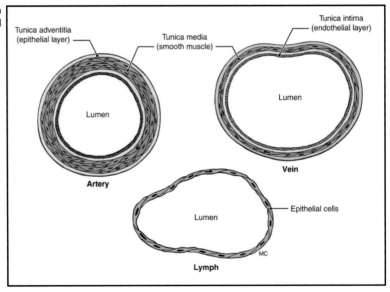

a large portion of muscle tissue and can regulate blood flow to specific organs. Elastic arteries are found as the major arteries of the trunk. Their elasticity can accommodate the large pressure increases that occur during the heart's contraction phase and maintain unidirectional blood flow during the heart's relaxation phase.

Veins return deoxygenated blood (except for the pulmonary vein which carries oxygenated blood) to the heart and have very little muscle. Blood flow toward the heart is supported by skeletal

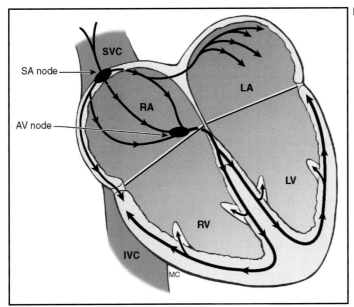

Figure 6-3. Cardiac conduction system.

muscle contraction creating pressure in veins. Lower pressures in the thorax produced during inspiration also assist in drawing blood toward the heart. Valves inside veins prevent back flow of blood.

Capillaries connect arteries (via arterioles) to veins (via venules) through networks of tiny vessels referred to as capillary beds. The exchange of gases, nutrients, hormones, and other materials to and from the blood takes place in these capillary beds.

Heart muscle requires oxygen and other nutrients, as all living tissues do. The *coronary arteries* branch from the base of the aorta and supply the entire myocardium. The left coronary artery is larger than the right and supplies a greater proportion of the heart. Congenital deformities of the coronary arteries pose a threat during vigorous exercise. Other pathology affecting the vascular system includes obstructive diseases, peripheral vascular disease, abnormal vasomotor responses, congenital vessel malformations, and aneurysms.

The heart has its own electrical conduction system that functions independently of the nervous system. The heartbeat begins as an electrical discharge, which causes a wave of muscular contraction. First, a small area in the heart called the *sinoatrial (SA) node* on the right atrium depolarizes (electrically discharges) and spreads an electric impulse through pathways of special myocardial fibers throughout the 2 atria, causing them to contract and move blood into the respective ventricles. When the depolarization impulse reaches the *atrioventricular (AV) node* between the atria and ventricles, the signal propagates into the ventricular walls by way of several additional myocardial fibers called the *AV Bundle (Bundle of His)*, bundle branches, and Purkinje fibers (Figure 6-3). This signal goes down the septum between the ventricles and to the apex of the heart and then causes ventricular contraction from "bottom up." The contraction of the ventricles pushes blood from the left ventricle into the aorta and from the right ventricle into the pulmonary artery. Pathology affecting the heart's conduction system changes the rhythm, pattern, or effectiveness of contraction.

Diastole refers to the period when the atria and the ventricles are both relaxed, as opposed to *systole*, which is the coordinated contraction of the atria and ventricles. During diastole, blood flows into and through the atria to the ventricles. At least 70% of ventricular filling occurs during diastole and the remaining ventricular capacity is filled during atrial contraction.

Atrial contraction (atrial systole) slightly precedes ventricular contraction (ventricular systole) to produce an efficient flow of blood through and out from the heart. Atrial contraction begins with SA node depolarization. This contraction increases pressure in both atria (Figure 6-4A), and blood is forced from both atria down into the ventricles. During ventricular contraction, the mitral

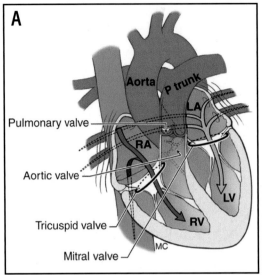
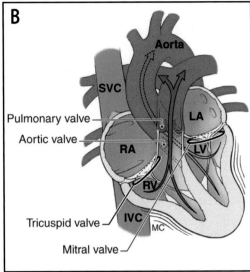

Figure 6-4. (A) Schematic of heart valves during ventricular diastole. (B) Schematic of heart valves during ventricular systole.

valve closes off the left atria and the aortic valve opens to allow blood to be pumped into the aortic artery. Simultaneously, ventricular contraction causes the tricuspid valve to close off the right atria and opens the pulmonary valve to allow blood to flow into the pulmonary artery (Figure 6-4B). As the ventricles relax, the aortic and pulmonary valves close, and the next cardiac contraction begins.

The amount of blood pumped into the aorta during a single ventricular contraction is the *stroke volume*. Stroke volume multiplied by heart rate (HR) (beats per minute) yields *cardiac output*, which is the volume of blood pumped from the heart per minute. Because of its role in providing circulation to the entire body, the left ventricle is larger than the right ventricle.

Table 6-1 lists the basic blood cells, their functions, and their normal values as measured through an analysis of a blood sample called a complete blood count. Most blood cells form in the red bone marrow of the long bones and flat bones. Production of red blood cells (RBCs) is stimulated by the hormone erythropoietin, which is released by the kidney. RBCs are biconcave in shape, which provides a greater surface area for transporting oxygen to the tissues. The number of circulating RBCs determines the viscosity of the blood. Increased numbers of RBCs increases the viscosity of the blood, causing the heart to have to work harder and increasing the risk for blood clots. As mentioned in Chapter 3, blood doping and the use of erythropoietin as a performance enhancer can lead to increased blood viscosity. Many diseases and pathological states affect the production and function of red blood cells and platelets. Leukocytes (white blood cells) play a critical role in the body's defense system and were discussed in Chapter 4.

Blood pressure (BP), the pressure that the blood exerts against the arterial walls, maintains perfusion of oxygen into the organs. Maintenance of BP within a certain range is crucial. If BP falls too low, the brain suffers from lack of oxygen. Conversely, over time high BP will damage the fragile capillaries. Table 6-2 summarizes some of the basic factors and mechanisms that affect BP.

Responses and Adaptations to Exercise

Exercising muscles require a large amount of oxygen. To meet the demand, HR and respiration rate both increase significantly once exercise begins, which produces stress on the heart. Left ventricular mass and volume increase as an adaptive response to regular aerobic exercise over weeks to months. These changes are adaptations to the increased cardiac demand, greater venous return, and increased oxygen demand from the body that occur with aerobic exercise. These adaptations lead to increases in HR and stroke volume, which in turn produce greater cardiac output.[7] Resistance

Table 6-1. Blood Cells and Their Functions

CELL TYPE	FUNCTION/COMMENTS
Red blood cells (erythrocytes)	Transport oxygen, remove carbon dioxide
White blood cells (lymphocytes)	Phagocytosis, mediate immune system response (useful in assessing inflammation/infection; may be low in endurance athletes)
Platelets (thrombocytes)	Clotting (sometimes elevated in athletes especially if dehydrated)
Hemoglobin (Hgb)	Oxygen-carrying molecule influenced by iron
Hematocrit (Hct)	Sometimes elevated in athletes especially if dehydrated
Mean cell volume (MCV)	Measurement of average size of RBC
Reticulocyte count	Percentage of young RBCs available to grow

Table 6-2. Basic Factors Affecting Blood Pressure

FACTOR	EFFECT ON BLOOD PRESSURE	MECHANISM
Decreased blood volume	Decrease	Inadequate fluid within vascular system to maintain pressure
Widespread vasodilation	Decrease	Systemic capacity exceeds fluid volume
Increased extracellular fluid	Increase	Higher BP needed to diffuse nutrients against the increased pressure gradient in capillaries
Renal failure	Increase	Higher BP needed to diffuse fluids against the increased pressure gradient in kidney capillaries

exercise also increases the muscle mass of the left ventricle as an adaption to increased resistance to blood flow. Oxygen demand, however, does not increase substantially with resistance training (relative to aerobic exercise), so the volume of the left ventricle does not change significantly.

Preparticipation Screening

Appropriate preparticipation screening can identify individuals who may be at risk for a cardiac event.[3,7] In 1996, the AHA published a set of 12 minimal components that should be included in a preparticipation screening examination.[7,8] These same components have recently been recommended by the 36th Bethesda Conference sponsored by the American College of Cardiology in its "Task Force 1: Preparticipation Screening and Diagnosis of Cardiovascular Disease in Athletes"[9] and the multi-association team physician consensus statement regarding care of master (age ≥ 50 years) athletes.[10] This report provides medical guidance for persons who wish to participate in sports but who have cardiac conditions. This has since been updated in 2014 to now have a set of 14 elements for a cardiovascular screen.[11] The full conference report is available at the American College of Cardiology website (https://www.acc.org/latest-in-cardiology/articles/2014/09/15/14/24/acc-aha-release-recommendations-for-congenital-and-genetic-heart-disease-screenings-in-youth).

The 14 AHA components fall into 3 categories: family medical history, personal medical history, and physical examination (Table 6-3). Preparticipation screening for cardiovascular conditions has been incorporated into the fourth edition of the *Preparticipation Physical Examination* monograph

Table 6-3. American Heart Association Minimal Components for Preparticipation Physical Examinations

FAMILY MEDICAL HISTORY	Premature death of a relative
	Living relative younger than 50 years diagnosed with heart disease or other cardiac conditions (ie, hypertrophic cardiomyopathy, long QT syndrome, Marfan syndrome, or clinically important arrhythmias)
PERSONAL HISTORY	Heart murmur
	Hypertension
	Unusual fatigue
	Exertional syncope (fainting)
	Excessive exertional dyspnea
	Exertional chest pain
PHYSICAL EXAMINATION	Resting heart rate
	Blood pressure
	Auscultation of the heart in supine and standing
	Assessment of femoral pulses
	Observation for signs of Marfan syndrome (see Table 6-4)

assembled by several medical and sports medicine associations and endorsed by the National Athletic Trainers' Association.[12] The screening is often performed with simple questionnaires, such as the Physical Activity Readiness Questionnaire or the Health/Fitness Facility Preparticipation Screening Questionnaire.[3] Positive responses to questions that cover the AHA's family and personal history components, particularly if these symptoms have ever interrupted a workout, may identify up to 50% of at-risk athletes. Medical examination during preparticipation screening should include auscultation of the heart and lungs and resting BP. Any murmur detected on auscultation warrants referral to a physician for further work-up. Of note, all diastolic murmurs require clearance by a specialist prior to clearance. If any abnormalities are suspected, follow-up medical testing by electrocardiogram (ECG), echocardiogram, electron-beam computed tomography scanning, cardiac magnetic resonance imaging, coronary artery angiography, or exercise (cardiac stress) testing may be required to rule out potential causes for sudden cardiac death.[13]

An ECG detects the electric activity of the heart and is used to identify pathology of the heart's electrical system. The ECG trace line has several waves; each subsequent wave is identified by the letters P, Q, R, S, and T (Figure 6-5). Each wave represents a specific heart action. The *P wave* is atrial depolarization; the *QRS segment* is ventricular depolarization, which hides atrial repolarization; and the *T wave* is ventricular repolarization. The *PR interval* represents the propagation of depolarization from the SA node in the atria through the AV node. The *QT interval* represents the ventricular depolarization-repolarization cycle.

There is some controversy as to whether preparticipation screening should include ECGs, echocardiograms, and other types of cardiac testing. Organizations or institutions considering adding these types of tests to routine preparticipation screening should carefully consider the current literature on the topic.[5,9,14-18] ECG is useful in identifying individuals with ventricular arrhythmias, ECG pattern changes that occur with hypertrophic cardiomyopathy, and long QT syndrome. The ECG is a somewhat affordable test on a per-athlete basis, but large-scale annual screening of all United States high school athletes may be cost prohibitive because of the large number of athletes in America,[15] although some models predict lower, less prohibitive costs.[19] Other countries such as

Table 6-4. Signs of Marfan Syndrome

Tall, thin body type

Arm span longer than height

Disproportionately long legs

Thoracic spine kyphosis

Sternum deformity (pectus carinatum, pectus excavatum)

Hyperlaxity in joints

Visual problems

Overlap of the thumb and fifth digit when wrapping the fingers around the wrist

Any 2 signs warrant medical referral for cardiac screening.

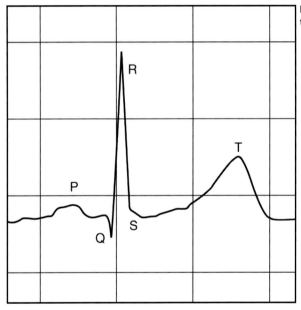

Figure 6-5. The normal electrocardiogram traceline.

Italy that have national health and medical programs are able to deliver ECG screening at very low cost and have incorporated it into routine preparticipation examinations for many years.[5]

ECGs may produce a large number of false-positive test results when used in asymptomatic people, which means that the test shows an abnormal response although no actual pathology exists.[16,20,21] False-positive results and the subsequent follow-up testing can lead to undue mental stress and unnecessary financial burden on the individual and their family. The false-positive issue is complex because the sensitivity of the test varies for different types of cardiac pathology,[21] and even the detection of a true pathological condition may not mean the person is at increased risk for sudden death. To decrease the false-positive rate, recently developed "modern" ECG interpretation criteria should be used and the test should be interpreted by an experienced cardiologist or sports medicine physician.[5,14,21,22] The use of additional medical tests such as echocardiogram and cardiovascular magnetic resonance imaging with other clinical criteria is another strategy to improve interpretation of ECG.[23] An ECG is not useful for identifying coronary artery deformities or disease or other structural abnormalities that do not affect the conduction system of the heart.

The echocardiogram, which uses ultrasonic technology to create an image of the heart, is useful in identifying thickening of the left ventricular wall caused by hypertrophic cardiomyopathy as well as other structural deformities including valve disorders and dilated cardiomyopathy.[9]

Unfortunately, as with ECG, echocardiograms are cost prohibitive for routine screening of all sports participants and may be best used as additional testing after the medical history or clinical signs suggest cardiac pathology.[15] Children in a family with a history of hypertrophic cardiomyopathy, however, should receive an annual echocardiogram for monitoring and primary prevention because of their substantially increased risk, regardless of their participation in organized athletics.[9] In other countries such as Italy, the gold standard for cardiovascular testing is not a resting echocardiogram but a stress echocardiogram. Various collegiate and professional organizations around the world have adopted different criteria for the use of echocardiogram and whether it should be resting or stress-based.

Blood testing to screen for sickle cell trait is inexpensive and very reliable. These tests should be considered for all individuals with a family history of sickle cell trait or sickle cell disease.

Athletic trainers should discuss the use of these cardiovascular screening tests with their team physicians. The decision to include these tests in the standard preparticipation physical examination is both a philosophical and financial one. Because many of the potential causes of sudden cardiac death are known to occur within specific populations (eg, risk of sickle cell trait is much higher among Black individuals), it may be prudent to base these decisions on the relevant characteristics and signs of the patients being screened. A protocol for cardiovascular screening that includes actions to be taken after a positive test result or suspicion of cardiovascular problems should be thoroughly discussed, written in detail, appropriately vetted by the relevant medical and administrative authorities, and communicated with athletes and their families well before using them in preparticipation examinations to avoid later confusion or disagreements.

SIGNS AND SYMPTOMS

Chest Pain (Angina)

Chest pain is the principal symptom of cardiac pathology. Cardiac pain originates from the myocardium when it is deprived of oxygen (myocardial ischemia). Anything that damages or causes inflammation in the myocardium can produce cardiac pain. Angina also occurs when the blood supply to the heart is inadequate to meet the demand of the work it is doing.

Cardiac pain typically occurs over the left chest and radiates to the left neck, shoulder, or arm. The pain may be described as a severe pressure in the chest that worsens with physical exertion. Autonomic system responses, such as diaphoresis or pallor, appearing with angina are signs of a cardiac emergency. See Algorithm 6-1 for clinical decision making related to chest pain.

There are 3 different types of chest pain that based on the presence of "(1) substernal pain, (2) provoked by exertion, or (3) relieved by rest or nitroglycerin." Typical angina has all 3 characteristics, atypical angina has 2 of the 3 characteristics, and nonanginal pain has only 1 of the 3 characteristics.[24] This is important due to the risk assessment for CAD based on gender and age.

Dyspnea

Shortness of breath (dyspnea) can occur when cardiac output decreases. Most cardiac problems decrease the ability of the heart to pump blood to the body. As blood flow from the heart decreases, less oxygen is available to the body. To compensate for the falling oxygen level, the respiration rate increases to draw in more air. As a result, the patient feels "short of breath." This type of dyspnea improves with rest or nitroglycerin, which reduces oxygen demand, and worsens with activity, which increases oxygen demand.

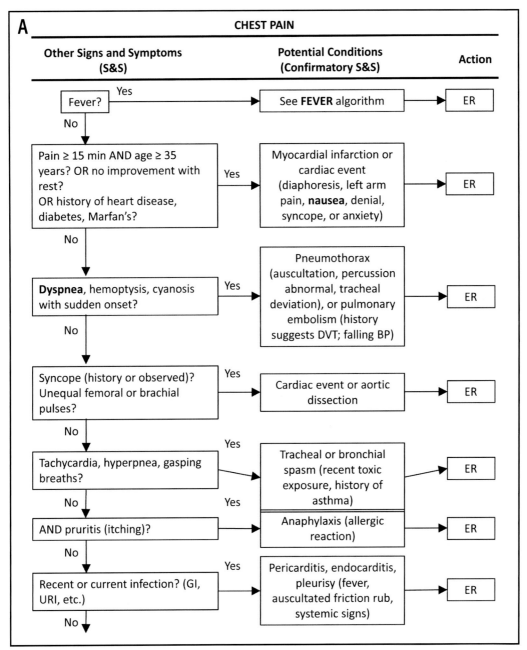

Algorithm 6-1. (A) *(continued)*

Fatigue

When cardiac output decreases and less blood is delivered to the body, the body adapts by limiting activity to lower the metabolic demand for energy and oxygen. The resulting effect is fatigue, a reduced capability to perform work. In the medical history, the person may report becoming easily fatigued by routine activities, which is a symptom of the heart's inability to keep up with the increased tissue demand for oxygen during those activities. This type of fatigue associated with heart failure gets progressively worse over the course of the day. As an athletic trainer, it is imperative to ask about fatigue with regards to Activities of Daily Living.

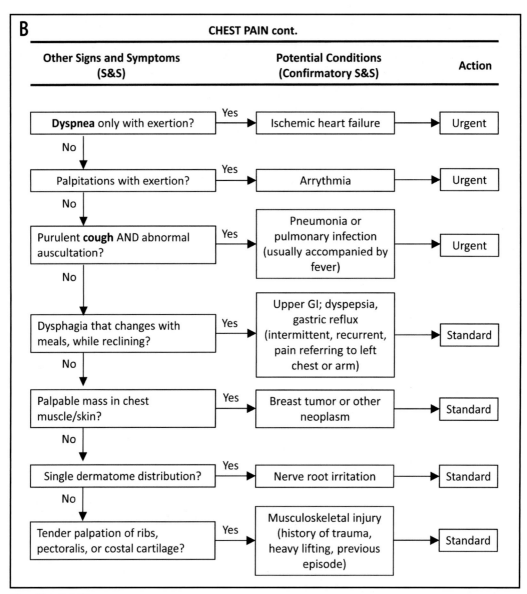

Algorithm 6-1. (B)

Palpitations

A palpitation is the sensation of "skipped beats" or the heart "fluttering" uncomfortably. Disturbances in the electrical activity that controls the heartbeat causes cardiac contractions of excessive rate or strength (arrhythmia); these irregular contractions are felt as palpitations. Palpitations accompanied by chest pain, dyspnea, fatigue, or light-headedness indicate a serious cardiac condition. Palpitations can also be caused by metabolic changes, hemodynamic changes, supplement use, and psychological disturbances.

Syncope

Syncope, or fainting, is a complete loss of consciousness and postural tone resulting from a sudden reduction in the brain's blood supply. Reduction in blood flow results in reduced oxygen. Brain activity decreases very quickly when its oxygen supply falls too low, causing loss of consciousness and motor control. Unexplained syncope indicates a serious heart problem and requires emergency medical care.

There are 3 primary causes of syncope. The first cause is sudden, widespread peripheral vaso-dilation, causing what is known as *orthostatic* syncope. Rapid perfusion of the extremities decreases blood to the brain because there is not enough blood to fill all of the body's vessels to their capacity at the same time. When the capacity of the vascular system increases but the amount of fluid in the blood remains the same, the pressure in the system decreases. Widespread vasodilation in the extremities thus causes a rapid drop in BP, which leads to syncope.

The second cause of syncope is increased *intracranial pressure*. The increased pressure in the cranium exceeds the pressure in the blood vessels and prevents adequate blood flow to the brain. The most common cause of increased intracranial pressure is intracranial bleeding from a head injury.

The third cause of syncope is an acute reduction in cardiac output, called *heart failure*. As dis-cussed with dyspnea and fatigue, a decrease in cardiac output decreases the oxygen being delivered to the body. A sudden drop in cardiac output, usually caused by a medical emergency such as a heart attack (myocardial infarction [MI]), deprives the brain of oxygen and syncope occurs.

Claudication

Claudication, Latin for "limping," occurs when the blood flow to a lower limb is blocked. Consequently, oxygen does not reach the muscles in sufficient quantity to meet its metabolic demands. The result is muscular ischemia, pain, and decrease in function. Claudication produces cramps, aches, and unusual fatigue in the affected limb that is worsen with exertion and improved with rest. Of note, pseudo-claudication (or neurogenic claudication caused by stenosis in the lum-bar spine) presents similarly except the symptoms worsens with sitting and rest and improve with walking.

Skin and Nail Temperature, Color, and Appearance

Vasomotor disorders can cause the skin to become notably cool ("clammy"), from vasocon-striction, or hot, from vasodilation. The skin or nails may also change color, ranging from very pale (vasoconstriction, low BP) to bright red (vasodilatation, hypertension) to blue or purple (lack of oxygen in the affected tissue). Patients who are in shock or experiencing a severe cardiac event often have pale, clammy skin as a result of decreased BP and decreased blood flow to the skin. Some cardiovascular disorders cause ulcers or lesions on the skin, usually a sign of chronic tissue ischemia (lack of blood), and "clubbing" (rounding) of the fingertips and nails (Figure 6-6).

Edema

Edema, the abnormal accumulation of fluid in the interstitial spaces, occurs with chronic cardi-ac conditions, an increase in capillary pressure, a decrease in capillary osmotic pressure, an increase in capillary permeability, or venous or lymphatic obstruction. Fluid in the blood moves from the vessels into the surrounding tissues. Cardiac failure causes generalized edema, whereas edema from vascular occlusion occurs only in the part of the limb that is distal to the obstruction.

PAIN PATTERNS

Cardiac

As noted above, inflammation of heart tissue produces chest pain and can refer pain along the pathways of spinal nerves C3 through T4, predominantly on the left. Thus, pain of cardiac origin

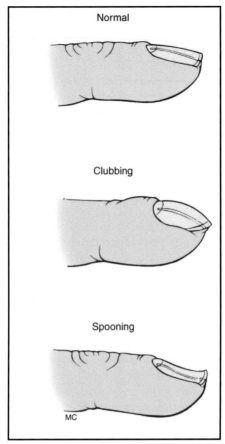

Figure 6-6. Clubbing and spooning of the fingernails.

can occur anywhere from the neck or throat to the medial side of the arm. As classically described, a "crushing" or pressure sensation begins in the chest and radiates into the arm (Figure 6-7).

Vascular

Vascular pain is described as a tearing, sharp, or throbbing sensation and occurs locally in the region of the affected vessel. Symptoms may appear in other tissues that are supplied by the vessel if blood supply to those tissues is affected.

MEDICAL HISTORY AND PHYSICAL EXAMINATION PROCEDURES

Family and Personal History

A history of sudden cardiac death under age 50 years in the immediate family is a strong risk factor for cardiovascular disease. A personal history of chronic physical inactivity, smoking, hypertension, high blood lipids (dyslipidemia), obesity, diabetes, Marfan syndrome, or connective tissue disorders also increases the risk of cardiovascular pathology.[2,3] Retrospective studies of sudden death among athletes have shown that many of them had reported a positive family history of cardiovascular disease and about 20% of them had experienced cardiovascular signs or symptoms before their fatal event, such as exertional angina, dyspnea, syncope, unusual fatigue, palpitations,

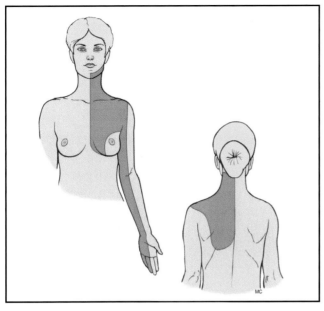

Figure 6-7. Cardiac pain pattern.

a known heart murmur, or increased BP.[25] A personal or family history of sickle cell trait or sickle cell disease also increases the risk of sudden death during exertion.

Symptoms

Angina is a hallmark sign of ischemic cardiac pathology. Pain of cardiac origin is either acute (sudden and severe) and constant or subacute (insidious and moderate) and recurrent. This pain is described as a crushing pressure in the chest. Chest pain that occurs during exertion also suggests cardiac pathology.[26] Up to 30% of people with sudden angina at rest have a MI (heart attack) within 3 months. Unexplained syncope, palpitations, or dyspnea, particularly occurring with chest pain or during exertion, requires a referral for medical examination.

Symptoms of vascular pathology include cramping, heaviness, weakness, swelling, pulsing, fatigue, or cold or cyanotic extremities. These symptoms invariably worsen with exertion and are relieved by rest.[27-31]

Inspection

Certain physical characteristics appear with some cardiovascular conditions. Individuals with Marfan syndrome, an abnormality of connective tissue, present with distinct physical characteristics (Table 6-4). These characteristics should be screened for during the preparticipation physical examination and during any evaluation involving cardiovascular symptoms. A lack of the normal thoracic kyphosis, or a deformed sternum (pectus carinatum or pectus excavatum), may be a sign of a congenital heart abnormality. Any notable deformity of the chest wall in a child should be further examined by a physician.

Heart Rate

HR, the number of heart beats per minute (bpm), can be palpated over the heart apex, at pulse-pressure sites (brachial, femoral, radial, posterior tibial, or dorsal pedis arteries), or at the carotid artery (Figure 6-8). When assessing HR, the rate (bpm), rhythm (regular vs irregular), and character (strong vs weak) should be reported (eg, "120 bpm, regular, and weak"). A normal heart beat is regular and strong. A weak or irregular ("skipping beats") heart beat indicates a potential cardiac emergency.

Figure 6-8. Location of pulse sites.

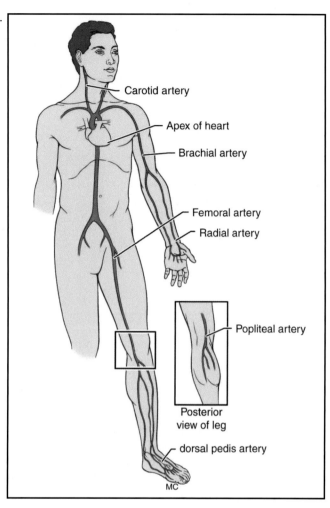

"Normal" HR in adults ranges between 60 and 100 bpm. Newborns have a HR ranging between 90 and 180 bpm. Children between ages 1 and 6 years have a HR between 70 and 140 bpm. Preadolescents between ages 10 and 14 years have a normal HR between 55 and 115 bpm. Adolescents' HR is approximately the same as adults.

A slow HR is called *bradycardia* and a fast HR is called *tachycardia*. Resting bradycardia (<60 bpm) can occur as an adaptation among trained persons and is not generally an indication of pathology; however, in the untrained person, this needs to be investigated further by a physician. A person with a resting HR above 100 bpm (tachycardia) should be examined and evaluated by a physician.

Table 6-5 describes how to assess HR. The radial artery is the most common site for assessing a patient's HR. The pulse should be palpated using the pads of the second and third fingers. There are several counting methods that can be used, depending on the characteristics of the pulse. If the rate and rhythm feel normal, the pulse can be counted for 15 seconds and the result multiplied by 4. Other methods include counting for 10 seconds and multiplying by 6 or 30 seconds and multiplying by 2. Each of these methods has some degree of error. Therefore, if the pulse rate is unusually fast or slow, the beats should be counted for a full 60 seconds. If the rhythm is irregular, the pulse should be assessed by auscultation, because the attempt to count palpated beats may be difficult.

Table 6-5. Assessment of Heart Rate and Respiration Rate

HEART RATE	
Step 1	Sit or stand facing your patient.
Step 2	Use your non-watch-bearing hand to grasp the patient's wrist, as if you are shaking hands (patient's right wrist with your right hand or the patient's left wrist with your left hand).
Step 3	Compress the radial artery with your index and middle fingers.
Step 4	Note whether the pulse is regular or irregular: • Regular: evenly spaced beats, may vary slightly with respiration • Regularly irregular: regular pattern overall with "skipped" beats • Irregularly irregular: chaotic, no real pattern, difficult to measure accurately
Step 5	Count the pulse for 15 seconds and multiply by 4.
Step 6	Count for a full minute if the pulse is irregular.
Step 7	Record the rate and rhythm.
Step 8	Interpretation: • Normal: between 60 and 100 beats per minute • Tachycardia: a pulse greater than 100 beats/minute; tachycardia is a normal response to stress or exercise. • Bradycardia: a pulse less than 60 beats/minute; athletes tend to be bradycardic at rest because of their level of conditioning.
RESPIRATION RATE	
Step 1	Best performed immediately after taking the patient's pulse, while still grasping the patient's wrist.
Step 2	Do NOT announce that you are measuring respirations.
Step 3	Without letting go of the patient's wrist, begin to observe the patient's breathing. Is it normal or labored?
Step 4	Count breaths for 1 full minute to yield the breaths/minute.
Step 5	Interpretation: • Normal: resting respiratory rates between 14 and 20 breaths/minute • Tachypnea: rapid respiration over 20 breaths/minute

Respiration Rate

The respiration rate for adults is normally 12 to 20 breaths per minute. Infants have a respiration rate of 30 to 60 breaths per minute, young children between 20 and 40 breaths per minute, and older children between 15 and 25 breaths per minute. Respiration at rest should be regular, moderate in depth, and require little effort. Forced or difficult respiration, obvious dyspnea, or rapid, shallow breaths are abnormal.

Table 6-5 describes the assessment of respiration rate. When assessing a patient's respiration rate, observe the chest or stomach rise and fall with each breath, noting rate, rhythm, depth, and effort. As with HR, respirations can be counted for 15 or 30 seconds and the result multiplied by

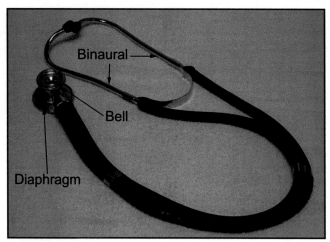

Figure 6-9. Stethoscope.

4 or 2, respectively. If rhythm or rate is abnormal, the respirations should be counted for a full 60 seconds. The following statement is an example of how to report an abnormal respiration rate: "Respiration rate is 22, irregular, shallow, and labored." Some individuals will unintentionally alter their breathing pattern if they know their breathing is being observed. For this reason, the athletic trainer should not announce that they are counting respirations. The respiration rate can be assessed while it appears that the athletic trainer is taking the HR.

Blood Pressure

Blood Pressure (BP) measures the pressure inside the arteries during systole and diastole. BP is usually measured at the brachial artery using a stethoscope (Figure 6-9) and a sphygmomanometer.[25] Table 6-6 outlines the steps that should be followed when measuring BP. The sounds used to determine systolic and diastolic BPs are referred to as *Korotkoff* sounds. The ease at which you hear these sounds can be influenced by a variety of factors including the quality of the stethoscope and the placement of the stethoscope diaphragm or bell over the brachial artery (Figure 6-10). Also, the stethoscope ear pieces should be placed in the ear at a slightly forward angle to match the ear canal. Raising the patient's arm up above their head before and while you inflate the cuff may be helpful in increasing the intensity of the Korotkoff sounds. Also, you can have the patient make a fist several times after you have inflated the cuff but before you begin the deflation process.

Proper selection of cuff size is important for accuracy in BP readings. Using a standard cuff on an obese patient or an athlete with a large upper arm will result in a false reading of hypertension (high BP). By the same token, using a standard cuff on a thin arm may result in false readings of hypotension (low BP). Large, pediatric, and thigh-size BP cuffs should be used when necessary. The ideal cuff size/length should be 80% of the patient's arm circumference and ideal width of at least 40%.[32]

Normally, in adults systolic BP ranges from 100 to 140 mm Hg and diastolic BP ranges from 70 to 90 mm Hg. Infants and young children have lower BP; at birth, systolic pressure is around 70 mm Hg, and a BP of 120/80 in a 10-year-old actually suggests hypertension. BP varies in children by body size (height and weight) in addition to age, making interpretation difficult, but BP in young children should be considerably lower than adult values. BP reaches adult levels in late adolescence. BP equal to or greater than 140/90 on consecutive days indicates chronic hypertension and needs further medical evaluation. Large differences in systolic BP (> 15 mm Hg) between lying, sitting, and standing suggests possible orthostatic hypotension, which may be caused by dehydration or other fluid loss (eg, hemorrhage).

Table 6-6. Assessment of Blood Pressure	
STEP 1	Position the patient so the antecubital crease is level with the heart.
STEP 2	Support the patient's arm with your arm or rest the arm on a table with the elbow slightly flexed.
STEP 3	Center the bladder of the cuff over the brachial artery, with the lower edge of the cuff resting approximately 2.5 cm or 2 finger widths above the antecubital crease.
STEP 4	Palpate the brachial artery in the area of the antecubital crease.
STEP 5	Place the bell of the stethoscope over the brachial artery (see Figure 6-10).
STEP 6	Inflate the cuff to approximately 200 mm Hg OR rapidly inflate the cuff until the radial pulse disappears and add 30 mm Hg to the value obtained. This latter method can avoid unnecessary discomfort for the patient. (If using the latter method, deflate the cuff and wait 15 to 30 seconds before actually measuring the BP.)
STEP 7	Release the pressure slowly at a rate of 2 to 3 mm Hg per second.
STEP 8	The level at which you consistently hear beats is the systolic pressure (read to the nearest 2 mm Hg).
STEP 9	Continue to lower the pressure until the sounds muffle and disappear. This is the diastolic pressure (also read to the nearest 2 mm Hg).
STEP 10	Quickly deflate the cuff to zero.
STEP 11	Record the blood pressure as systolic over diastolic (example: 120/70).

Auscultation

Auscultation involves using a stethoscope to listen to internal body sounds. Cardiac auscultation allows listening to heart sounds.[25,26,33] The athletic trainer's role with auscultation is to identify abnormal heart sounds rather than diagnose cardiac pathology. The ability to recognize abnormal sounds requires a fair amount of practice in listening to normal sounds. There are numerous websites that provide examples of normal and abnormal heart sounds; some are listed at the end of this chapter.

The normal, rhythmic "*lub-dub*" heart sounds are produced by the heart valves closing. The first sound, S_1 ("lub"), corresponds to the closing of the mitral and tricuspid valves with ventricular systole. The second sound, S_2 ("dub"), corresponds to the aortic and pulmonary valves closing after ventricular systole. Abnormal cardiac sounds include "extra" heart sounds (S_3 and S_4), muffled heart sounds, murmurs, or rubbing or hissing sounds caused by valve deformities. These sounds are produced by the changes in turbulence of blood flowing through narrowed or incompletely closed heart valves.

Cardiac auscultation is performed over 4 distinct listening zones, which correspond to the location of the 4 heart valves (Figure 6-11). The aortic listening zone (A) is located just to the right of the sternum in the second intercostal space. Moving just left of the sternum, the pulmonary listening zone (P) is located in the left, second intercostal space. Palpating down the left sternal border, the tricuspid zone (T) is located in the left, fourth or fifth intercostal space. The mitral listening zone (M) corresponds to the apex of the heart and is located in the left, fifth intercostal space in line

Figure 6-10. Stethoscope placement during blood pressure assessment.

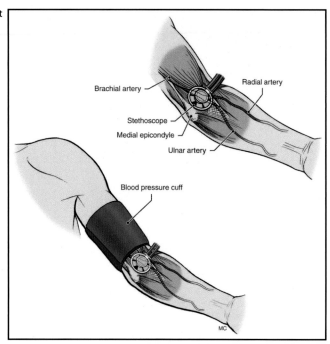

Figure 6-11. Cardiac auscultation listening zones.

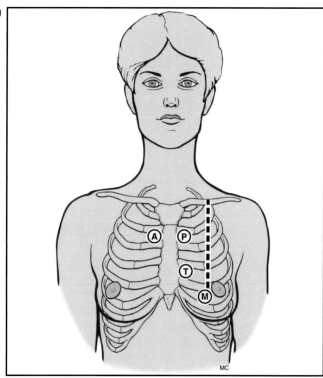

with the mid-clavicle. Auscultation should be performed with the patient in 3 different positions: supine, left-side lying, and sitting (Figures 6-12). Table 6-7 outlines the step-by-step procedures for performing cardiac auscultation.

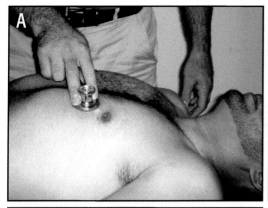
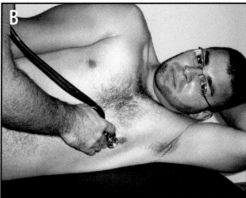
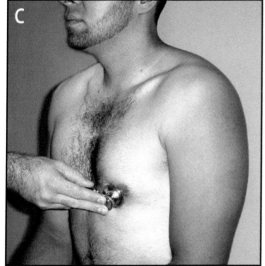

Figure 6-12. Patient positioning for cardiac auscultation. (A) Supine. (B) Sidelying. (C) Sitting.

Many stethoscopes include both a diaphragm and a bell (see Figure 6-9). The diaphragm is better suited for hearing the normal S_1 and S_2 sounds, as well as aortic murmurs. The bell is more sensitive to the high-pitched, abnormal S_3 and S_4 sounds, as well as some mitral valve disorders.

Auscultation can also be used to examine the major vessels, such as the abdominal aorta, brachial arteries, and femoral arteries. Normally, the sound of the heartbeat may be faintly detectable, accompanied by intermittent rushing sounds created by blood flowing through these large vessels. Abnormal vascular sounds, called *bruits*, include loud clicks, pounding, or continuous rather than intermittent rushing sounds. The turbulent blood flow in arteries that have been pathologically narrowed (atherosclerosis) or deformed (aneurysm) cause bruits.

Palpation

Arterial pulses can be palpated where major arteries are close to the skin (see Figure 6-8). Pulses may be absent or diminished in vascular occlusion syndromes. Aneurysms may be palpated as a "throbbing mass" on the affected artery. A palpable abdominal pulse wider than the normal aortic pulsation that extends 2 inches to either side of midline may indicate an aortic aneurysm.

Table 6-7. Cardiac Auscultation

STEP 1	Position patient in supine, males without shirt, females wearing sports bra.
STEP 2	Instruct the subject to breathe as normally as possible.
STEP 3	Locate the aortic listening zone (A) at the superior right sternal border in second intercostal space (as shown in Figure 6-11).
STEP 4	Carefully listen for the S_1 and S_2 ("lub-dub") heart sounds during several cardiac contraction cycles. Also listen for additional "beat" sounds (S_3 and S_4) or other abnormal sounds (murmurs, rubs, etc).
STEP 5	Move the stethoscope sequentially to auscultate the remaining 3 zones: • Pulmonary valve (P) at the superior left sternal border at the second intercostal space • Tricuspid valve (T) at the inferior left sternal border at the fourth or fifth intercostal space • Mitral valve (M) at the fifth intercostal space in midclavicular line An alternate technique can be used that starts with M (the apex of the heart) and moves sequentially through T, P, and A.
STEP 6	If no abnormal sounds are heard in supine, have the patient lie on the left side (see Figure 6-12B) and again auscultate the 4 listening zones. This position moves the apex of the heart closer to the chest wall, making mitral valve disorders more distinguishable.
STEP 7	If left side lying auscultation is normal, have the patient sit, lean for-ward, exhale completely, and hold their breath (ie, not inhale) (see Figure 6-12C). Again, listen to several heart cycles at each zone. Instruct the patient to breathe between zones.
STEP 8	With the patient sitting, instruct them to hold their breath and bear down as if emptying the bowels (Valsalva maneuver). Auscultate the heart apex (M). A "clicking" sound during this maneuver suggests potential mitral valve prolapse.

PATHOLOGY AND PATHOGENESIS

Sudden (Cardiac) Death

Exercise-induced death (defined as occurring during or within 1 hour of physical activity) is rare, ranging from 1 fatality in 50,000 to 200,000 males and 1 fatality in 200,000 to 769,000 females of high school or collegiate age.[25] The risk of sudden death during exercise increases with age and is highest in those who have undiagnosed heart disease.[10] Although SCD can occur in any sport, it has been reported most frequently in basketball and football.[34] Non-traumatic SCD usually presents symptoms within 1 hour of the onset of exercise or sports participation or shortly after the cessation of exercise. The most common causes of SCD in athletes are hypertrophic cardiomyopathy, congenital coronary artery anomalies, cardiac electrical and conduction abnormalities, trauma (commotio cordis), or acquired myocarditis.[2-4,7,25,35] Some contributing factors in SCD include high-intensity exercise, electrolyte imbalances from dehydration, high body temperature from exercise in extreme heat and humidity, sudden cessation of intense physical activity (causing vasodilation

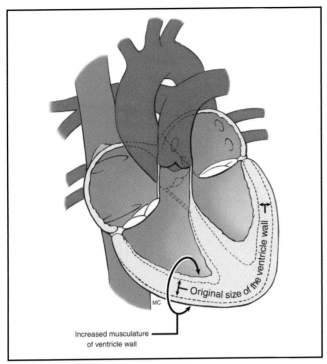

Figure 6-13. Cardiac hypertrophy.

and decreasing BP, similar to shock),[25] and the use of performance-enhancing substances or dietary supplements.[36] Other less common causes of sudden cardiac death include aortic rupture (Marfan syndrome), commotio cordis, aortic stenosis, congenital cerebrovascular deformities, pulmonary disease, peripheral embolism, and drug abuse.[7,25]

For secondary prevention of sudden cardiac arrest of any etiology, the National Athletic Trainers' Association (NATA), in cooperation with an inter-association task force, has issued consensus statements recommending that athletic trainers, coaches, school nurses, and team physicians be trained in first aid, cardiopulmonary resuscitation, and the use of automatic external defibrillators (AEDs).[37,38] Of note, new changes to the cardiopulmonary resuscitation algorithm going from ABC to CAB have shown the shift in philosophy on what to address with a patient wh may be experiencing a potential cardiac event. Emergency action plans should also be in place to ensure immediate access to an AED, as well as a coordinated plan for activating emergency medical services, initiating cardiopulmonary resuscitation, AED, and advanced cardiac life support services as soon as possible after recognizing a cardiac event.[39]

Hypertrophic Cardiomyopathy

Three locations of cardiac hypertrophy, or enlargement of the heart (Figure 6-13), are recognized: general cardiac hypertrophy (both ventricles), left ventricular hypertrophy, and right ventricular hypertrophy. *General cardiac hypertrophy* occurring in highly fit persons as an adaptation to strenuous aerobic exercise is not considered pathological. This so-called *"athlete's heart"* does not reduce the size of the left ventricle cavity and may in fact increase it.[40] By contrast, pathological enlargement of the heart is called *hypertrophic cardiomyopathy* and is associated with an asymmetrical enlargement of one ventricle. In this inheritable condition, abnormal myocardial fibers produce hypertrophy of the myocardium that is not evenly distributed in the ventricle wall and may decrease the ventricular cavity diameter.[23,41] These changes can cause obstruction of blood flowing through the heart and arrhythmias, particularly atrial fibrillation, because the abnormal fibers interrupt conduction pathways.[41] Eventually, progressive hypertrophic cardiomyopathy leads to heart failure, ischemic myocardial damage, or fatal arrhythmia as the tissue propagates and interferes with the heart's muscle function, vascular supply, or electrical system.[2,41]

Hypertrophic cardiomyopathy is the leading cause of sudden cardiac death in young, competitive athletes.[40] An estimated 1 in 500 young adults display signs of potential hypertrophic cardiomyopathy; however, not all of these people have cardiac pathology.[25] Identifying which are most at risk for a catastrophic event during sports is a challenge. Many people with hypertrophic cardiomyopathy have a family history of a close relative with sudden death under age 50 years, or a personal history of unexplained episodes of syncope, angina, or dyspnea.[41] A heart murmur that increases with a Valsalva maneuver (see Table 6-7) is sometimes auscultated at the lower left sternal border, medial to the apex of the heart. A left ventricular wall thickness of 15 mm or more measured on an echocardiogram after changes seen on an ECG results in the diagnosis of hypertrophic cardiomyopathy.[9,23,42] A definitive diagnosis requires an echocardiography or cardiac magnetic resonance imaging.[23] A comprehensive approach to screening and examination for hypertrophic cardiomyopathy has been described, including thorough personal and family history, genetic testing, imaging studies, and other clinical tests.[41]

Hypertrophic cardiomyopathy is treated through medications (β blockers) and activity restriction, and surgery is sometimes required. Risk of arrhythmia increases as cardiac demand increases. β blockers decrease the HR and the force of cardiac contractions, which decreases the risk of arrhythmia. β blockers also lead to exercise fatigue and decreased athletic performance; therefore, noncompliance with these medications is often a problem with competitive athletes.

The 36th Bethesda Conference classified sports for making return-to-play decisions in individuals who have a cardiovascular abnormality. Table 6-8 describes the classification system, which is based on the level of intensity and the potential for bodily collision. The 36th Bethesda Conference recommends that an athlete with hypertrophic cardiomyopathy be restricted from most competitive sports with the exception of Class IA, or low-intensity, sports. Some athletes and their parents may choose to ignore a physician's recommendation and accept the risk of a fatal cardiac event with continued participation. Under these circumstances, athletic trainers and physicians must counsel the athlete and parents of the potential risk in order for them to make an informed decision.[25,36]

Coronary Artery Anomalies

Congenital coronary artery anomalies are the second leading cause of SCD in young athletes.[7,43] The most common type of coronary artery anomaly involves the left main coronary artery being abnormally positioned such that it runs between the aortic and pulmonary trunks (Figure 6-14). As the aortic and pulmonary trunks expand with increased blood flow during exercise, they compress the left main coronary artery leading to ischemia of the myocardium and, eventually, fatal arrhythmia.

Unfortunately, patients with coronary artery anomalies may not experience symptoms prior to SCD. Resting and exercise ECGs are typically normal. This diagnosis is usually made with a high index of suspicion and can only be found on coronary angiography. Individuals who experience exertional syncope should be referred to a physician for follow-up. The 36th Bethesda Conference recommends that athletes who are diagnosed with coronary artery anomalies be restricted from all competitive sports.[43]

Disorders of the Myocardium and Coronary Artery Disease

Heart Failure

When cardiac output decreases because of an insufficient heart pump mechanism, the resulting condition is called *heart failure*. The types of heart failure are identified by the side of the heart that is affected (left or right) and whether the failure is acute or chronic. Acute heart failure is

Table 6-8. Sport Classifications

	CLASS A (< 40% MAXO$_2$)	CLASS B (40% TO 70% MAXO$_2$)	CLASS C (> 70% MAXO$_2$)
I. LOW (< 20% MVC)	Billiards, bowling, cricket, curling, golf, riflery, yoga	Baseball, softball, fencing, table tennis, volleyball	Badminton, cross-country skiing (classic technique), field hockey, orienteering, race walking, racquet-ball/squash, running (long distance), soccer
II. MODERATE (20% TO 50% MVC)	Archery, auto racing, diving, equestrian, motorcycling	American football, field events (jumping), figure skating, rodeoing, rugby, running (sprint), surfing, synchronized swim-ming, "ultra" racing	Basketball, ice hockey, cross-country skiing (skating technique), lacrosse, running (middle distance), swim-ming, team handball, tennis
III. HIGH (> 50% MVC)	Bobsledding/luge, field events (throwing), gymnastics, martial arts, sailing, sport climbing, water skiing, weight lifting, windsurfing	Body building, downhill skiing, skateboarding, snowboarding, wrestling	Boxing, canoeing/kayaking, cycling, decathlon, rowing, speed-skating, triathlon

MaxO$_2$ = maximum volume of oxygen (aerobic capacity); MVC = maximum voluntary contraction.

Reproduced with permission from Mitchell JH, Haskell W, Snell P, Van Camp SP. 36th Bethesda conference task force 8: classification of sport. *J Am Coll Cardiol*. 2005;45:1364-1367.

immediately life threatening, whereas chronic heart failure causes gradual but progressive failures in the body's organ systems. Table 6-9 summarizes the respective effects of these conditions.

Cor pulmonale is the term used for right heart failure that occurs as a consequence of pulmonary disease. The pulmonary disease increases pressure in the pulmonary vascular system. The increased pressure increases the workload on the right ventricle, which pumps blood through the pulmonary artery to the lungs. If the pressure rises high enough, such as occurs with a complete vascular occlusion in the lung, the right ventricle cannot push the blood into the lungs, resulting in acute right-sided heart failure. Signs and symptoms of cor pulmonale are similar to those of right heart failure plus signs of pulmonary disease (see Chapter 7). Typically, right heart failure also comes with left heart failure.

Myocardial Ischemia

Myocardial ischemia occurs when the oxygen needed by the myocardium of the heart exceeds the oxygen delivered by the blood in the coronary arteries, which comes off the aorta. This ischemic state causes *angina* (chest pain). In addition to angina, ischemic disorders affecting the myocardium usually exhibit typical cardiac signs and symptoms: fatigue, dyspnea, dizziness, and syncope. In a cardiac emergency, the vital signs (HR, respiration rate, BP) change rapidly. Of note, in diabetes, the typical angina and related symptoms may not be as apparent so a high index of suspicion for cardiac pathology is warranted.

Figure 6-14. Coronary artery anomaly. (A) Normal anterior coronary artery. (B) Abnormal course of the anterior coronary artery, running between the aorta and the pulmonary artery.

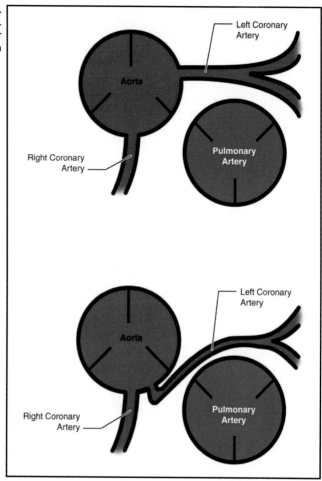

Anything that limits myocardial blood supply causes angina. For example, if CAD obstructs the coronary arteries, the associated myocardium becomes ischemic and dies, a condition called MI. A significant proportion of MIs are caused by moderate to heavy activity, such as manual labor or athletics. CAD, including arteriosclerosis, comprises the majority of cardiac deaths among physically active persons over 35 years of age.[10] For this reason, angina accompanied by other cardiac signs and symptoms, particularly changes in vital signs, warrants activation of the emergency action plan and immediate referral.

Arrhythmogenic Right Ventricular Dysplasia

Arrhythmogenic right ventricular dysplasia (ARVD) is fatty infiltration (penetration) and fibrosis of the myocardium of the right ventricle. ARVD has a genetic component (most commonly reported by the Italians) and can produce ventricular tachycardia or life-threatening ventricular arrhythmia.[42] Persons with ARVD may have a history of cardiac signs and symptoms upon exertion and should be excluded from participation in most sports.[44]

Valve Disorders

The heart valves can be affected by congenital deformities or acquired disease. Two deformities are *stenosis* (narrowing) that restricts blood flow through the valve (Figure 6-15) and structural malformations that do not allow the valve to close completely. Valve disorders cause murmurs from turbulent blood flow through the deformed valve on auscultation. Heart valve disorders are often

Table 6-9. Types of Heart Failure, Mechanisms, and Signs

LOCATION	MECHANISM	SIGNS
Acute left	Failure to deliver blood to the body Pulmonary edema Typical pathology: myocardial infarction	Dyspnea, pink frothy pulmonary edema and sputum, cyanosis, hypotension
Chronic left	Failure to deliver blood to the body Pulmonary edema Typical pathology: cardiomyopathy	Dyspnea with exertion and during sleep, unusual fatigue, tachycardia, cool skin, cyanosis, pulmonary edema
Acute right	Usually with pulmonary embolism Failure to deliver blood to lungs Systemic edema Typical pathology: acute cor pulmonale (pulmonary embolism)	Cool skin, hypotension, cyanosis
Chronic right	Failure to deliver blood to lungs Systemic edema Typical pathology: chronic pulmonary disease	Dyspnea, fatigue, abdominal discomfort, decreased appetite, peripheral edema

present with other cardiac or systemic diseases. Infection can also damage the heart valves, particularly in children.

Generally, people who have valve disorders with normal HRs and rhythm, normal heart size, and normal cardiac function are not excluded from participating in sports or other physical activity.[45] Decisions related to the participation of people who have more severe valve deformities that cause electrical (arrhythmia) or structural changes (hypertrophy) or affect heart function depend on the severity of the disorder and the person's chosen activity.[45]

Mitral valve prolapse is the most common valve disorder. Mitral valve prolapse is a deformity of the mitral valve leaflets that prevents it from closing completely. The leaflets bulge back into the left atrium during ventricular systole.[42] As a result, blood flows back into the left atrium, decreasing the flow of blood into the aorta (see Figure 6-15). This backflow varies depending on the severity of the deformity. For many people, mitral valve prolapse causes no functional problem. Mitral valve prolapse is usually first detected during cardiac auscultation and may be heard as a mid-systolic click or a mitral regurgitation murmur. The condition can be further diagnosed through an echocardiogram. Individuals who have mitral valve prolapse without syncope, family history of sudden death, arrhythmia, substantial back flow, or a previous cardiac-related event can participate in sports without restriction.[36]

Figure 6-15. Common valvular disorders.

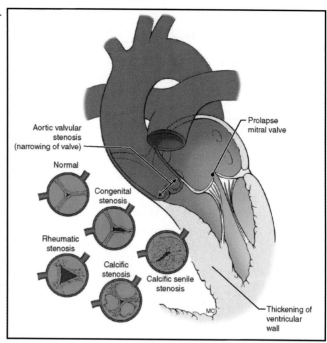

Cardiac Conduction Disorders

Conduction disorders (problems with the heart's electrical system) result in arrhythmia.[44,46] Pathological arrhythmia is produced by abnormal or blocked conduction pathways, leading to ventricular fibrillation and acute heart failure. Benign atrial arrhythmia occurs in some highly fit persons as a result of exercise-induced resting bradycardia, although the presence of atrial fibrillation, particularly during exercise or other physical exertion, requires medical examination to rule out cardiac abnormalities.[44,47] Arrhythmias are diagnosed by ECG. Common benign arrhythmias include sinus bradycardia, asymptomatic first degree AV block and second degree type I AV block.

Most people with a clinically significant arrhythmia have exertional palpitations or exertional syncope.[47] Syncope during exercise is highly suggestive of significant cardiac arrhythmia.[48] Patients with symptomatic arrhythmia should be excluded from sports competition or heavy physical activity for at least 6 months and cleared by ECG before returning. Qualification for sports depends on the type and severity of the arrhythmia.[48]

Paroxysmal Supraventricular Tachycardia

An intermittently occurring very rapid resting HR, exceeding 150 bpm, is called paroxysmal supraventricular tachycardia (*PSVT*). The etiology of PSVT is a defect in the discharge pattern of the SA node, atria, or AV node that causes a dramatic increase in HR. This condition is most common in children and may also be observed in adolescents. An attack of PSVT is usually accompanied by palpitations, anxiety, dyspnea, chest pain or tightness, and possibly syncope. Physical examination reveals a very rapid, but regular and strong, HR. The HR returns to normal between attacks. An ECG monitor may have to be worn for 24 hours or longer to detect this syndrome because the ECG trace is normal between attacks.

PSVT may last for several minutes or several hours and is generally not dangerous or life threatening but may be uncomfortable and frightening to the individual. Use of nicotine, caffeine, alcohol, or drugs may precipitate an attack. Mild PSVT may spontaneously remit and require no treatment. A longer attack may be interrupted by the patient performing a Valsalva maneuver, which is holding the breath and contracting the abdominal muscles as if having a bowel movement. The increased abdominal pressure stimulates pressure receptors in the blood vessels, which generate an autonomic signal to decrease HR. A strong cough or using a ice towel to the face may have the same effect. Electrical shock, medications, or surgery to disrupt the electrical pathway or implant a pacemaker may be necessary in extreme cases.

Long Q-T Syndrome

The Q-T interval on an ECG is a measure of the time it takes for the ventricles to depolarize and repolarize. About 1 in 10,000 people inherit a condition in which the Q-T interval is longer than normal.[7] This increase in the timing of the depolarization-repolarization cycle interferes with the heart's contraction and can lead to a fatal ventricular tachycardia when HR increases, as occurs with exercise.[42,46] Many people are asymptomatic until the arrhythmia occurs, but others will have a history of exertional syncope. Approximately 30% will have a family history of SCD or actual diagnosis of long Q-T syndrome.[7] Diagnosis can be made by ECG before or after symptoms appear. A person with long Q-T syndrome requires medication to control HR, avoidance of physically stressful activity, including sports, and sometimes a pacemaker.[35] β-blockers are the most commonly prescribed medications for long Q-T syndrome.

Wolfe-Parkinson-White Syndrome

Wolfe-Parkinson-White syndrome involves an accessory conduction pathway between the atria and ventricles.[42,46] The accessory pathway conducts more rapidly than the AV node, and the result is that one of the ventricles depolarizes slightly before the other. Atrial fibrillation may occur when a premature atrial depolarization stimulates the additional pathway, which conducts the depolarization in reverse back to the atria. This condition causes the depolarization to circulate in a loop between the atria and the additional pathway, one stimulating the other, resulting in atrial fibrillation. Less common but more severely, the premature atrial depolarization may bypass the AV node into the ventricles, which creates a depolarization that goes back to the atria through the additional pathway and then down the AV node to the ventricles again. The result is a loop of depolarization that causes ventricular fibrillation, which is fatal unless defibrillation occurs within minutes. The presence of exertional syncope or cardiac symptoms increases the risk for ventricular fibrillation. These individuals should undergo a 12-lead ECG, exercise testing, and an echocardiogram to rule out other cardiovascular abnormalities. The syndrome is treated with medication to limit heart rate and surgery to obliterate the additional conduction pathway. Surgery is necessary for individuals who have multiple accessory pathways or demonstrate ventricular rates greater than 240 bpm. Athletes may continue participation in all sports if they have no history of palpitations or structural abnormalities and they do not present with tachycardia.

Marfan Syndrome

Marfan syndrome is an inherited connective tissue disorder associated with increased risk for SCD.[42] Most individuals (80% to 90%) with Marfan syndrome develop potentially fatal deformities in the aorta.[43] The clinical diagnosis of Marfan syndrome is based on the distinct physical characteristics presented in Table 6-4.[42] Definitive diagnosis can be made through echocardiographic measurement of aortic root dimension. The 36th Bethesda Conference recommended that athletes with Marfan syndrome can participate in competitive sports (Class IA or IIA only) if "they do not have one or more of the following: (1) aortic root dilation, (2) moderate to severe mitral regurgitation, or (3) family history of dissection or sudden death in a Marfan relative."[49]

Commotio Cordis

A sudden traumatic blow to the chest that occurs during the vulnerable phase of cardiac repolarization can induce a severe ventricular arrhythmia called *commotio cordis*.[35,42,44,50] Commotio cordis was associated with 130 deaths during the time period of 1998 to 2001, with the average age of victims being 13 years. This life-threatening condition can occur in any sport. It has been reported most frequently in baseball, softball, ice hockey, football, and lacrosse due to sudden physical contact or projectiles such as balls or hockey pucks.[50]

Life-saving efforts should focus on immediate access to an AED. Commotio cordis has a very low rate of resuscitation (15%), unless defibrillation by an AED occurs within 2 minutes of onset.[7] The NATA has published an official statement on commotio cordis that includes suggestions for preventing this condition,[51] as well as an official statement about AED accessibility and emergency planning.[52] Coaches should make sure that all protective equipment fits properly and that young athletes are instructed on the proper techniques for avoiding blows to the chest. For example, young baseball and softball athletes should be instructed to turn away from an inside pitch rather than turn into it.

Hypertension

Hypertension is defined as a resting BP greater than 140/90 on 2 or more consecutive occasions in athletes older than 18 years old.[53] In people below 18 years of age, hypertension is defined as >95th percentile average for systolic or diastolic pressure based on sex, age, and height.[54] Optimal BP is less than 120/80. Prehypertension is defined as a systolic pressure of 120 to 139 mm Hg with a diastolic pressure of 80 to 90 mm Hg. People with prehypertension are at risk for developing hypertension. Prehypertension is not considered a pathological state but is used to identify people at risk for development of hypertension. Individuals with prehypertension should be counseled to make modifications in their diet, to participate in regular exercise, and to avoid sodium and alcohol.

The pathological condition of hypertension is currently categorized into 2 stages. Stage I hypertension is defined as a systolic BP of 140 to 159 mm Hg or diastolic BP of 90 to 99 mm Hg.[55] Stage II hypertension is defined as systolic BP of 141 mm Hg or greater or diastolic BP of 100 mm Hg or greater.[53]

Primary ("essential") arterial hypertension often has unknown pathogenesis, but genetic, behavioral, and environmental factors (eg, urban living, diet, obesity, chronic stress, smoking, alcohol, and drug use—including many performance-enhancing substances) contribute to the condition.[56] Secondary hypertension is the result of another medical condition, most often a renal, hormonal, or metabolic disorder.

Many people with hypertension are asymptomatic, although some experience frequent occipital headaches and epistaxis (nosebleed). A headache can occur when diastolic pressure exceeds 120 mm Hg. Hypertension headaches are usually mild, present on waking, and are relieved by mild activity. Extreme BP responses during exercise (systolic pressure of 240 mm Hg or greater) may be a sign of severe cardiovascular pathology.[57]

Long-term complications of hypertension include heart disease, stroke, retinal damage, renal failure, and peripheral vascular disease. The constant high pressure eventually damages those vessels and the associated tissues. In addition, the left ventricle becomes hypertrophied as an adaptation to the increased work of pumping blood in the highly pressurized system. Left ventricular hypertrophy, if hypertension remains unaddressed, increases the risk of ischemic heart damage, arrhythmia, and heart failure.

People with mild to moderate hypertension without associated organ damage or heart disease need not be restricted from participating in sports but should be approved to do so by their personal physician, be closely monitored, and be fully reevaluated every 2 to 3 months to ensure that their hypertension remains controlled.[55,56] Severe hypertension requires avoidance of strenuous sports that require high-load muscle contraction (eg, power lifting, gymnastics, snow skiing, cycling) until it is controlled by lifestyle or medication and organ damage has been assessed.[53,55,56]

A variety of medications are used to manage hypertension. Angiotensin-converting enzymes inhibitors, Angiotensin II receptor blockers and calcium channel blockers that are prescribed for hypertension have no particular precautions relative to exercise restrictions. Patients taking diuretics to limit plasma volume, thus reducing BP, need to be monitored during activity for dehydration.

All diuretics are banned substances in organized competitive athletics because they can mask the presence of other banned substances such as anabolic steroids. These patients may also require potassium supplementation to avoid hypokalemia (low potassium levels), which can decrease blood flow to muscles and cause serious muscle damage during intense exercise. β blockers (which are banned in some sports) limit maximum HRs, so HR should be monitored during exercise.

Regular aerobic exercise at 60% to 70% of maximum HR has been shown to decrease resting BP, particularly for patients with mild hypertension.[53] All patients with controlled hypertension should participate in a regular exercise program under the guidance of their physician.

Disorders of the Blood

Anemia is described as a hemoglobin level or red blood cell (RBC) volume (hematocrit) that is lower than 95% of people of the same age. For adults, this means hemoglobin levels of less than 13 g/100 dL in men and less than 11.5 g/100 dL in women. Since the hemoglobin in RBC carries oxygen, anemia limits work capacity because it limits the amount of oxygen that is available.[58] Therefore, anemia affects physical performance.

Primary risk factors for anemia include malnutrition and chronic disease. Other risk factors are intense physical training (damages RBCs), prolonged use of analgesics (impairs RBC formation), family history, heavy menstruation (depletes RBCs), and medical treatments such as chemotherapy and radiation (destroys RBCs). Anemia produces pallor, swollen tongue, spooning (thin, concave) nails (see Figure 6-6), scaly lips with fissures at the edges, fatigue, and impaired attention.

Dilutional anemia, also known as "sports anemia" or "pseudoanemia," is common among highly fit individuals. Exercise increases blood plasma volume but does not affect RBC production. In these individuals, blood tests may show anemia because the RBC count looks low relative to blood volume. Dilutional anemia produces no symptoms and does not affect performance because the absolute number of RBCs is normal, so the amount of oxygen being delivered is unaffected. Once the athlete stops his exercise for 1-2 weeks, their anemia resolves.

Most studies indicate that exercise neither causes nor exacerbates true anemia. Chronic blood loss in physically active women, most often through a combination of menstruation, increased stress, intense exercise, and oral contraceptives, will lead to laboratory tests showing low blood iron. Low iron levels are not equivalent to anemia but can lead to anemia if uncorrected because hemoglobin requires iron. Mild iron deficiency alone will not affect physical performance.

Sickle Cell Disease and Sickle Cell Trait

Sickle cell disease is an inherited condition that produces abnormally shaped RBCs (sickle shaped) that inhibit the binding of oxygen[59] and can lead to life-threatening events.[60] Individuals who inherit 2 genes of sickle hemoglobin (one from each parent) are said to have sickle cell disease or sickle cell anemia. The result, like all types of true anemia, is decreased oxygen delivery. Because of the extreme deficiency in oxygen delivery and the corresponding limitation of performance capacity, these individuals will rarely participate in competitive or recreational sports. They may participate in low-impact, moderate duration, low- to moderate-intensity exercise and activities, including walking, calisthenics, swimming, and golf,[61] but should avoid contact and collision sports and probably avoid high-intensity or prolonged (>20 minutes) exercise or activities.[62] Avoiding extreme environmental temperatures and maintaining appropriate hydration during activity are important for prevention of acute sickle cell crisis.[62]

Individuals who inherit one sickle hemoglobin gene and one normal gene are said to have the *sickle cell trait (SCT)*. Approximately 300 million people worldwide[60] and between 8% and 10% of Blacks carry the genetic SCT, and about 1% develop sickle cell anemia.[59] The relative risk of sudden death is 27 times higher among people of African descent who carry the SCT than among persons of African descent without the trait and 40 times higher than the risk in other races. Sudden death in individuals with SCT is usually caused by emboli, because sickled cells tend to clot easily or by sickle cell crises, which lead to widespread vascular occlusion, organ infarction, shock, and death.

Table 6-10. Distinguishing Characteristics of Exertional Sickling

MUSCLE WEAKNESS AND/OR CRAMPING	Muscle weakness is greater in exertional sickling, whereas muscle pain is greater with heat cramps
	Muscles appear normal with exertional sickling as compared to obvious spasms observed with heat cramps
RESPIRATIONS	Exertional sickling will produce tachypnea due to lactic acidosis; however, still able to move air effectively
	Asthmatic will demonstrate reduced air flow
COLLAPSE	Individuals with exertional sickling will "slump" to the ground
	Individuals with sudden cardiac arrest collapse suddenly
	Individuals with heat cramps "pull up" or "hobble" off the field/court
LEVEL OF CONSCIOUSNESS	Individuals with exertional sickling will still be conscious and able to talk after slumping to the ground
	Individuals with sudden cardiac arrest will be unconscious and nonresponsive
RECTAL TEMPERATURE	Individuals with exertional sickling will have rectal temperatures < 103°F (39.4°C)
	Exertional heat stroke associated with rectal temperatures > 104°F (40°C)

Adapted from O'Connor FG, Bergeron MF, Cantrell J, et al. ACSM and CHAMP summit on sickle cell trait: mitigating risks for warfighters and athletes. *Med Sci Sports Exerc*. 2012;44(11):2045-2056.

Sickle cell crises that occur in athletes or other physically active individuals with SCT are typically associated with intense exercise; therefore, these events are referred to as exertional sickling.[63-65]

Signs and symptoms of exertional sickling include muscle pain, cramping and weakness in the lower extremity and low back; inability to catch one's breath during or immediately after an exercise bout; fatigue; and difficulty recovering from an exercise bout.[64,65] Risk for exertional sickling is greater during exercise in hot and high-altitude environments. Other risk factors include dehydration and asthma. The clinical presentation of exertional sickling can mimic that of heat illness, cardiac arrest, or asthma.[63] Knowledge of an individual's SCT status can help in the differentiation of exertional sickling. Table 6-10 outlines specific characteristics that can help athletic trainers differentiate exertional sickling from heat illness, asthma, or cardiac arrest. The NATA has issued a consensus statement entitled "Sickle Cell Trait and the Athlete" that outlines identification of exertional sickling risk and preventive measures.[66]

Individuals who present with signs and symptoms of exertional sickling should be immediately removed from activity and treated with rest, high-flow supplemental oxygen (15 L/min) with a non-rebreather mask, hydration, and cooling (as needed).[64,65] Collapse with exertional sickling is a medical emergency and requires immediate transport to the nearest hospital.

Prevention of exertional sickling should focus on educating athletes, coaches, parents, and all health care professionals about the signs and symptoms of sickling, as well as the importance of proper hydration and acclimatization to exercise intensity and hot, humid environments. Supplemental oxygen should be available during all practices and games. Athletes with SCT should be given longer rest periods between exercise bouts and possibly excluded from timed performance trials (ie, mile run, serial sprints).[64, 65]

SCT is also a risk factor for acute exertional rhabdomyolysis, which is a sudden metabolic breakdown of skeletal muscle that usually occurs during vigorous exercise in hot, humid weather.[60,67,68]

In this condition, myoglobin (a muscle protein) and enzymes from the damaged muscle enter the blood stream. Acute renal failure, shock, and death may result as the proteins and enzymes block the glomeruli, the functional units of the kidneys.[60,68]

Despite these increased risks, individuals with SCT are not restricted from participation in physical activity and sports, although increased attention to proper acclimatization, maintaining adequate hydration, and close monitoring in hot weather, as well as the standard precautions for exercising in the heat (eg, adjusting intensity and duration of activity, wearing loose-fitting clothing, frequent breaks,) are needed.[61] Effective management of exertional sickling requires early recognition and immediate referral. Preventative efforts should focus on gradual acclimatization to hot or high-altitude environments and proper hydration.

Hemophilia

Hemophilia is a genetic disorder that impairs the ability of the blood to clot.[69] Several types of hemophilia exist. The types depend on the clotting factors that are deficient (Table 6-11). Most types of hemophilia are extremely rare. Some types of hemophilia, such as types A and B, are more common and lead to prolonged, severe blood loss with even minor injuries, and are therefore dangerous for competitive athletes. The general recommendation for individuals with the severe types of hemophilia is to avoid collision sports and some contact sports, thus decreasing the risk of injury,[70] but decisions about sports participation should be made on a case-by-case basis with guidance and oversight from the managing physician.[71,72] Furthermore, regular replacement of blood clotting factors is recommended to prevent severe hemorrhaging during sports participation,[69] and treatment regimens that are tailored to the person and desired activities and lifestyle may be required.[71] Prolonged bleeding also means that individuals with hemophilia may take longer than expected to recover from injuries.[70]

Vascular Disorders

Trauma

Repeated blunt trauma, as may occur in the hand and fingers from repeatedly catching a ball, can damage the capillaries and arterioles, producing ischemia distal to the injury.[30,73,74] Symptoms occur in the affected region and include hypersensitivity to cold, numbness, and pallor.[30,73] This condition is treated with rest, padding, and avoidance of cold. Medications to produce vasodilation may also be required.

Occlusion Syndromes

Occlusion of arteries can be caused by mechanical pressure, inflammation, or blood clots. Common sites of occlusion include the subclavian, axillary, popliteal, and femoral arteries.[28,31] Chronic arterial occlusion produces intermittent muscle cramps, diminished distal pulses, bruits on auscultation, dystrophic (yellow, scaly) skin and nails, ulcerations of the skin, and loss of hair in a distal area. Acute arterial occlusion produces the "5 Ps": pain, pallor, pulselessness, paresthesia, and paralysis distal to the occlusion. There are several occlusion syndromes common in physically active populations (Box 6-1).

Thoracic Outlet Syndrome

Thoracic outlet syndrome is defined as clinical presentation (signs/symptoms) caused by compression of the neurovascular bundle by various structures, either between the scalene muscles, between the clavicle/first rib, or by the pectoralis minor tendon near the coracoid process.[74] The compression can either be neurogenic (95%), venous (2-3%), arterial (1%), or mixed. The patient's history usually reveals repetitive strenuous overhead activity (eg, throwing, swimming, or racquet sports) or prolonged postures involving scapular protraction (eg, deskwork). Symptoms include diffuse arm aching that increases with exertion, paresthesia that increases at night, easy fatigability of

Table 6-11. Types of Bleeding Disorders Caused by Deficiencies in Clotting Factors (Most Common Disorders Listed First)

CLOTTING FACTOR	DISORDERS	CHARACTERISTICS	TREATMENT
VIII	Hemophilia A	X-linked recessive trait: affects men, very rarely affects women 80% of all hemophilia cases	Desmopression acetate (DDAVP) to stimulate release of clotting factors from blood vessel walls Factor VIII infusion at the first sign of bleeding Plasma and plasma concentrates More severe cases may require prophylactic factor VIII
IX	Hemophilia B (Christmas disease)	X-linked recessive trait Second most common type of hemophilia	Factor IX infusion at the first sign of bleeding Plasma and plasma concentrates
von Willebrand	von Willebrand disease	Autosomal dominant trait, affects 1% to 2% of the population Abnormal von Willebrand protein affects platelet function	DDAVP to stimulate release of clotting factors, including von Willebrand, from blood vessel walls
I (fibrinogen)	Afibrinogenesis Hypofibrinogenesis Dysfibrinogenesis	Autosomal recessive trait Very rare: only 200 known cases	Cryoprecipitate Plasma
II (prothrombin)	Hypoprothrombinemia Dysprothrombinemia	Autosomal recessive trait or acquired from severe vitamin K deficiency or liver disease Inherited condition is very rare: only 30 known cases	Plasma Prothrombin complex concentrates (PCCs)
V	Parahemophilia Owren's disease	Autosomal recessive trait Very rare: only 150 known cases Factor V accelerates thrombin activity; deficiency slows clot formation	Plasma, only useful when bleeding because factor V breaks down very quickly

(continued)

Table 6-11 (continued). Types of Bleeding Disorders Caused by Deficiencies in Clotting Factors (Most Common Disorders Listed First)

CLOTTING FACTOR	DISORDERS	CHARACTERISTICS	TREATMENT
VII (proconvertin)	Factor VII deficiency	Autosomal recessive trait, extremely rare Is also rarely acquired when using Couma-din, an anticoagulant	Plasma, only useful when bleeding because factor VII breaks down very quickly
X (Stuart-Prower)	Factor X deficiency	Autosomal recessive trait Extremely rare: only 50 known cases	Plasma, only useful when bleeding because factor X breaks down very quickly PCCs for bleeding episodes
XI	Hemophilia C Plasma thromboplastic antecedent Rosenthal syndrome	Autosomal recessive trait Very rare: only 200 known cases Usually discovered with excessive bleeding during surgery	Plasma Fresh frozen factor X concentrate Fibrin glue to create a clot during surgery DDAVP
XII (Hageman)	Factor XII deficiency	Autosomal recessive trait, very rare Does NOT cause excessive bleeding	Typically, no treatment is required
XIII (fibrin stabilizing factor)	Factor XIII deficiency	Autosomal recessive trait, exceptionally rare Clot forms, but is very weak because factor XIII cross-links fibrin Very severe bleeding	Plasma Cryoprecipitate Fresh frozen factor XIII concentrate

the limb, and intermittent swelling of the limb.[31] Clinical signs vary, but distal temperature changes and cyanosis are common. In addition, diminished distal (radial) pulse during clinical tests, such as Adson's test, military bracing, Allen's test, or repeated clenching of the fist with the hand overhead, may be positive if the artery is involved.[74]

Other vascular occlusion syndromes can also occur.[74] Acute (traumatic) or chronic (exertional) *compartment syndromes* can occlude an artery in the affected compartment. Compartment syndrome of the anterior compartment of the lower leg produces weak dorsiflexion and foot drop in more severe cases, numbness of the first web space (between toes 1 and 2), and weak or absent dorsal pedis pulse.[74] Buerger's disease (*thromboangiitis obliterans*) is a condition associated with tobacco use, producing segmental inflammation and occlusion of arterioles and resulting in signs of

---

Box 6-1: The 5 Ps of Ocular Occlusion

1. Pain
2. Pallor
3. Pulselessness
4. Paresthesia
5. Paralysis

---

occlusion simultaneously in the upper and lower extremities that subside with cessation of tobacco use.[28] An *iliac artery compression syndrome* that produces lower limb symptoms and impairs performance has been described in cyclists and other endurance athletes in sports requiring prolonged lower limb exertion (eg, runners, cross-country skiers).[74,75]

Deep Vein Thrombosis and Pulmonary Embolism

Deep vein thrombosis (*DVT*) and *pulmonary embolism* can occur after casting or other immobilization, after surgery, or in a hypercoagulable state that may be the result of age (>60 years), an inherited blood clotting abnormality, a disease such as cancer, a pathological state such as obesity, tobacco smoking, the use of oral contraceptives, or prolonged sitting (eg, long airplane flights).[76] Injury of the vascular endothelium, venous stasis or pooling of blood, and hypercoagulability comprise the "*Virchow's triad*" of risk factors for developing thrombosis.[76] Extreme effort or exertion may damage venous walls sufficiently enough to result in formation of a thrombus, particularly in the axillary or subclavian vein of throwers.[74] As blood pools in large veins or is stimulated chemically or mechanically by local vascular injury, the cells clot together to form a mass called a *thrombus*, usually resulting in venous swelling called *thrombophlebitis*. The presence of a thrombus in a vein is called *thrombosis*. A thrombus that has broken free from its origin and moves through the circulation is called an *embolus*.

The classically described signs and symptoms of DVT in the lower extremity are severe calf tenderness, distended veins, distal edema, and pain with passive dorsiflexion (*Homan's sign*). Fewer than one-third of the patients who have DVT, however, actually exhibit these symptoms. Diagnosis is made by Doppler ultrasound, which uses high-frequency sound waves to measure blood flow velocity; abnormally slow blood flow in a vein indicates occlusion. Of note, a high index of suspicion is needed to suspect a DVT. Using Well's Criteria can help guide the necessary testing required. To prevent DVT, particularly for patients with immobilized or casted lower extremities, walking or active range of motion exercises requiring muscle contraction should be performed several times a day. If such activity is not possible, treatments such as medication (anticoagulants) and intermittent compression may be used. Compression stockings are also often used to prevent DVT.

Pulmonary embolism occurs when an embolus travels to a lung, and blocks a blood vessel and the blood flow to a portion of the lung, which can cause necrosis of lung tissue. This condition presents with chest pain, dyspnea, cough, hemoptysis (bloody sputum with cough), diaphoresis, anxiety, and hyperpnea (more than 20 breaths per minute). A pulmonary embolism is a medical emergency **911** because, if it affects a large lung segment, it can produce syncope, shock, and death. Most cases will resolve if treated appropriately with hospitalization and anticoagulants. In some cases, anticoagulant medications may be taken for lifetime after the occurrence of the pulmonary embolism. Return to play decisions for DVT and pulmonary embolism depends on various factors including risk factors, age, recurrence, and sport. This decision will likely be made with a multispecialty team including the team physician, a hematologist, cardiologist, and/or pulmonologist. Anticoagulant medications have significantly improved over the last decade which has altered the management of these clots in athletes.

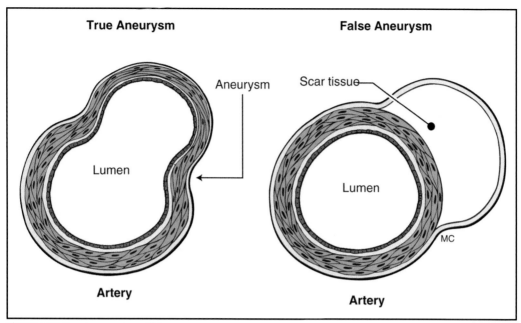

Figure 6-16. True aneurysm and false aneurysm.

Aneurysm

An aneurysm is a weakness in the wall of a blood vessel, usually a result of arteriosclerosis, genetics, or infection, which causes a local dilation or bulging of all layers of the vessel wall (Figure 6-16).[28] Aneurysms produce pulsing pain, auscultated bruits, and asymmetrical distal pulses. Aneurysms are susceptible to rupture, which may cause severe internal hemorrhage, shock, and death if untreated. Common sites at which aneurysms develop include the aorta (common in Marfan syndrome and smokers), the iliac artery, the subclavian artery, the axillary artery, and the cerebral arteries.[28,73,74]

A *false aneurysm* can occur after trauma in sports or other physical activity. In a false aneurysm, the wall of the vessel tears and causes a hematoma that subsequently develops into a fibrous scar (see Figure 6-13). The interior diameter (lumen) of the vessel is unchanged and blood flow is unaffected.[28] Symptoms are caused by the bulging scar compressing nearby anatomical structures, such as nerves or other vessels. History typically includes a local traumatic injury that has not resolved as expected. A painful, pulsatile mass is often palpable at the site of the false aneurysm, but pulses distal to the injury are normal.[27,28] Rest is usually all that is needed, although occasionally surgical excision is required.

Headaches

Headaches can be caused by several neurovascular problems. A *migraine headache* causes intense throbbing pain, usually unilaterally, with associated symptoms of nausea, vomiting, photophobia (aversion to light), and phonophobia (aversion to sound). Many who suffer migraines have a positive family history. The causes and mechanisms of migraine headaches are poorly understood but may be related to alterations in the neurotransmitter serotonin, inflammatory effects on the trigeminal nerve complex, and hormonal variations.

A *cluster headache* is an intense, gnawing pain that is deep and non-throbbing in nature, occurring unilaterally around one eye. Lacrimation (tearing), rhinorrhea ("runny nose") or nasal congestion, diaphoresis, unilateral pupillary constriction (miosis), ptosis (drooping eyelid), and psychomotor agitation may also be present as a result of trigeminal nerve and parasympathetic involvement.[77]

A cluster headache episode lasts up to 45 minutes and may recur on a daily basis; the defining characteristic is the recurrence of the headache across several days followed by a long period with no headache. Common exacerbating factors include psychoemotional stress and alcohol or tobacco use. Similar to migraines, the etiology and pathophysiology of cluster headaches are not well understood but may be related to neurovascular, hormonal, or autonomic nervous system abnormalities.

A *toxic vascular headache* presents diffuse, throbbing, severe pain over the entire crown of the head; this type of headache is never unilateral. Etiology includes infection (usually accompanied by fever), caffeine abuse or withdrawal, alcohol abuse or withdrawal (hangover), hypoxia, hypoglycemia (low blood sugar), and metabolic disorders.

 People with vascular headaches are awake and alert, have no fever, and demonstrate a negative neurological examination (see Chapters 1 and 13). Treatment consists of rest in a quiet, dark room and prescription medication if the headaches are recurrent and disabling. If other systemic signs occur simultaneously with a severe headache, urgent medical attention is required.

PEDIATRIC CONCERNS

Chest Pain

Chest pain in a child is rarely due to cardiac pathology. Chest pain is usually attributable to a musculoskeletal condition or a specific injury or other event.[26] Asthma, depression, anxiety disorders, hyperventilation, autoimmune disease, anemia, school or family stress, or physical abuse may also cause chest pain. Children with a family history of heart disease who have chest pain, however, should be referred for medical examination.[26]

Congenital Heart Conditions

The most common congenital heart problems are septal wall defects and vascular anomalies. These disorders are often detected and surgically corrected during infancy, but subtle cases occasionally go undetected. Some children with congenital heart conditions have a history of frequent illnesses, delayed growth, intolerance to activity, malaise, and other signs of chronic disease. Signs of potential cardiac pathology include digital clubbing, cyanosis, syncope, fatigue, dyspnea, and auscultated pericardial rub, murmurs, or clicks.[26]

Most congenital heart conditions are not adversely affected by exercise and do not prevent participation in sports.[78] Some exceptions are hypertrophic cardiomyopathy, congenital coronary artery anomalies, cardiac complications of Marfan syndrome, myocarditis, and major heart-vascular malformations.[43] Each child who has a heart condition requires an individual treatment plan. Physical activity should be restricted only to the extent that it is medically necessary. In general, baseline and annual exercise testing with ECG and BP monitoring should be conducted to ascertain progression of disease as the child matures.[43] The 36th Bethesda Conference guidelines should be consulted when making decisions regarding sports participation.

SUMMARY

The hallmark of cardiac pathology is chest pain, or angina, with referred pain into the left upper arm, anterior throat, face, jaw, or posterior chest wall. Other symptoms associated with cardiac pathology include dyspnea, fatigue, palpitations, and syncope. Clinical signs include cyanosis; edema; diaphoresis; clubbing of fingers and toes; dystrophic (yellow, scaly) nails; changes in rate, rhythm, or character of heartbeat; auscultated murmurs; and changes in BP. Symptoms of vascular pathology include changes in skin temperature; numbness, cramping, or pain with activity; and limb fatigue during activity. Associated signs are localized skin pallor or cyanosis; distal edema; changes in the rate, rhythm, or character of distal pulses; dilated or distended veins; and palpable pulsatile masses.

A thorough preparticipation physical exam can play an important role in identifying individuals who might have a potentially serious cardiovascular condition. When planning these examinations, athletic trainers should ensure that the AHA minimal components are included in both the history and physical examination portions of the screening. Athletic trainers should also be diligent in following up on all potential cardiovascular conditions identified through the preparticipation physical examination.

CASE STUDY

Tiffany, a 16-year-old Black female basketball athlete, is carried into your athletic training facility by her coaches. The coaches explain that they were conducting conditioning drills outside on the track when Tiffany fainted. She had been complaining throughout the drills, but this was natural for Tiffany. When she fainted, they knew that they needed to bring her to you. She is conscious now and complaining of dizziness, chest pains, and shortness of breath.

As you begin your physical examination, you find that her pulse is 98, weak, and irregular; blood pressure is 150/80; respirations are 24, rapid, shallow, and labored.

As you question her further, Tiffany tells you that she fainted once before when she was in middle school. She said it happened during basketball practice. Her mother took her to the doctor, but he didn't find anything wrong with her.

Critical Thinking Questions

1. Based on Tiffany's complaints and your initial physical examination, what conditions would you include in your differential diagnosis? Why?
2. What steps will you take in managing Tiffany's condition?
3. What are the potential risks for Tiffany?

REFERENCES

1. National Athletic Trainers' Association. *Athletic Training Education Competencies.* 5th ed. The Commission on Accreditation of Athletic Training Education; 2011.
2. NIH Consensus Development Panel on Physical Activity and Cardiovascular Health. Physical activity and cardiovascular health. *JAMA.* 1996;276:241-246.
3. American College of Sports Medicine and American Heart Association. Recommendations for cardiovascular screening, staffing, and emergency policies at health/fitness facilities. *Med Sci Sports Exerc.* 1998;30:1009-1018.
4. Thompson PD, Balady GJ, Chaitman BR, Clark LT, Levine BD, Myerburg RJ. 36th Bethesda Conference Task Force 6: coronary artery disease. *J Am Coll Cardiol.* 2005;45:1348-1353.
5. Corrado D, Drezner J, Basso C, Pelliccia A, Thiene G. Strategies for the prevention of sudden cardiac death during sports. *Eur J Cardiovasc Prev Rehabil.* 2011;18:197-208.
6. Campbell RM, Berger S, Drezner J. Sudden cardiac arrest in children and young athletes: the importance of a detailed personal and family history in the pre-participation evaluation. *Br J Sports Med.* 2009;43:336-341.
7. Koester MC. A review of sudden cardiac death in young athletes and strategies for preparticipation cardiovascular screening. *J Athl Train.* 2001;36:197-204.
8. Maron BJ, Thompson PD, Puffer JC, et al. Cardiovascular preparticipation screening of competitive athletes: a statement for health professionals from the Sudden Death Committee (clinical cardiology) and Congenital Cardiac Defects Committee (cardiovascular disease in the young), American Heart Association. *Circulation.* 1996;94:850-856.

9. Maron BJ, Douglas PS, Graham TP, Nishimura RA, Thompson PD. 36th Bethesda Conference Task Force 1: preparticipation screening and diagnosis of cardiovascular disease in athletes. *J Am Coll Cardiol*. 2005;45:1322-1326.

10. 1American Academy of Family Physicians, American Academy of Orthopaedic Surgeons, American College of Sports Medicine, American Medical Society for Sports Medicine, American Orthopaedic Society for Sports Medicine, American Osteopathic Academy of Sports Medicine, Kibler WB, Putukian M. Selected issues for the master athlete and the team physician: a consensus statement. *Med Sci Sports Exerc*. 2010;42:820-833.

11. Maron BJ, Levine BD, Washington RL, et al. Eligibility and Disqualification Recommendations for Competitive Athletes with Cardiovascular Abnormalities: Task Force 2: Preparticipation Screening for Cardiovascular Disease in Competitive Athletes. *Circulation*. 2015;132(22):267-272.

12. American Academy of Family Physicians, American Academy of Pediatrics, American College of Sports Medicine, American Medical Society for Sports Medicine, American Orthopaedic Society for Sports Medicine, American Osteopathic Academy of Sports Medicine, Bernhardt DT, Roberts WO, eds. *PPE Preparticipation Physical Evaluation*. 4th ed. American Academy of Pediatrics; 2010.

13. Terry GC, Kyle JM, Ellis JM, Cantwell J, Courson R, Medlin R. Sudden cardiac arrest in athletic medicine. *J Athl Train*. 2001;36:205-209.

14. Corrado D, Pelliccia A, Heidbuchel H, et al. Recommendations for interpretation of 12-lead electrocardiogram in the athlete. *Eur Heart J*. 2010;31:243-259.

15. Maron BJ, Thompson PD, Ackerman MJ, et al. Recommendations and considerations related to preparticipation screening for cardiovascular abnormalities in competitive athletes: 2007 update: a scientific statement from the American Heart Association Council on Nutrition, Physical Activity, and Metabolism: endorsed by the American College of Cardiology Foundation. *Circulation*. 2007;115:1643-1455.

16. Rodday AM, Triedman JK, Alexander ME, et al. Electrocardiogram screening for disorders that cause sudden cardiac death in asymptomatic children: a meta-analysis. *Pediatrics*. 2012;129:e999-e1010.

17. Estes NA 3rd, Link MS. Preparticipation athletic screening including an electrocardiogram: an unproven strategy for prevention of sudden cardiac death in the athlete. *Prog Cardiovasc Dis*. 2012;54:451-454.

18. Asif IM, Drezner JA. Sudden cardiac death and preparticipation screening: the debate continues-in support of electrocardiogram-inclusive preparticipation screening. *Prog Cardiovasc Dis*. 2012;54:445-450.

19. Wheeler MT, Heidenreich PA, Froelicher VF, Hlatky MA, Ashley EA. Cost-effectiveness of preparticipation screening for prevention of sudden cardiac death in young athletes. *Ann Intern Med*. 2010;152:276-286.

20. O'Connor DP, Knoblauch MA. Electrocardiogram testing during athletic preparticipation physical examinations. *J Athl Train*. 2010;45:265-272.

21. Lawless CE, Best TM. Electrocardiograms in athletes: interpretation and diagnostic accuracy. *Med Sci Sports Exerc*. 2008;40:787-798.

22. Drezner JA, Ackerman MJ, Anderson J, et al. Electrocardiographic interpretation in athletes: the 'Seattle Criteria'. *J Sports Med*. 2013;47:122-124.

23. Pelliccia A, Maron MS, Maron BJ. Assessment of left ventricular hypertrophy in a trained athlete: differential diagnosis of physiologic athlete's heart from pathologic hypertrophy. *Prog Cardiovasc Dis*. 2012;54:387-396.

24. Cayley WE. Diagnosing the Cause of Chest Pain. *Am Fam Physician*. 2005;72(10):2012-2021.

25. Maron BJ. Cardiovascular risks to young persons on the athletic field. *Ann Intern Med*. 1998;129:379-386.

26. Anzai AK. Adolescent chest pain. *Am Fam Physician*. 1996;53:1682-1690.

27. Bandy WD, Strong L, Roberts T, Dyer R. False aneurysm—a complication following an inversion ankle sprain: a case report. *J Orthop Sports Phys Ther*. 1996;23(4):272-279.

28. Cohn SL, Taylor WC. Vascular problems of the lower extremity in athletes. *Clin Sports Med*. 1990;9:449-470.

29. Karas SE. Thoracic outlet syndrome. *Clin Sports Med*. 1990;9:297-310.

30. Rettig AC. Neurovascular injuries in the wrists and hands of athletes. *Clin Sports Med*. 1990;9:389-417.

31. Sotta RR. Vascular problems in the proximal upper extremity. *Clin Sports Med*. 1990;9:379-388.

32. Smith L. New AHA Recommendations for Blood Pressure Measurement. *Am Fam Physician*. 2005;72(7):1391-1398.

33. Barrett MJ, Ayub B, Martinez MW. Cardiac auscultation in sports medicine: strategies to improve clinical care. *Curr Sports Med Rep*. 2012;11:78-84.

34. Maron BJ, Zipes DP. 36th Bethesda Conference Introduction: recommendations for competitive athletes with cardiovascular abnormalities—general considerations. *J Am Coll Cardiol*. 2005;45:1318-1321.

35. Link MS, Mark Estes NA 3rd. Sudden cardiac death in athletes. *Prog Cardiovasc Dis*. 2008;51(1):44-57.

36. Estes NAM, III, Kloner R. 36th Bethesda Conference Task Force 9: drugs and performance-enhancing substances. *J Am Coll Cardiol*. 2005;45:1368-1369.

37. Drezner JA, Courson RW, Roberts WO, Mosesso VN, Link MS, Maron BJ. Inter-association Task Force recommendations on emergency preparedness and management of sudden cardiac arrest in high school and college athletic programs: a consensus statement. *J Athl Train*. 2007;42:143-158.

38. Casa DJ, Anderson SA, Baker L, et al. The inter-association task force for preventing sudden death in collegiate conditioning sessions: best practices recommendations. *J Athl Train*. 2012;47:477-480.

39. Andersen J, Courson RW, Kleiner DM, McLoda TA. National Athletic Trainers' Association Position Statement: Emergency planning in athletics. *J Athl Train.* 2002;37:99-104.

40. Maron BJ. Hypertrophic cardiomyopathy: practical steps for preventing sudden death. *Phys Sportsmed.* 2002;30(1):19-24.

41. Maron BJ, Maron MS. Hypertrophic cardiomyopathy. *Lancet.* 2013;381:242-255.

42. Mason PK, Mounsey JP. Common issues in sports cardiology. *Clin Sports Med.* 2005;24:463-476.

43. Graham TP, Driscoll DJ, Gersony WM, Newburger JW, Rocchini A, Towbin JA. 36th Bethesda Conference Task Force 2: congenital heart disease. *J Am Coll Cardiol.* 2005;45:1326-1333.

44. Link MS, Estes NA. Athletes and arrhythmias. *J Cardiovasc Electrophysiol.* 2010;21(10):1184-1189.

45. Bonow RO, Cheitlin MD, Crawford MH, Douglas PS. 36th Bethesda Conference Task Force 3: valvular heart disease. *J Am Coll Cardiol.* 2005;45:1334-1340.

46. Stoebner R, Bellin DA, Haigney MC. Cardiac electrophysiology and the athlete: a primer for the sports clinician. *Curr Sports Med Rep.* 2012;11:70-77.

47. Lampert R. Evaluation and management of arrhythmia in the athletic patient. *Prog Cardiovasc Dis.* 2012;54:423-431.

48. Zipes DP, Ackerman MJ, Estes NAM III, Grant AO, Myerburg RJ, Van Hare G. 36th Bethesda Conference Task Force 7: arrhythmias. *J Am Coll Cardiol.* 2005;45:1354-1365.

49. Maron BJ, Ackerman MJ, Nishimura RA, Pyeritz RE, Towbin JA, Udelson JE. 36th Bethesda Conference Task Force 4: HCM and other cardiomyopathies, mitral valve prolapse, myocarditis, and Marfan syndrome. *J Am Coll Cardiol.* 2005;45:1340-1345.

50. Maron BJ, Estes NAM III, Link MS. 36th Bethesda Conference Task Force 11: commotio cordis. *J Am Coll Cardiol.* 2005;45:1371-1373.

51. National Athletic Trainers' Association. Official Statement from the National Athletic Trainers' Association on commotio cordis. Available at http://www.nata.org/publicinformation/files/ASTFstmt.pdf. Accessed September 30, 2005.

52. National Athletic Trainers' Association. Official Statement—Automated External Defibrillators. Available at http://www.nata.org/sites/default/files/AutomatedExternalDefibrillators.pdf. Accessed July 8, 2013.

53. Kaplan NM, Gidding SS. 36th Bethesda Conference Task Force 5: systemic hypertension. *J Am Coll Cardiol.* 2005;45:1346-1348.

54. Moyer VA; U.S. Preventive Services Task Force. Screening for primary hypertension in children and adolescents: U.S. Preventive Services Task Force recommendation statement. *Pediatrics.* 2013;132:907-914.

55. Bruno RM, Cartoni G, Taddei S. Hypertension in special populations: athletes. *Future Cardiol.* 2011;7:571-584.

56. Leddy JJ, Izzo J. Hypertension in athletes. *J Clin Hypertens (Greenwich).* 2009;11:226-233.

57. Palatini P. Exaggerated blood pressure response to exercise: pathophysiologic mechanisms and clinical relevance. *J Sports Med Phys Fitness.* 1998;38(1):1-9.

58. Chatard J, Mujika I, Guy C, Lacour J. Anaemia and iron deficiency in athletes: practical recommendations for treatment. *Sports Med.* 1999;27(4):229-240.

59. Jones JD, Kleiner DM. Awareness and identification of athletes with sickle cell disorders at historically black colleges and universities. *J Athl Train.* 1996;31:220-222.

60. Tsaras G, Owusu-Ansah A, Boateng FO, Amoateng-Adjepong Y. Complications associated with sickle cell trait: a brief narrative review. *Am J Med.* 2009;122:507-512.

61. Al-Rimawi H, Jallad S. Sport participation in adolescents with sickle cell disease. *Pediatr Endocrinol Rev.* 2008;6(Suppl 1):214-216.

62. Connes P, Machado R, Hue O, Reid H. Exercise limitation, exercise testing and exercise recommendations in sickle cell anemia. *Clin Hemorheol Microcirc.* 2011;49:151-163.

63. O'Connor FG, Bergeron MF, Cantrell J, et al. ACSM and CHAMP summit on sickle cell trait: mitigating risks for warfighters and athletes. *Med Sci Sports Exerc.* 2012;44:2045-2056.

64. Casa DJ, Guskiewicz KM, Anderson SA, et al. National Athletic Trainers' Association position statement: preventing sudden death in sports. *J Athl Train.* 2012;47:96-118.

65. Casa DJ, Almquist J, Anderson SA, et al. The Inter-Association Task Force for Preventing Sudden Death in Secondary School Athletics Programs: Best Practices Recommendations. *J Athl Train.* 2013;48(4):546-553.

66. National Athletic Trainers' Association. Consensus Statement—Sickle Cell Trait and the Athlete. Available at http://www.nata.org/sites/default/files/SickleCellTraitAndTheAthlete.pdf. Accessed July 30, 2013.

67. Cleary MA. Sickle cell trait and exertional rhabdomyolysis. *Athl Ther Today.* 2003;8(5):66-67.

68. Harrelson GL, Fincher AL, Robinson JB. Acute exertional rhabdomyolysis and its relationship to sickle cell trait. *J Athl Train.* 1995;30:309-312.

69. Fiala KA, Ritenour DM. Medical care for athletes with hemophilia. *Athl Ther Today.* 2004;9:16-19.

70. Buzzard BM. Sports and hemophilia: antagonist or protagonist. *Clin Orthop Relat Res.* 1996;328:25-30.

71. Petrini P, Seuser A. Haemophilia care in adolescents—compliance and lifestyle issues. *Haemophilia.* 2009;15(Suppl 1):15-19.

72. Morris PJ. Physical activity recommendations for children and adolescents with chronic disease. *Curr Sports Med Rep.* 2008;7:353-358.
73. Thompson RW, Driskill M. Neurovascular problems in the athlete's shoulder. Clin Sports Med. 2008;27:789-802.
74. Sanders RJ, Hammond SL, Rao NM. Diagnosis of thoracic outlet syndrome. *J Vasc Surg.* 2007;46(3):601.
75. Lim CS, Gohel MS, Shepherd AC, Davies AH. Iliac artery compression in cyclists: mechanisms, diagnosis and treatment. *Eur J Vasc Endovasc Surg.* 2009;38:180-186.
76. Grabowski G, Whiteside WK, Kanwisher M. Venous thrombosis in athletes. *J Am Acad Orthop Surg.* 2013;21:108-117.
77. Garten CE. Headaches and athletes. *Athl Ther Today.* 2005;10:28-29.
78. Committee on Sports and Fitness. Medical conditions affecting sports participation. *Pediatrics.* 2001;107:1205-1209.

ONLINE RESOURCES

Heart Sounds

◊ **The Auscultation Assistant**

  ¤ www.med.ucla.edu/wilkes/intro.html

◊ **Barrett MJ, Ayub B, Martinez MW29 ("Innocent Murmur" and "Hypertropic Cardiomyopathy")**

  ¤ http://links.lww.com/CSMR/A1 and http://links.lww.com/CSMR/A2

◊ **Blaufuss Multimedia Heart Sounds and Cardiac Arrhythmia**

  ¤ www.blaufuss.org/

◊ **Easy Auscultation**

  ¤ http://www.easyauscultation.com/heart-sounds

◊ **Practical Clinical Skills**

  ¤ http://www.practicalclinicalskills.com/heart-sounds-murmurs.aspx

NATA Statements

◊ **NATA Consensus Statement: Preventing Sudden Death in Secondary School Athletics**

  ¤ http://www.nata.org/sites/default/files/preventing-sudden-death.pdf

◊ **NATA Consensus Statement: Sickle Cell Trait and the Athlete**

  ¤ http://www.nata.org/sites/default/files/SickleCellTraitAndTheAthlete.pdf

◊ **NATA Official Statement on Automatic External Defibrillators**

  ¤ http://www.nata.org/sites/default/files/AutomatedExternalDefibrillators.pdf

◊ **NATA Official Statement on Commotio Cordis**

  ¤ http://www.nata.org/sites/default/files/CommotioCordis.pdf

◊ **NATA Official Statement: Preventing Sudden Death in Sports**

  ¤ http://www.nata.org/sites/default/files/Preventing-Sudden-Death-Position-Statement_2.pdf

◊ **The Inter-Association Task Force for Preventing Sudden Death in Collegiate Conditioning Sessions: Best Practices Recommendations**

  ¤ http://www.nata.org/sites/default/files/preventingsuddendeath-consensusstatement.pdf

Others

◊ **The Cardiomyopathy Association**
  ¤ http://www.cardiomyopathy.org/html/which_card_hcm.htm
◊ **Hypertrophic Cardiomyopathy Association**
  ¤ https://www.4hcm.org/
◊ **The National Marfan Foundation**
  ¤ www.marfan.org

Please visit www.routledge.com/9781630917234
to access additional material.

CHAPTER 7

Pulmonary System

CHAPTER OUTLINE AND OBJECTIVES

Introduction

Review of Anatomy, Physiology, and Pathogenesis

◊ Describe basic pulmonary anatomy and function.

◊ Review pathophysiological mechanisms of the pulmonary system.

◊ Describe the response of the pulmonary system to exercise.

Signs and Symptoms

◊ Identify the general signs and symptoms of pulmonary pathology.

Pain Patterns

◊ Identify the referred pain patterns associated with pulmonary pathology.

Medical History and Physical Examination Procedures

◊ Discuss medical history results that are relevant to pulmonary pathology.

◊ Perform physical examination procedures and interpret findings relevant to injury or illness involving the pulmonary system.

  ¤ Family and Personal History

  ¤ Inspection

  ¤ Palpation

  ¤ Respiration Rate and Depth

  ¤ Heart Rate

  ¤ Blood Pressure

  ¤ Percussion

  ¤ Auscultation

Bhojani RA, O'Connor DP, Fincher AL. *Clinical Pathology for Athletic Trainers: Recognizing Systemic Disease, Fourth Edition* (pp 161-198).
© 2022 Taylor & Francis Group.

- ¤ Pulse Oximetry
- ¤ Peak Expiratory Flow Rate

Therapeutic Interventions for Pulmonary Pathology

- ◊ Explain the indications, application, and treatment parameters for supplemental oxygen administration for emergency pulmonary conditions.
- ◊ Explain the indications, application, and treatment parameters for administering a nebulizer treatment for a patient with asthma.
- ◊ Explain the indications, application, and treatment parameters for the use of a metered dose inhaler in treating asthma.
- ◊ Explain the therapeutic strategies for preventing and treating acute asthma attacks.

Pathology and Pathogenesis

- ◊ Explain the strategies that should be used to prevent acute asthma attacks.
- ◊ Discuss the etiology, signs, symptoms, management, medical referral guidelines and, when appropriate, return-to-participation guidelines for asthma attacks.
- ◊ Discuss the etiology, signs, symptoms, management, medical referral guidelines and, when appropriate, return-to-participation guidelines for respiratory infections.
  - ¤ Upper Respiratory Infections
  - ¤ Lower Respiratory Infections
    - • Acute Bronchitis
    - • Influenza
    - • Pneumonia
- ◊ Discuss the etiology, signs, symptoms, management, medical referral guidelines and, when appropriate, return-to-participation guidelines for pathology associated with pulmonary obstruction.
  - ¤ Chronic Obstructive Pulmonary Disease
  - ¤ Chronic Bronchitis
- ◊ Discuss the etiology, signs, symptoms, management, medical referral guidelines and, when appropriate, return-to-participation guidelines for pulmonary pathology associated with trauma.
  - ¤ Atelectasis
  - ¤ Drowning and Near-Drowning
  - ¤ Flail Chest Injury
  - ¤ Pneumothorax, Tension Pneumothorax, and Hemothorax
  - ¤ Pneumomediastinum
- ◊ Discuss the risk factors, signs, symptoms, treatment, and prognosis associated with lung cancer.

Pediatric Concerns

- ◊ Discuss the common pulmonary disorders that affect children.
  - ¤ Asthma in Children
  - ¤ Cystic Fibrosis
  - ¤ Neuromuscular Diseases
  - ¤ Scoliosis
  - ¤ Pertussis (Whooping Cough)

Summary

Case Study

◊ Develop critical-thinking and clinical decision-making skills.

Online Resources

This chapter addresses the following knowledge and skills from the *Athletic Training Education Competencies, Fifth Edition*[1]:

Content Area	Knowledge and Skills
Prevention and Health Promotion (PHP)	16, 17b
Clinical Examination and Diagnosis (CE)	1-3, 7, 13, 15-19, 20a-d, g, 21j, 22
Acute Care of Injuries and Illnesses (AC)	5-7, 15-18, 31-33, 36i
Therapeutic Interventions (TI)	28, 30

INTRODUCTION

The pulmonary system extracts oxygen from the air and exchanges it with carbon dioxide in the blood, thus performing a critical, life-sustaining function.[2] Disorders of the pulmonary system can significantly affect normal physical functioning, as well as athletic performance. For example, close to 25 million people have asthma, many of whom regularly participate in physical activity. Athletic trainers are likely to encounter pulmonary conditions ranging from upper respiratory infections to potentially life-threatening injuries and diseases involving the airways and lungs.

This chapter will review the normal anatomy and physiology of the pulmonary system, as well as discuss the pathophysiology associated with the common pulmonary conditions. The clinical presentation of these conditions will be discussed, along with the appropriate assessment procedures that should be used, such as percussion, auscultation, pulse oximetry, and the measurement of peak expiratory flow rate. Also, the pharmacologic and other therapeutic treatment strategies for the common pulmonary conditions will be described. Lastly, the guidelines for physician referral and emergency transport will be outlined, along with the criteria for return-to-participation decisions.

REVIEW OF ANATOMY, PHYSIOLOGY, AND PATHOGENESIS

The lungs, consisting of the bronchi, alveoli, and a rich blood supply, are the primary organs of the pulmonary system (Figure 7-1). Air enters the nasopharynx, passes down the trachea and through the bronchi and bronchioles, and arrives in the alveoli. The capillary-rich alveoli, the terminal units of the respiratory pathway, exchange gases between the air and the blood. The other airway structures are physiological "dead space" because they do not participate in *respiration* (gas exchange). In some pulmonary disorders, the amount of this physiological dead space in the lung increases and creates a functional (ie, nonanatomic) obstruction to respiration.[2]

The upper airway, primarily the nasopharynx, adds warmth and moisture as it filters the incoming air.[2,3] Mucus and tiny hair-like projections (*cilia*) that cover the upper airway and bronchi serve to filter the incoming air. Particles in the air are trapped by the mucus, moved upward by the cilia, and expelled by coughing.

Figure 7-1. Schematic representation of the anatomy of the lungs.

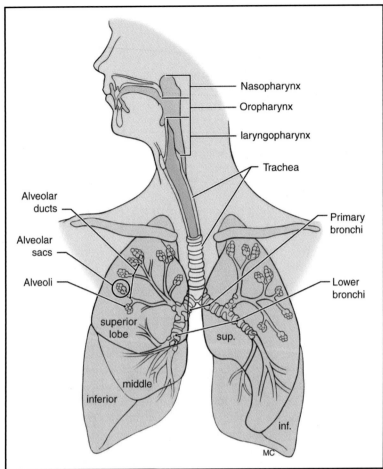

During the process called *ventilation*, air moves into and out of the lungs as an effect of pressure changing within the thorax in accordance with a principal of physics called Boyle's law. Boyle's law states that the relation between the volume and the pressure of a gas is constant: as volume increases, pressure decreases, and vice versa. During inspiration, as the diaphragm and external intercostal muscles contract, the thorax's circumference expands. The visceral and parietal pleura that line the lungs and thorax maintain a negative pressure in the interpleural space—the space between the 2 pleura. Thus, when the thorax expands, this negative pressure in the interpleural space expands the lungs by keeping the lungs close to the wall of the thorax. As the pressure inside the thorax falls below atmospheric pressure, the lungs draw in air. Boyle's law demonstrates the effect: a given volume of air at atmospheric pressure will flow toward lower pressure, which occurs when the lungs expand to increase their volume. Expiration of air occurs as elastic recoil of the ribcage compresses the lungs and alveolar pressure exceeds atmospheric pressure.[3]

Therefore, inspiration requires active muscle contraction, whereas expiration occurs passively, although some muscles can cause forceful expiration if needed.[3] Accessory inspiratory muscles include the abdominals, sternocleidomastoid, and scalenes and can include the serratus anterior, pectoralis muscles, and upper trapezius as the task of inhalation becomes more difficult. Accessory muscles of ventilation are not normally active during quiet breathing but do become active as oxygen demand or the work of breathing increases, as occurs during exercise.[3]

Oxygen and carbon dioxide are exchanged in the alveoli by diffusion in a process called respiration (Figure 7-2). The rate of diffusion varies depending on the difference in the partial pressures of the gases at the alveolar wall. The diffusing capacity can be calculated as the volume of the gas

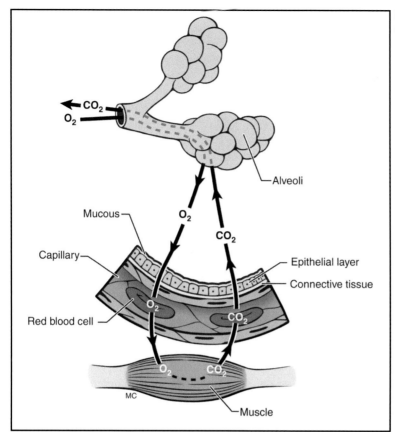

Figure 7-2. Diffusion of gases across the alveolar wall.

entering the blood divided by the difference between the partial pressure of the gas in the alveoli and the partial pressure of the gas in the blood. Oxygen's partial pressure in the atmosphere (and therefore in the alveoli) is greater than its pressure in the alveolar capillaries, so oxygen moves into the blood across the single-celled walls of the alveoli.[2] Likewise, carbon dioxide moves into the alveoli because the partial pressure of carbon dioxide in the capillaries is greater than the pressure in the atmosphere (and the alveoli).[2]

Many complex mechanisms affect pulmonary gas exchange. When either ventilation or blood flow to the lungs is disrupted, the process of binding oxygen to hemoglobin is impaired. The amount of oxygen in the blood decreases rapidly when this occurs, leading to hypoxemia, tissue hypoxia, and other severe physiological and metabolic consequences.

Ventilation is regulated by several mechanisms. The first mechanism involves regions of the medulla oblongata that are sensitive to carbon dioxide and pH levels in the blood.[3] Low pH indicates chemical acidity and high pH indicates alkalinity. Carbon dioxide, and most metabolic byproducts in the blood, are acidic and thereby decrease blood pH. The low pH stimulates the breathing center in the medulla oblongata, which increases ventilation rate and depth to expel the acidic waste products and rebalance pH.[2,3]

The second mechanism involves receptors that are sensitive to pressure, called *baroreceptors*, in the aorta and carotid arteries; these receptors detect changes in blood pressure. *Chemoreceptors* in the same areas detect decreases in blood oxygen levels. These 2 types of receptors act in concert to increase ventilation to maintain blood oxygen concentration.[2,3]

The third mechanism involves several processes in the nervous system. Stretch receptors in the intercostal muscles cause inspiration to stop and expiration to begin.[3] Neurons controlling the ventilation muscles (diaphragm, intercostals, and accessory muscles) travel through the phrenic nerve (from nerve roots C3-5), cranial nerve XI (sternocleidomastoid), and the segmental thoracic nerves that supply the intercostal muscles.[3] Regions of the pons in the brainstem also contribute to the rate and depth of respiration. Damage to the spinal cord above vertebral level C3 or C4 disrupts these neural pathways and usually necessitates the use of a ventilator. The neurological signal for voluntary control of breathing is passed from the brain through the corticospinal tracts to the diaphragm and intercostal neurons.[2]

Both ventilation and respiration are affected by exercise. First, the lungs receive more blood as heart rate and stroke volume (ie, cardiac output) increases. Next, during exercise the muscles use more oxygen, and the partial pressure of oxygen in the pulmonary vessels decreases. As a consequence, more of the oxygen in the inhaled air diffuses into the alveolar capillaries and is made available to the body. Third, the acid and buffering carbon dioxide produced by vigorously exercising muscles causes a reflexive increase in ventilation when the chemoreceptors of the carotid bodies are stimulated. Last, to meet the growing oxygen demand, the rate of ventilation increases; this increase occurs nearly immediately at the onset of exercise.[2]

Signs and Symptoms

Dyspnea

Dyspnea is a breathlessness or shortness of breath that occurs as blood oxygen level decreases. Airway obstruction, metabolic imbalances, psychological stress such as anxiety, mechanical restriction of the lungs, cardiac pathology, or pulmonary disease can cause dyspnea.[4]

Dyspnea produced when in the supine position is called *orthopnea*. Orthopnea is a sign of fluid shift into the lungs, enlarged abdominal organs pushing on the diaphragm, or left-sided heart failure.[4] See Algorithm 7-1 for clinical decision making related to dyspnea.

Cough

A *cough* is a reflex contraction of the diaphragm that forces a blast of air from the lungs to eliminate an irritation in the airway.[3] A dry, nonproductive cough is most often caused by allergic reactions to environmental irritants. A cough producing clear sputum, consisting primarily of watery mucus, suggests an upper airway irritation. *Purulent* sputum, containing pus, or opaque sputum is a sign of lower respiratory infection.[4,5] See Algorithm 7-2 for clinical decision making related to cough.

Hemoptysis

Hemoptysis is the coughing up of blood or blood-stained sputum (mucus from the respiratory tract). This is a sign of injury or illness involving the trachea, larynx, bronchi or lungs and requires prompt medical attention.[4-6]

Cyanosis

Cyanosis is a bluish tint in the fingernails, lips, face, and mucous membranes that occurs when oxygen saturation in arterial blood decreases below 85%.[3,4] Sudden onset of cyanosis indicates hypoxemia and is a medical emergency.

Wheezing

Wheezing produces a high-pitched, whistling sound when air moves through narrowed or constricted airways. Although wheezing can occur during both inhalation and exhalation, it is more common during exhalation. Wheezing during inhalation and exhalation suggests a more serious airway obstruction than wheezing during exhalation only. Wheezing is a common sign associated with asthma.

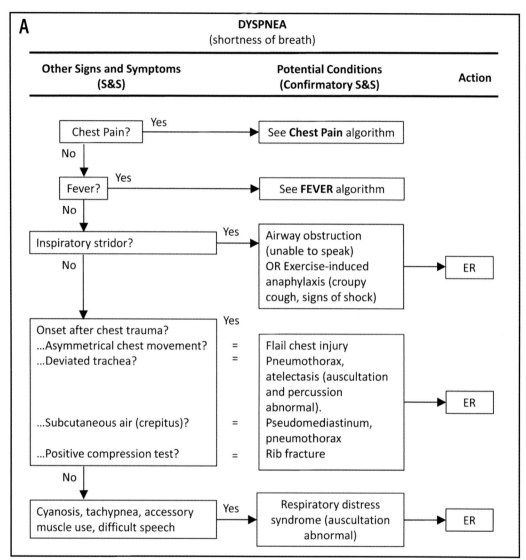

Algorithm 7-1. (A) *(continued)*

Chest Pain or Tightness

Although chest pain is most commonly associated with cardiovascular pathology, individuals experiencing a respiratory disorder will also complain of chest pain or tightness.

PAIN PATTERNS

Pain from pathology in the pulmonary system rarely occurs without accompanying signs and symptoms, including coughing, wheezing, sore throat, and dyspnea. Pulmonary structures can refer pain to the chest, neck, and shoulders, as seen in Figure 7-3.

Lung

Tumors in the apex of the lung (Pancoast tumor) may compress the brachial plexus and vascular structures, causing pain and vascular symptoms (numbness, pallor, cramping) in the ipsilateral

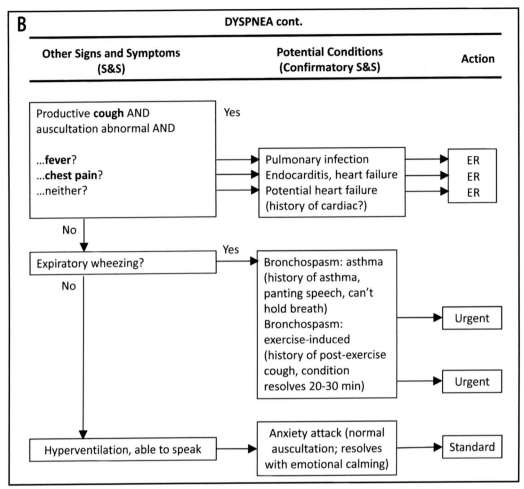

Algorithm 7-1. (B)

upper extremity. Tumors can also compress the bronchi, causing cough, dyspnea, or chest pain. Lung tissue usually does not produce pain until inflammation affects the parietal pleura.[7]

Tracheobronchial

The trachea and proximal bronchial tree will refer pain to the overlying cutaneous areas.

Diaphragm

Diaphragmatic pain usually refers to the ipsilateral shoulder but may also occur in the neck, ribs, or spine.[6] Abdominal hemorrhage is characterized by a similar pain referral pattern, resulting from irritation of the central diaphragm (see Chapter 8).

Pleurisy

Pleural pain, or *pleurisy*, results from inflammation of the parietal pleura. Inflamed pleura creates sharp, stabbing pain over the affected area that worsens with coughing or deep inspiration.[4,6,7] Pleurisy can occur with trauma, infection, tumors, or pulmonary disease.

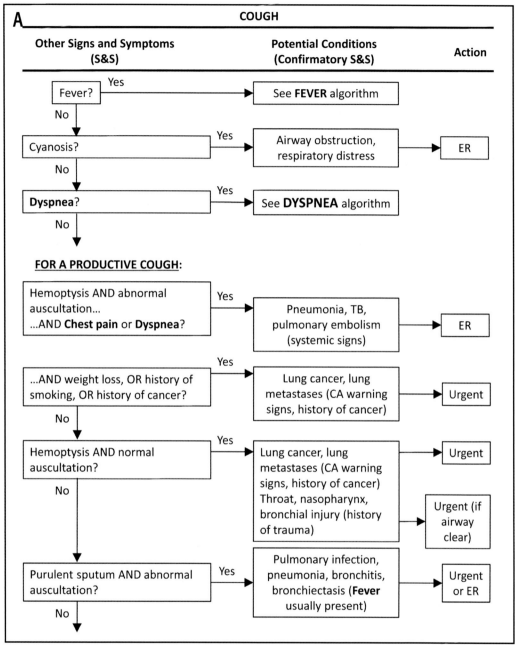

Algorithm 7-2. (A) *(continued)*

MEDICAL HISTORY AND PHYSICAL EXAMINATION PROCEDURES

Family and Personal History

Cigarette smoking is a strong risk factor for virtually all acquired pulmonary disorders. A careful history can reveal a previously undetected chronic pulmonary disorder (intermittent symptoms with respiration, coughing, or wheezing) or infection (fever, recent infection, fatigue). Personal

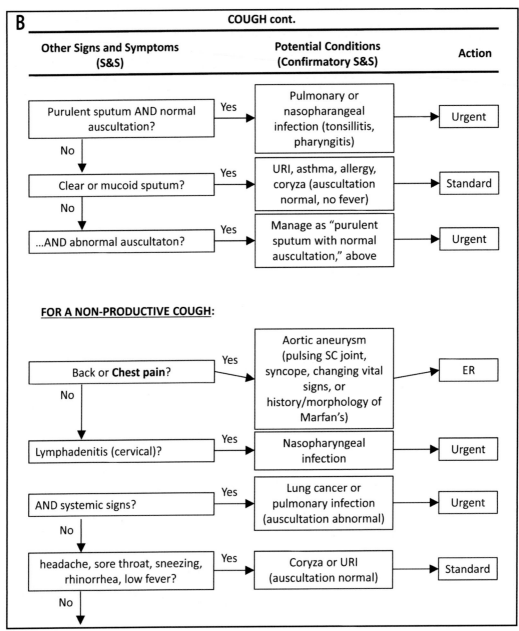

Algorithm 7-2. (B) (continued)

history questions should include information on allergies. Injury history that includes blunt trauma to the chest or sudden deceleration, particularly when accompanied by dyspnea, suggests a pneumothorax or other lung injury.[8]

Dyspnea, cough, chest tightness, wheezing, and decreased capacity for exercise (because of impairment of gas exchange) are common pulmonary symptoms. These symptoms may change with physical activity, deep breaths, speaking, or laughing.[9-11]

Inspection

Visual inspection of the patient during the history portion of the examination can reveal valuable clues related to a possible respiratory condition. Signs of potential respiratory pathology

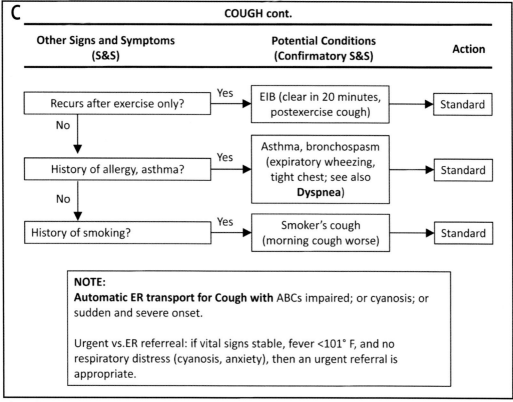

Algorithm 7-2. (C)

can include tachypnea, cyanosis, abnormal breathing patterns, or the use of accessory respiratory muscles. The rib cage and spinal column should be visually inspected for obvious deformities or asymmetries that affect inspiration, such as pectus excavatum (Figure 7-4A), pectus carinatum (Figure 7-4B), scoliosis, or displaced rib fractures. Obesity can also restrict rib cage expansion and diaphragm contraction, thus hindering breathing.[5] The rib cage should move symmetrically during inspiration and expiration. Any abnormal breathing patterns (eg, Cheyne-Stokes respiration, Kussmaul's respirations) should also be noted. The Cheyne-Stokes breathing pattern present as alternating patterns of hypernea and apnea and are associated with brain injury, heart failure, renal failure, and drug-induced respiratory depression.[12] The Kussmaul breathing pattern occurs secondary to metabolic acidosis and presents as deep breathing, with either a rapid or slow, gasping rate.[12]

Palpation

With the patient in a sitting or supine position, the mechanics of breathing can be evaluated by palpating the motion of the rib cage. Bilateral palpation should be conducted at the superior, anterior, inferior, and posterior aspects of the rib cage. With normal inspiration, the rib cage moves symmetrically and the ribs and abdomen rise together. Examples of abnormal patterns include the following: the abdomen rising first; no movement of the rib cage; excessive use of accessory breathing muscles (sternocleidomastoid, abdominals, levator scapula, trapezius, pectoralis major and minor, serratus anterior); or asymmetrical expansion or contraction of the rib cage.[6] Palpation can also reveal *crepitus*, a subcutaneous grinding sensation, which indicates air leaking into the subcutaneous tissues, or *fremitus*, a subtle vibration with breathing, suggesting pulmonary or pleural edema.[8]

Any areas of reported pain or tenderness should also be palpated. If a fracture is suspected, the ribs should be palpated for point tenderness, deformity, or crepitus. The rib compression test can be

Figure 7-3. Pain patterns of pulmonary structures.

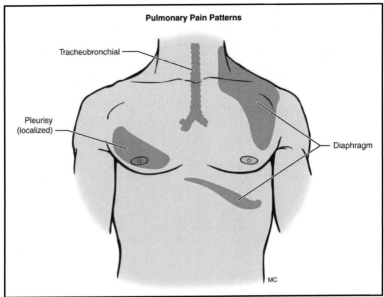

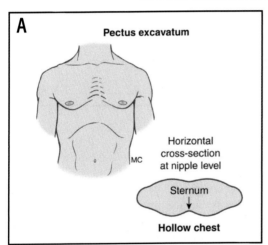

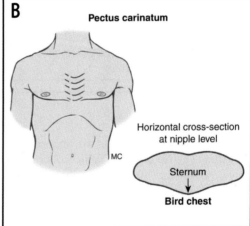

Figure 7-4. (A) Pectus excavatum. (B) Pectus carinatum.

used to assess for possible rib fracture. If pain is produced with anteroposterior compression of the thorax, a lateral rib fracture should be suspected (Figure 7-5A). Conversely, pain produced by lateral compression of the thorax suggests an anterior or posterior rib fracture (Figure 7-5B).

Respiration Rate and Depth

Breathing patterns are described by rate, depth, effort, and regularity. Normal breathing in adults is 12 to 20 breaths per minute, shallow, relatively effortless, and regular. Adolescents' (12 to 18 years) and children's (6 to 12 years) breathing is more rapid (ranging from 12 to 30 breaths per minute). Changes in any of these parameters may suggest pulmonary impairment.

The relative length of inspiration and expiration is one to one; both phases last about the same amount of time.[2] In people with obstructive pulmonary disorders, such as asthma, the expiration phase is significantly longer than inspiration.[5]

An increased rate (over 20 breaths per minute) or depth (over 750 mL) of ventilation is called *hyperpnea*. An increase in breathing rate without an increase in depth, known as *hyperventilation*, rapidly decreases the partial pressure of carbon dioxide in the blood and increases pH, producing a

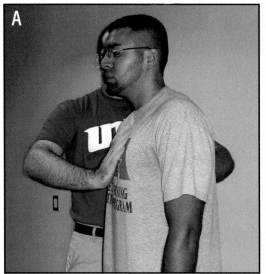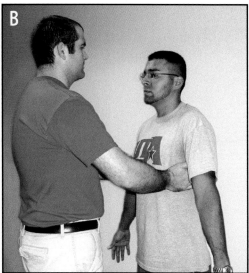

Figure 7-5. (A) Anterior compression test for a lateral rib fracture. (B) Lateral compression test for an anterior or posterior rib fracture.

state called respiratory alkalosis. Hyperventilation can be triggered by acidosis, in which the blood pH has increased due to a metabolic disorder, such as diabetes mellitus (see Chapter 9), or various psychological states, such as anxiety or panic.

Hyperpnea associated with metabolic acidosis is a medical emergency; psychogenic hyperventilation is not. Having a person hold their breath can discern metabolic hyperpnea from hyperventilation. Individuals with metabolic hyperpnea have difficulty holding their breath because that worsens their hypoxemia. In addition, other pulmonary signs, such as cyanosis and chest pain, are usually present. Psychogenic hyperventilation improves when the breath is held because it allows the carbon dioxide concentration and pH to return to normal.

Heart Rate

See Chapter 6. In general, the heart rate and respiration rate both increase and decrease together. Thus, a pulmonary condition that increases respiration rate will usually also increase the heart rate.

Blood Pressure

See Chapter 6. As the amount of oxygen in the blood decreases, the blood pressure increases to maintain the delivery of oxygen to the tissues.

Percussion

Percussion plays an important part in the evaluation of pulmonary pathology, particularly those conditions caused by physical trauma. The skill of percussion requires practice not just with the technique, but also in listening for and identifying the different types of normal and abnormal sounds. Percussion can help identify tissues as fluid filled, air filled, or solid. When possible, athletic trainers should include percussion in their clinical examination of pulmonary conditions. However, because of the crowd noise associated with many sporting events, it may not be feasible to perform percussion as part of a sideline examination.

When performing pulmonary percussion, the right-handed examiner should hyperextend the third finger of the left hand (hand positions would be reversed for a left-handed examiner). The volar surface of the distal interphalangeal (DIP) joint is then placed on the surface to be percussed. The rest of the third finger, as well as all of the remaining fingers, should not touch the patient

Figure 7-6. Hand posture for pulmonary percussion.

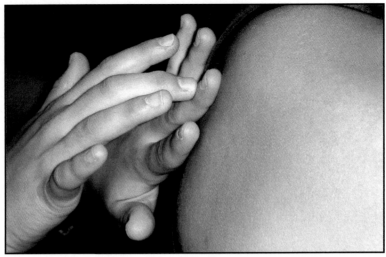

(Figure 7-6). The third finger of the examiner's right hand is used to apply the percussing blows. Position the right wrist in slight hyperextension, with the third finger flexed at the metacarpopha-langeal and proximal interphalangeal joints. The tip of the third finger should be used to strike the DIP joint of the left hand. Striking with the pad of the finger is incorrect and will dampen the sound. The percussing blow should be performed with a quick tapping motion. The technique can be prac-ticed on a variety of surfaces that can provide examples of normal and abnormal sounds. Percussing the anterior thigh will produce a flat or dull sound, which might equate to the sounds produced by pleural effusion. Percussing your own puffed out cheek will produce a hollow, tympanic sound that might equate to the sounds heard when percussing over a pneumothorax (collapsed lung). If you feel as though you cannot hear the percussion sounds well and need to "turn up the volume," press more firmly with the DIP surface of the left hand rather than striking harder with the right hand.

When percussing the thorax and lungs, the examiner should follow the numbered percussion sites illustrated in Figure 7-7, tapping at least twice at each site. It is important to alternate between contralateral, matched sites to compare percussion sounds.[5]

Hyperresonance, percussion creating a sound like a tympanic drum, indicates an abnormal air space in the thorax, as occurs with pneumothorax.[8] Pulmonary edema, pleural edema, and hemo-thorax produces a dull thud rather than the normal hollow sound over the lungs.[5] Areas of the thorax that do not sound normal to percussion should be auscultated.[5]

Auscultation

Auscultation of the lungs provides valuable information regarding the flow of air through the respiratory system. When auscultating the lungs, the examiner should follow the same pat-tern as that used for percussion (see Figure 7-7). Also, as with percussion, auscultation should be performed alternating between contralateral, matched sites.[5,13] The diaphragm of the stethoscope should be placed firmly against the skin, with the examiner listening to at least one full breath at each site. Instruct the patient to take deep breaths with the mouth open. If the patient begins to feel lightheaded or dizzy from the continuous deep breathing, have them take a short break before completing the exam.

When listening to breath sounds, it is important to note the sound's pitch and intensity, as well as the duration or length of the inspiratory and expiratory phases of breathing. There are 3 main types of normal breath sounds: vesicular, bronchial, and bronchovesicular. The *vesicular* breath sounds, described as "swooshing" sounds, can be heard over most of the anterior and posterior thorax (Figure 7-8), and are characterized by a low pitch, soft intensity, and a longer inspiration phase.[14,15] Normal *bronchial* breath sounds can be heard over the trachea (see Figure 7-8A) and sound hollow

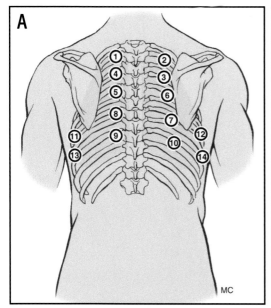 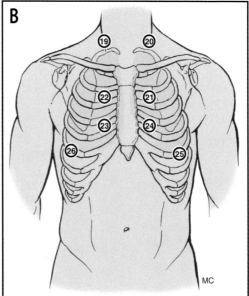

Figure 7-7. (A) Pattern of pulmonary percussion and auscultation: posterior. (B) Pattern of pulmonary percussion and auscultation: anterior.

or like wind rushing through a metallic tube or pipe. They have a higher pitch, louder intensity, and longer expiratory phase.[15,16] *Bronchovesicular* breath sounds are detectable within the first and second intercostal spaces anteriorly and between the scapulae posteriorly (see Figure 7-8).[16] The inspiratory and expiratory phases of bronchovesicular breath sounds are fairly equal in duration, with intensity and pitch between that of vesicular and bronchial sounds.[16] Bronchovesicular sounds are similar to vesicular sounds on inspiration and bronchial sounds on expiration.[5] Normal breath sounds, when heard outside their normal anatomical regions, are considered abnormal.[5]

Clearly heard spoken sounds (*bronchophony*), whispered sounds (*whispered pectoriloquy*), or high-pitched but intelligible spoken sounds (*egophony*) with auscultation are all abnormal.[5] These conditions occur when the lung and pleura are so inflamed and filled with exudate that they become "consolidated"—dense and solid rather than spongy and aerated—which means they can no longer exchange gases.

Inflammation of the pleura, obstruction of a bronchus, atelectasis, and pneumothorax can all cause "decreased breath sounds," in which the normal breath sounds are less audible or absent.[5,6] A complete absence of the normal breath sounds is, of course, also abnormal and warrants emergency referral.

Adventitious sounds are heard in addition to, or superimposed over, normal breath sounds and can include crackles, rhonchi, stridor, wheezes, and pulmonary friction rub.[5] Table 7-1 provides a summary of the adventitious sounds and their associated pathology. There are 2 types of *crackles*: fine (high-pitched) and course (low-pitched). When present, crackles are heard during inspiration and sounds similar to "crinkling plastic wrap."[17] This sound can be simulated by rubbing strands of hair between 2 fingers near your ear.[16,17] *Rhonchi* are low-pitched, continuous, rumbling sounds auscultated during either inspiration or expiration, although they tend to be more predominant during expiration.[16,17] The sound produced by rhonchi has been described as a "hoarse moan" or "deep snore"[16] and indicates an incomplete obstruction of bronchi or lower trachea producing turbulent air.[5,6] *Stridor* is a high-pitched, raspy sound that is audible on inspiration, often even without a stethoscope. Stridor is caused by a sudden and nearly complete obstruction of the airway by a foreign object or inflammation.[5] Stridor is a medical emergency. Stridor that occurs with coughing is called *croup*.[4] A pleural "*friction rub*" can be auscultated when the visceral and parietal pleura

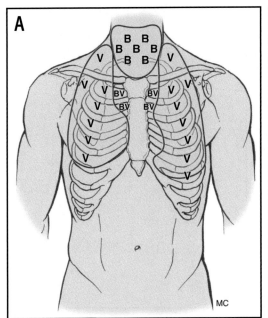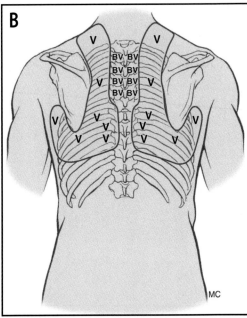

Figure 7-8. (A) Location of breath sounds: anterior. (B) Location of breath sounds: posterior. B = bronchial; BV = bronchovesicular; V = vesicular.

become inflamed. A friction rub sounds like a creaking or a clicking at the end of inspiration and is most commonly auscultated over the posterior and lateral thorax.[5] The sound produced by friction rubs has also been described as "skin rubbing against wet leather."[17] In addition, pain from the inflamed pleura may cause the person to pause during inspiration and expiration.

Pulse Oximetry

A *pulse oximeter* can be used to monitor a patient's respiratory function by measuring the oxygen saturation in peripheral blood vessels (SpO_2). The SpO_2 is the percentage of hemoglobin that is saturated with oxygen. The pulse oximeter uses a clothespin-like design to attach a probe and sensor to opposite sides of a fingertip (Figure 7-9). The probe emits 2 lights with different wavelengths: red and infrared. The sensor, which is positioned opposite of the probe, detects the amount of red and infrared light that passes through the capillary bed. Oxygenated hemoglobin and deoxygenated hemoglobin absorb the 2 lights differently, which allows the sensor microprocessor within the oximeter to calculate a percentage of oxygen saturation.[18]

Most fingertip pulse oximeters provide both pulse and SpO_2 values. To ensure accuracy of the measurements, the pulse reading from the oximeter should be compared to a manual assessment of the radial pulse.[19] If the 2 pulse values do not match, the oximeter should be repositioned on the fingertip. Table 7-2 provides a summary of the steps to be followed when using a pulse oximeter to measure oxygen saturation. Oxygen saturation levels of 95% or greater are considered normal. SpO_2 levels less than 90% would indicate the need for supplemental oxygen.

Peak Expiratory Flow Rate

Peak expiratory flow rate (PEFR) is the volume of air that can be exhaled in one breath. PEFR is typically measured in liters per minute (L/min) and provides an indicator of airway function. A hand-held spirometer or *peak flow meter* can be used to measure PEFR and, in turn, monitor airway function (Figure 7-10). Peak flow meters are commonly used in the assessment and management

Table 7-1. Summary of Adventitious Breath Sounds

ADVENTITIOUS SOUND	DESCRIPTION OF SOUND	DURATION	PATHOLOGY
Crackles	Sounds like "crinkling plastic wrap" or "rubbing strands of hair between 2 fingers near the ear"	Inspiration	Atelectasis; pulmonary edema, pulmonary fibrosis
Rhonchi	"Snoring" sound	Inspiration or expiration; more predominant with expiration	Chronic bronchitis
Stridor	High-pitched, raspy	Inspiration	Life-threatening airway obstruction
Wheezes	High-pitched, whistling sound	Inspiration or expiration	Narrowed airways; asthma (predominantly expiration)
Friction rub	Creaking; "rubbing two pieces of leather together"	End of inspiration	Pleural inflammation; pleurisy

of asthma patients. Table 7-3 outlines the steps to follow when instructing a patient to use a peak flow meter.

Once a baseline PEFR measure is established (best of 3 attempts), PEFR measures can be taken and compared to baseline each day immediately before physical activity. For people with moderate to severe asthma, a PEFR less than 80% of personal best indicates an impending acute bronchospasm or asthma attack.[20-22] Prescribed medication (bronchodilators) may be used to restore PEFR to near baseline value. If the medication does not restore PEFR, as indicated by repeating the test, the person is held out of vigorous physical activity for that day.[21] If PEFR falls below 50% despite taking medication, the person should be transported for emergency medical care.

THERAPEUTIC INTERVENTIONS FOR PULMONARY PATHOLOGY

Injury or illness involving the pulmonary system can significantly affect a patient's ability to maintain normal respirations, which in turn can affect their ability to sustain adequate oxygenation of the body's tissues. There are several therapeutic interventions that athletic trainers can use or assist their patients in using to improve airway function during immediate care of an emergent pulmonary disorder.

Supplemental Oxygen

Several of the injuries and illnesses described later in this chapter involve conditions in which the normal respiratory functions are compromised (eg, acute asthma attack, pneumothorax), which can lead to reduced oxygenation of the tissues in the body. In these emergent situations, administering supplemental oxygen can help improve the oxygen saturation of tissues prior to transport of the patient to an emergency facility.

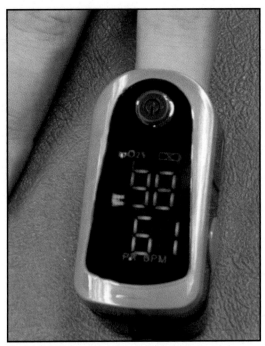

Figure 7-9. Pulse oximeter.

There are 2 sizes of oxygen tanks that are recommended for use in prehospital settings (athletic training room; athletic sideline, field or court): D (360 L) and E (625L). A regulator is attached to the top of the oxygen tank and includes a pressure gauge, a valve to reduce the pressure, and a flow meter (Figure 7-11).[23] Table 7-4 describes the steps that should be followed when administering supplemental oxygen. There are 3 types of delivery devices that can be used when administering supplemental oxygen: the nasal cannula (Figure 7-12A), which delivers low-flow oxygen (2 to 6 L/m); the non-rebreather mask (Figure 7-12B), which delivers high-flow oxygen (10 to 15 L/m); and the bag valve mask, which also delivers high-flow oxygen. Each of these devices delivers a set amount of oxygen, also referred to as the fraction of inspired oxygen or FiO_2. The nasal cannula delivers 25% to 40% of FiO_2, while the non-rebreather mask and bag valve mask deliver 60% to 90% and 100%, respectively.

Administration of Metered Dose Inhaler

Metered Dose Inhalers (MDIs) are used to administer medications directly to the tissues within the airways. Most important, an MDI can be used to administer a β_2 agonist drug (bronchodilator) to reduce the bronchial spasms associated with an acute asthma attack. The procedures for using a β_2 agonist MDI, also referred to as a "rescue inhaler," are described in Table 7-5. Athletic trainers should be familiar with the use of these devices and be able to assist a patient with their use when necessary.

Nebulizer Treatment

Nebulizers can also be used to administer medication to the airway tissues when managing an acute asthma attack. If a nebulizer treatment is included in a patient's asthma action plan, athletic trainers should be able to assemble the unit and assist the patient in the treatment (Table 7-6).

Table 7-2. Steps for Using a Pulse Oximeter to Measure Oxygen Saturation	
STEP 1	Make sure the fingertip to be used is warm and has good circulation.
STEP 2	Remove any dirt or fingernail polish from the finger because this can interfere with accurate measurement.
STEP 3	Place the pulse oximeter securely on the fingertip.
STEP 4	Check that the pulse reading on the oximeter corresponds to a manual assessment of the radial pulse. If not, reposition oximeter on fingertip.
STEP 5	Allow the oximeter to "settle" for 5 minutes.
STEP 6	The oximeter should be repositioned every 1 to 2 hours if being used continuously.

Adapted with permission from Booker R. Pulse oximetry. *Nursing Stand.* 2008;22(30):39-41.

PATHOLOGY AND PATHOGENESIS

Pathology of the pulmonary system can affect the interstitial lung tissue, the wall of the thorax, or the bronchi. Pulmonary pathology may be caused by environmental influences, trauma, genetic factors, or immune responses. Table 7-7 outlines the mechanisms and signs and symptoms of the major pulmonary disorders.

Asthma

Asthma is a chronic inflammatory disease of the airways that is associated with intermittent acute bronchospasms. Airway obstruction results from the combined effects of inflammation, bronchospasm, and swelling within the airways.[22] The National Athletic Trainers' Association has issued a detailed position statement regarding the recognition, evaluation, and management of asthma in athletes, including exercise-induced asthma.[22] Table 7-8 summarizes the recommendations of the National Athletic Trainers' Association position statement.

Asthma affects approximately 25 million people in the United States and 300 million worldwide.[24] Asthma causes epithelial cell damage and fibrous changes in the bronchioles, which can lead to a chronic reduction in airflow.

Clinical signs and symptoms of asthma include dyspnea, coughing, wheezing, chest tightness, prolonged expiration, panting speech, which may also be accompanied by leaning forward to assist breathing, cyanosis, and, in severe cases, seizure.[21] Hyperpnea and tachycardia occur when there is significant obstruction, as breathing becomes increasingly more difficult and hypoxemia increases.[21] Auscultation will reveal decreased breath sounds and expiratory wheezes.

Asthmatic bronchospasm may be precipitated by allergens (see Chapter 4), respiratory infections, cold or dry air, drugs (especially aspirin or nonsteroidal anti-inflammatory drugs [NSAIDs]), and certain emotional states.[10,20,25,26] Goals of asthma treatment include limiting bronchial inflammation, controlling symptoms, preventing exacerbation, maintaining normal pulmonary function, and limiting the side effects of medication.[20,27]

Strategies for the pharmacologic management of asthma focus on the use of anti-inflammatory medications (corticosteroids, mast cell stabilizers, and antileukotrienes) to control the underlying chronic inflammation and provide long-term control and bronchodilators (short-acting β_2-agonists) to provide quick relief from acute bronchospasm.[22,25] Long-acting β_2-agonists are often used in

Figure 7-10. Peak flow meters.

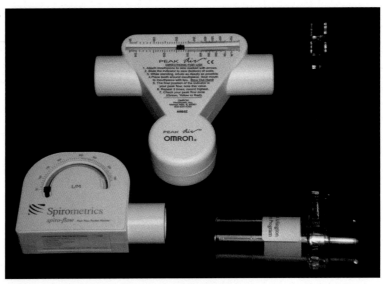

Table 7-3. Steps for Instructing a Patient in the Use of a Peak Flow Meter

STEP 1	Reset dial to zero.
STEP 2	Instruct the patient to take as deep a breath as possible.
STEP 3	Instruct the patient to put the mouthpiece in the mouth and form a tight seal with the lips.
STEP 4	Instruct the patient to blow out as hard and as fast as possible.
STEP 5	Record the peak expiratory flow reading.
STEP 6	Complete a total of 3 trials if establishing baseline. (Baseline is the best of the 3 attempts.)
STEP 7	Calculate functional zones • Green zone (PEFR ≥ 80% of baseline): no restrictions in activity • Yellow zone (PEFR 50% to 80%): modify activity • Red zone (PEFR < 50%): no activity; medical referral

PEFR = peak expiratory flow rate.

combination with a corticosteroid to assist with the long-term control of the chronic inflammation. It is important that patients with asthma and athletic trainers understand the difference between these different types of medication and the role each plays in the overall asthma treatment strategy. While anti-inflammatories should be taken on a daily basis, short-acting bronchodilators should be used on an as-needed basis. Noncompliance with the maintenance medications can lead to more frequent acute attacks and more scarring within the lungs. Likewise, inappropriate use of an anti-inflammatory to treat an acute asthma attack can lead to serious consequences. Confusion between the "rescue" medication (short-acting β_2-agonists) and the long-term management medications (anti-inflammatories and long-acting β_2-agonists) can be compounded when multiple medications are delivered by an inhaler. Athletic trainers should be familiar with the asthma drugs used by their

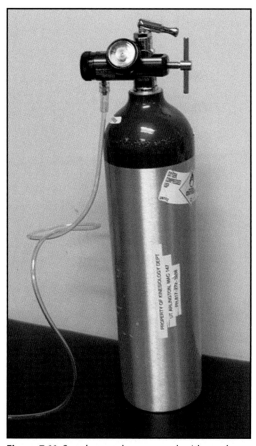

Figure 7-11. Supplemental oxygen tank with regulator.

patients and play an active role in ensuring their proper use. The common asthma drugs and their routes of delivery are discussed more thoroughly in Chapter 3.

Athletic trainers should have a written Asthma Action Plan for each of their patients who has asthma. The plan should be developed by the patient's physician and should outline the plan of care for both long-term management and the treatment strategy for acute asthma attacks. Table 7-9 outlines the components that should be included in a written asthma action plan. The physician's treatment strategy for acute asthma attacks may include administration of a short-acting bronchodilator via MDI and/or nebulizer, as well as administration of a corticosteroid, and possibly supplemental oxygen. The athletic trainer should be familiar with all aspects of the recommended treatment strategy, as well as the criteria for emergency transport.

To manage an acute asthma attack, the patient should be in a seated position (lying down will increase dyspnea), take deep breaths, and exhale through pursed lips, which increases pressure throughout the airway. An attempt should be made to calm the person emotionally. Administration of a short-acting β_2 agonist, if prescribed, is indicated. The onset of action for short-acting β_2 agonists is 5 to 15 minutes and up to 3 doses can be administered during a 1-hour period. Recovery should occur gradually and in less than 1 hour. PEFR measures should be taken before and after doses of asthma medication to monitor improvement in pulmonary function. A pulse oximeter can be used to monitor oxygen saturation during recovery. Administration of supplemental oxygen would be indicated for SpO_2 less than 92%.[28] Severe attacks that do not respond to these measures should be treated as an emergency and transported to the local emergency room.

911

Table 7-4. Steps for Administering Supplemental Oxygen

STEP 1	Assemble the tank and regulator.
STEP 2	Line up the regulator pins with the holes on the tank stem. Hand-tighten the regulator.
STEP 3	Check the tank pressure by turning the valve stem one complete turn. • 2000 psi: 100% full • 1500 psi: 75% full • 1000 psi: 50% full • 500 psi: 25% full (TANK SHOULD BE REFILLED)
STEP 4	Select the appropriate delivery device (eg, non-rebreather mask, nasal cannula, bag valve mask).
STEP 5	Attach the oxygen tubing from the mask or cannula to the regulator.
STEP 6	Adjust the oxygen flow rate to the appropriate setting. • Non-rebreather mask: 10 to 15 l/min • Bag valve mask: 15 l/min • Nasal cannula: 2 to 4 l/min
STEP 7	Apply the mask or cannula to the patient's face and adjust for proper fit.
STEP 8	When terminating the oxygen administration, remove the mask from the patient's face BEFORE turning off the oxygen.
STEP 9	Turn off oxygen.
STEP 10	Relieve the pressure in the regulator.

A severe asthma attack can produce pneumothorax, acute right-sided heart failure, hypoxemia, and metabolic collapse.[21] Signs of pending respiratory failure warrant immediate activation of the emergency action plan.[28] These signs include the use of accessory muscles for breathing, cyanosis, confusion, sweating, and poor air movement.[28]

Exercise-Induced Bronchospasm

Exercise-induced bronchospasm (EIB), which is also known as exercise-induced asthma, is more common than asthma, affecting approximately 15% of the population; 90% of people with asthma and 35% to 40% of people with allergies experience EIB.[10,29-31] EIB occurs 5 or 10 minutes into an exercise session and becomes progressively worse as activity continues. Spontaneous recovery occurs 30 to 60 minutes after stopping exercise.[9-11,29,32] In contrast to asthma, EIB that is not associated with asthma does not produce chronic inflammation in the bronchioles.

Cool or dry air and breathing through the mouth during vigorous exercise have been identified as factors that may exacerbate EIB. Allergens, infection, or pollution have also been identified as potential triggers.[11,29-31] Symptoms include unusual dyspnea and central chest pain or tightness during exercise.[9-11,29] Coughing after strenuous exercise is another common sign of EIB, which may also be accompanied by an ache in the gut. Syncope and cyanosis may appear if air flow into the lungs is significantly obstructed, producing hypoxemia.[9-11,29]

Diagnosis is made by measuring the amount of air that can be moved from the lungs in 1 second before and after exercise on a treadmill or cycle ergometer. EIB is identified if the post-exercise

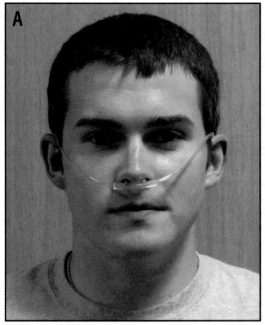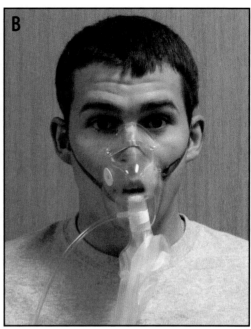

Figure 7-12. (A) Administration of supplemental oxygen with nasal cannula. (B) Administration of supplemental oxygen with non-rebreather mask.

value is more than 15% below the pre-exercise value.[30] Preventive treatment involves control of underlying asthma (if present), preventive medication, and environmental precautions, mainly avoiding cold, dry air during exercise.[9] In addition, a prolonged warm-up (60 minutes before competition, exercise for 10 to 15 minutes at 50% maximal heart rate, rest 15 minutes before beginning full exercise session) induces mild EIB followed by a refractory period during which EIB will not recur.[11,29,32] If control of onset of bronchospasm cannot be obtained, switching sports or exercising in a humid, warm environments may be indicated.[9] Bronchodilators, either oral or inhaled, can effectively control EIB but have undesired side effects for physical activity, such as anxiety, tremor, and tachycardia. In addition, many of these medications are banned by competitive athletic associations.[11,29]

Acute EIB is managed much like an acute asthma attack. The person is removed from exercise, reassured emotionally, evaluated to rule out exercise-induced anaphylaxis (see Chapter 4), and monitored until symptoms resolve. EIB that persists for more than 60 minutes or produces syncope or cyanosis at any time is an emergency.

Upper Respiratory Infections

Several types of viruses produce upper respiratory infections (URIs).[33-37] For example, most common colds (*coryza*) are the result of infection by a rhinovirus.[35,37] URIs produce a common set of signs and symptoms, including rhinitis, rhinorrhea, sore throat, nonproductive cough, sneeze, headache, malaise, chills, low-grade fever, laryngitis, and arthralgia.[26,28,35] The number of coughs, sneezes, and need to blow the nose per day can be used to track progression of an URI because their frequency decreases as recovery occurs.[36] Most cases of URIs last approximately 7 to 10 days, with some persistent symptoms such as cough lasting 3 to 4 weeks.

Ear and sinus infections are 2 complications that may arise from URIs. Acute sinusitis will present with a similar clinical picture to the common cold, often making it difficult to differentiate the 2 infections. Differentiating symptoms of sinusitis can include tooth pain, facial or sinus pressure and pain, nasal congestion or discharge, and foul breath.[39]

Table 7-5. Procedures for Using a Typical Metered Dose Inhaler

STEP 1	Prepare the MDI according to the directions on the container (eg, suspensions must be shaken before use to obtain a consistent dose with each use).
STEP 2	Hold the inhaler upright and tip the head back slightly to facilitate flow of drug into the lungs.
STEP 3	Exhale slowly.
STEP 4	Place the inhaler (or spacer with inhaler attached) in mouth and seal the lips securely around the mouthpiece of the inhaler (or spacer).
STEP 5	Press down on the inhaler to release the medication and at the same time take a slow, deep inhalation.
STEP 6	Hold the breath for about 10 seconds before exhaling.
STEP 7	If another puff is needed of a quick-relief inhaler, wait about 1 minute before taking the second puff. This will give time for the first puff to begin working and may improve the effectiveness of the second puff.
STEP 8	When using a corticosteroid, rinse mouth out with water.

Reproduced with permission from Houglam JE, Harrelson GL. *Principles of Pharmacology for Athletic Trainers*. 2nd ed. Thorofare, NJ: SLACK Incorporated; 2011.

Table 7-6. Procedures for Delivering a Nebulizer Treatment

STEP 1	Assemble the nebulizer according to the manufacturer's instructions.
STEP 2	Carefully pour the appropriate amount of medication into the medicine cup.
STEP 3	Attach the hose and mouthpiece (or mask) to the medicine cup.
STEP 4	Turn on the nebulizer.
STEP 5	Instruct the patient to put the mouthpiece in the mouth and form tight seal with lips (or place mask over mouth and nose, forming a tight seal against the face).
STEP 6	Instruct the patient to breathe in and out slowly through the mouth, without removing the mouthpiece from the mouth (or mask from the face). Patient should continue this breathing pattern until the medication is completely gone (about 15 to 20 minutes).
STEP 7	Turn off nebulizer.
STEP 8	Rinse the medicine cup and mouthpiece (or mask) with warm water and let air dry.
STEP 9	Instruct the patient to rinse out the mouth to remove any medication residue.
STEP 10	Disassemble nebulizer for storage.

Table 7-7. Types of Major Pulmonary Pathology

PATHOLOGY	MECHANISM	SIGNS AND SYMPTOMS
Atelectasis	Bronchial obstruction	Dyspnea, cough, hemoptysis, diminished breath sounds or crackles
Pneumothorax	Puncture of the pleura (as with rib fracture) or sudden increase in lung pressure leading to collapse of the pleural space and retraction of the lung	Acute chest pain, hyperpnea, decreased or absent breath sounds, hyperresonance on percussion, subcutaneous crepitus, contralateral tracheal shift
Asthma	Intermittent bronchospasm, causing bronchial obstruction; swelling within airways; increased mucous production	Anxiety, dyspnea, coughing, wheezing, chest tightness or pain, panting speech, cyanosis
Exercise-induced bronchospasm	Bronchospasm caused by environmental irritants (eg, cold, allergens) and exercise	Dyspnea, coughing, chest tightness or pain, abdominal discomfort
Upper respiratory infections	Viral infection affecting the upper respiratory structures	Rhinitis, rhinorrhea, sore throat, nonproductive cough, sneeze, headache, malaise, chills, low-grade fever, laryngitis, and arthralgia
Influenza	Influenza virus (A, B, C)	
Acute bronchitis	Viral (most common) or bacterial infection of the lower respiratory structures (bronchi, bronchioles, alveoli, lungs)	Fever, cough (may begin as unproductive progressing to productive), sore throat, wheezing
Pneumonia	Bacterial, viral or fungal infection of the lower respiratory structures	Productive cough, dyspnea, pleuritic chest pain, fever, myalgia, malaise, tachypnea, and tachycardia
Chronic obstructive pulmonary disease	Lower airway obstruction caused by mechanical insufficiency, bronchospasm, or inflammation	Cough, dyspnea, barrel chest, signs of chronic illness
Lung cancer	Chronic chemical or mechanical irritation of lung tissue	Cough, weight loss, fatigue, various pulmonary symptoms
Cystic fibrosis	Genetic abnormality of exocrine glands, causing blockage of the airway and intestines	Cough, wasting, signs of pulmonary infection

Table 7-8. Recommendations From the National Athletic Trainers' Association Position Statement Regarding the Management of Asthma in Athletes

During the preparticipation examination, athletes should be screened for asthma.

The athletic trainer should be aware of the signs and symptoms that are suggestive of asthma, including chest tightness, coughing, shortness of breath, wheezing, and limitation of physical activity due to breathing difficulty.

Pulmonary testing may be indicated for athletes with a history of asthma or athletes in whom the diagnosis of asthma cannot be excluded by medical history alone.

An Asthma Action Plan should be incorporated into the overall emergency plan of a sports medicine service.

Athletes who have asthma should have a rescue inhaler available at all times, and the athletic trainer should have access to a nebulizer for emergencies.

Alternate workout sites should be considered when possible to avoid allergens that may trigger an asthma attack.

Patients with asthma should have regular follow-up visits with their physician to monitor and modify the individualized treatment regimen.

Athletic trainers should be familiar with the pharmacological interventions used in the treatment of asthma.

Proper warm-up may provide a refractory period lasting up to 2 hours.

Athletes should be educated about asthma, including the signs and symptoms, potential triggers, proper use of spirometry, pharmacological and non-pharmacological supportive treatments, use of metered dose inhalers and nebulizers, and that asthma need not limit participation in sports and other physical activities.

Athletic trainers should be aware of other medical conditions that may mimic the signs of asthma, including vocal cord dysfunction and other upper respiratory diseases.

Patients with asthma should be encouraged to exercise.

Athletic trainers should be able to differentiate between restricted, banned, and permitted asthma medications relative to participation in organized competitive sports.

URIs are contagious, spreading from person to person through contact with an infected person's respiratory secretions.[35] Hand-to-hand contact after touching the mouth, nose, or eyes appears to be the most efficient mode of transmission.[36] The virus is active for at least 8 days following the initial infection, during which the person may transmit the virus; communicability is highest in the first 72 hours.[36,37] Frequent hand washing and avoidance of persons known to have a URI can prevent its spread. For the most effective hand washing, you should continuously scrub your hands for approximately 20 seconds, or the time it takes to sing one verse of the "Happy Birthday" song.

Recognition of URIs and support of the immune system with rest, fluids, and nutrition can limit the duration of the infection. Antibiotics, which are effective against bacterial infections, usually have no role in the treatment of a viral URI. Over-the-counter medications can be used to treat the symptoms and therefore reduce the individual's discomfort during the course of the infection.

Analgesics such as acetaminophen and ibuprofen are effective in treating the headache and fever associated with URIs. Aspirin should not be used by children and adolescents younger than 18 years because of the risk of developing Reye's syndrome. Although rare, Reye's syndrome has been

Table 7-9. Components of a Written Asthma Action Plan

Physician's name and contact information.

The long-term and quick-relief medications (names and doses) that the patient has been prescribed.

Personal best PEFR value and ranges for green, yellow, and red zones.

Physician's instructions for managing patient's acute asthma attack, to include rescue inhaler (number puffs/dose, time between doses, number of doses), nebulizer, and supplemental oxygen.

Criteria for seeking emergency medical support.

Return-to-participation criteria.

PEFR = peak expiratory flow rate.

reported in children who had viral infections and ingested aspirin. This potentially life-threatening illness is signaled by altered mental status and severe vomiting.

Antihistamines are effective in treating a runny nose and sneezing. Daytime dosing or dosing in individuals who need to remain alert should include loratadine (Claritin), fexofenadine (Allegra), or other second-generation antihistamines (see Chapter 3). Because diphenhydramine (Benadryl) is known to produce drowsiness, it is a better choice for antihistamine bedtime dosing.

An antitussive, like dextromethorphan, can be used to suppress a dry, hacking cough. Sucking on cough drops containing dextromethorphan or menthol can also suppress the cough and provide some anesthetic relief to a sore throat. Codeine and hydrocodone are generally more effective in cough suppression; however, they have a higher potential for dependency and are only available by prescription. Of note, antitussives and expectorants have been shown to be no more effective than placebo for cough.[40]

Decongestants are effective in reducing nasal congestion and are available in oral form, as well as in sprays, inhalers, and drops. Pseudoephedrine is a common oral nasal decongestant and can provide relief within 30 minutes of dosing. Nasal decongestant sprays should be used only for a short period of time (3 to 5 days) because they can result in rebound congestion. Also, some nasal decongestants are banned by certain drug-testing authorities. Also, zinc acetate or gluconate as well as *Lactobacilus casei* has also been shown to reduce symptom duration if started within 3 days of symptom onset.[40]

Because of the multitude of symptoms associated with URIs, many individuals choose a multi-symptom reliever product such as Tylenol Cold and Sinus or NyQuil, which may contain a pain reliever, antihistamine, decongestant, and cough suppressant. The specific antihistamine included in the product determines whether it is better suited for daytime or nighttime dosing (as discussed in Chapter 3). Although these medications are more convenient than taking several different medications, they can be associated with adverse reactions when taken with other medications. For example, taking an NSAID along with a multi-symptom cold product containing ibuprofen can lead to gastric discomfort due to the additive effect of taking 2 NSAIDs. Athletes should be aware that some multi-symptom cold relievers containing decongestants may cause them to fail a drug test. Also of note when treating athletes, athletic trainers should be aware that taking systemic antihistamines and decongestants can contribute to heat-related illnesses.

Athletes who are experiencing symptoms of URI should limit their activities until the fever resolves to avoid fatigue and dehydration and to prevent infecting their teammates.[35,36] Some physicians use the "neck rule" in determining return-to-play in individuals with an URI. Individuals with symptoms above the neck only (eg, runny nose, sore throat) and no fever may return to activity. People with below-the-neck symptoms (eg, cough, body aches) or fever should not exercise until 24 hours after the symptoms are gone.[38,39] If no evidence of cardiac, pulmonary, gastrointestinal, or other systemic involvement appears, full activity can resume within a few days.[33,35,37,41]

Influenza

Influenza, or "flu," is often incorrectly used as a general term for a URI but more correctly describes a disease caused by the influenza virus from the Orthomyxoviridae family. Influenza infections occur annually, usually beginning in the fall, peaking in winter, and lasting into early spring. The influenza virus occurs in 3 recognized strains, called A, B, and C; the A strain is the one most commonly associated with large seasonal outbreaks of flu. The A strain of the influenza virus mutates slightly each year, appearing as variants or strains, rendering vaccination programs only partially effective. As discussed in Chapter 4, vaccination is the injection of deactivated virus antigens, which stimulates antibody formation. The antibodies then recognize the virus on infection and can mount a more effective immune response.

The influenza virus travels from person to person in respiratory secretions that are either inhaled as airborne droplets or picked up by touching contaminated objects. After an *incubation* (time between infection and appearance of symptoms) period of 2 days, fever, myalgia, headache, and upper respiratory symptoms (rhinitis, rhinorrhea, sore throat, sneezing) appear. As infection progresses, a productive cough (ie, with sputum, signifying a lower respiratory infection) develops, as well as pharyngitis, conjunctivitis, and nausea.

The active stage lasts 2 to 3 days, followed by a reduction in fever, diaphoresis, and fatigue (ie, "breaking" fever) that may last several additional days. Secondary infections of the respiratory tract with additional bacteria or viruses may coexist, producing hemoptysis, recurrent fever, purulent sputum, or progressive dyspnea. As mentioned above, aspirin is not recommended for use among children and adolescents with viral infections because of the risk of developing Reye's syndrome.

Treatment for influenza is generally supportive to address the symptoms. The use of an expectorant, such as guaifenesin, can help thin mucus secretions, allowing them to be removed from the respiratory tract by coughing. Nausea is a common side effect reported by some individuals when taking guaifenesin. Maintaining hydration can also help thin mucus secretions. The body's immune response is the primary mechanism by which the infection is addressed. People with weaker immune responses, including young children and older people, cannot fight the viral infection as effectively. As a result, influenza can be fatal in these groups; hospitalization is often required to maintain hydration.

Occasionally, antiviral medications are used prophylactically to prevent the spread of the influenza virus throughout an athletic team or to reduce the duration of the virus when administered at the first sign of symptoms. Amantadine (Symmetrel) and rimantadine (Flumadine) are both effective in preventing and reducing the duration of influenza A. Zahamivir (Relenza) is effective in treating both influenza A and B. Possible side effects associated with these medications include nausea, nervousness, anxiety, lightheadedness, and insomnia.

Return-to-participation criteria for patients recovering from the influenza virus are similar to those used for URIs. Using the neck rule, patients can return to some level of activity once they are fever free and do not have any symptoms below the neck. It should be understood that even well-conditioned athletes will not be able to return directly to the same intensity of workouts that they were participating in prior to their bout with the flu. They will continue to experience fatigue for some time because of the catabolism and energy deficit that occurred during their body's immune response to the invading influenza virus. Return-to-participation will require a gradual increase in intensity and duration.

Lower Respiratory Infections

The lower respiratory system includes the trachea, bronchi, bronchioles, alveoli, and lungs. Lower respiratory infections often occur secondary to infections of the upper respiratory system, and if left untreated, can compromise the normal functioning of the respiratory system. Acute bronchitis and pneumonia, which are the 2 most common lower respiratory infections, are discussed later. While the influenza virus can also involve the structures of the lower respiratory system, it is typically viewed as an upper respiratory infection, which is why it was discussed in the previous section.

Acute Bronchitis

Acute bronchitis is the most common lower respiratory infection.[42] It occurs most frequently a result of an infection or chemical irritant that produces an inflammatory response; viral infection is the most common cause.[31,42] Acute bronchitis is typically preceded by a URI that includes symptoms of nasal congestion, sore throat, myalgias, and malaise.[42,43] Early signs and symptoms include fever, nonproductive cough, sore throat, and musculoskeletal chest pain from violent and persistent coughing. Acute bronchitis progresses to a productive cough, wheezing, and systemic signs of infection, such as fever. Cough suppressants, rest, and hydration are the usual course of treatment; antibiotics should be prescribed only if a bacterial organism is identified.[31] Athletes should consume at least 3 to 4 liters of fluids to maintain hydration and reduce the viscosity of respiratory secretions.[42] Patients who experience wheezing may be prescribed a β_2 agonist inhaler; those whose cough persists may be given an inhaled corticosteroid.[43]

If neglected, the edema and irritation produced by acute bronchitis provide an ideal environment to produce a severe bronchial infection. The chronic cough can also lead to hemoptysis that may appear as blood-tinged sputum.[42] Return-to-participation decisions are made based on the same neck rule discussed above regarding URIs.

Pneumonia

Pneumonia can be bacterial, viral, or fungal; however, the *Streptococcus pneumoniae* bacterium is the most common cause. Signs and symptoms of pneumonia will typically include a productive cough, dyspnea, pleuritic chest pain, fever, myalgia, malaise, tachypnea, and tachycardia.[44,45] Pulmonary auscultation will usually reveal crackles, whereas percussion will produce dullness. Because pneumonia is commonly bacterial in origin, patients suspected of having this lower respiratory infection should be referred to a physician for definitive diagnosis. A chest X-ray will usually show some degree of infiltrates in the lungs (eg, fluid, exudate) with pneumonia. Treatment includes antibiotics, rest, fluids, antipyretics, and analgesics.[45] The use of low-flow supplemental oxygen via a nasal cannula would also be recommended for any patients who present with $SpO_2 < 92\%$. Return-to-participation criteria would be similar to that for acute bronchitis; however, the recovery period would typically be lengthier.

Chronic Obstructive Pulmonary Disease

Chronic obstructive pulmonary disease is a classification for diseases involving partially blocked airways. Examples of Chronic obstructive pulmonary disease include bronchitis, emphysema, and cystic fibrosis.[5,46] Obstruction caused by mechanical insufficiency, bronchospasm, or inflammation traps air in the lower airway, increasing residual volume (the air remaining in the lungs) and decreasing the volume of air exchanged during ventilation, called vital capacity. These effects mean that less fresh air is available for gas exchange. In addition, carbon dioxide concentration increases and oxygen concentration decreases in the lungs, thus decreasing the diffusion gradient for these gases between the alveoli and capillaries and impairing gas exchange.[46]

Chronic bronchitis is caused by prolonged or repeated exposure to irritants that inflame the bronchial mucous membranes. The chronic inflammation decreases the functional diameter of the bronchi and impairs airflow. As the distal bronchioles become completely obstructed, air is trapped in the alveoli. This causes hypoxemia and cyanosis because the trapped air is quickly depleted of oxygen and causes pulmonary hypertension because the hypoxemia causes vasoconstriction of the pulmonary vasculature. Right ventricular hypertrophy develops in response to the pulmonary hypertension (*cor pulmonale*), which in turn leads to the development of peripheral edema as blood return to the heart is impaired.

Wheezing and dyspnea appear, and fever may develop. The cough associated with chronic bronchitis is more productive in the mornings and evenings; the cough is an attempt to clear the airway of mucus and other fluids produced by the inflammation. A cough that is present 3 months per year for 2 consecutive years and accompanied by reduced expiratory capacity with no other medical explanation suggests chronic bronchitis.[46]

Emphysema, a complication of chronic pulmonary disease and prolonged smoking, is not likely to be encountered in physically active people.[46] Emphysema is a chronic inflammatory reaction to chemicals in smoke that destroys the alveolar walls, capillaries, and lung elasticity and decreases the lung area that is available for gas exchange. The signs and symptoms are dyspnea, increased breathing effort, a barrel-chested (hyperinflated) appearance, and signs of infection and cor pulmonale. The lung damage in emphysema is irreversible and prognosis for recovery is poor.

Disorders of the Lung and Thorax

Atelectasis

Atelectasis (pronounced at-uh-LECK-ta-sis) is the collapse of a lung segment's alveoli; it is not itself a disease but rather is a consequence of disease or injury. Atelectasis is usually a result of a complete obstruction by an object or mucus lodged in the bronchi (Figure 7-13).[2] Atelectasis leads to pulmonary hypertension and cor pulmonale and increases risk for development of pneumonia. Patients who are bedridden are most at risk, but lung injury such as a severe blow to the thorax can also cause atelectasis. The signs of atelectasis are dyspnea, cough, and hemoptysis. Auscultation may detect diminished breath sounds or rales in the affected area. Depending on the amount of tissue damage, full recovery or return to sports can take a long time.[47]

Drowning and Near-Drowning

Drowning causes many deaths each year among children, adolescents, and young adults. Water aspiration, when water is inhaled into the lungs, physically damages lung tissue, leading to atelectasis and infection. In addition, a drowning victim may asphyxiate—die from respiratory and ventilatory failure—because of a reflex spasm of the larynx.[48] Among near-drowning survivors, neurological and renal complications are the most obvious and disabling consequences. Time of immersion and temperature of the water determines the extent of tissue damage in these systems.

The inability to breathe underwater causes *anoxia*, a lack of oxygen, which produces severe, irreversible neurological and renal damage within minutes. Cold water temperatures, however, allow for longer immersion because of the mammalian diving reflex, which reduces metabolic demand.[48] A drowning rescue should continue resuscitation efforts until advanced medical care is obtained. While 90% of those rescued while drowning survive, 20% have permanent complications. Rapid, progressive respiratory failure can occur 12 to 24 hours after a near-drowning incident, so all such victims should be transported to a hospital for evaluation and observation.

Flail Chest Injury

A "flail chest" results from multiple anterior or posterior rib fractures, creating a free-floating segment of rib cage (Figure 7-14). The affected region collapses on inspiration and bulges on expiration, referred to as "paradoxical excursion" of the chest. Flail chest injury is a medical emergency and is often accompanied by pneumothorax (collapsed lung).

Pneumothorax, Tension Pneumothorax, and Hemothorax

Pneumothorax, or a "collapsed lung," is the medical term for the presence of air in the pleural space, resulting either from a sudden increase in lung pressure or trauma causing pleural injury,

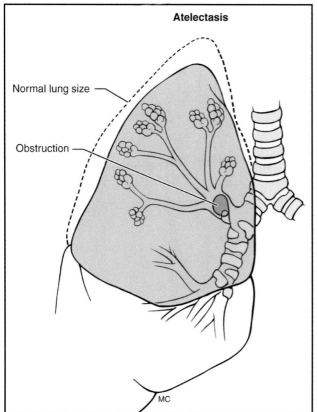

Figure 7-13. Atelectasis.

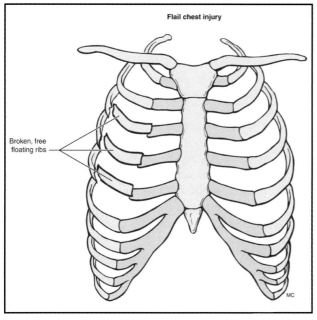

Figure 7-14. Flail chest injury.

Figure 7-15. Pneumothorax.

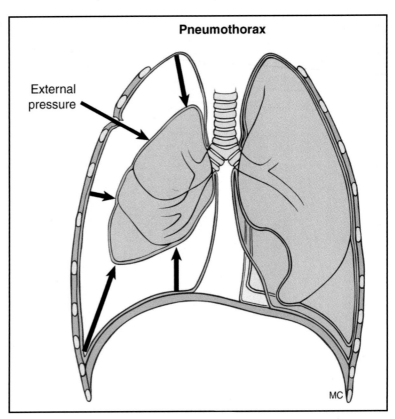

Pneumothorax

External pressure

MC

such as a rib fracture.[2,8,47,49] The negative pressure in the pleural space that holds the lungs inflated is lost, and the lung retracts toward the bronchial tree (Figure 7-15). Without the negative pleural pressure, the lung cannot reinflate when the thorax expands.

Symptoms of pneumothorax include acute pleuritic chest pain and dyspnea. Signs including hyperpnea, decreased or absent breath sounds on auscultation, crepitus (palpable subcutaneous air in the thorax), and hyperresonance on percussion may be noted over the affected lung.[8,47,49] If the pleural space continues to collect air, a *tension pneumothorax* results, in which the intrathoracic pressure increases rapidly with respect to the environment (Figure 7-16). The trachea and mediastinum (the chest compartment that contains the heart and other structures) may deviate to the side opposite the collapsed lung and the thorax may twist asymmetrically.[47] If uncorrected, the pressure from the tension pneumothorax occludes the major vessels and compresses the heart, resulting in death. Treatment requires decompression with a chest tube, inserted surgically through the thorax wall. The tube provides an outlet to relieve the pressure of the air in the thorax.

Suspected pneumothorax is treated by splinting the thorax by hugging a pillow, calming the patient to control coughing or gasping for air, monitoring vital signs, sealing any open wounds with an occlusive dressing, and providing immediate emergency transport.[49] Returning to sports after pneumothorax (not tension pneumothorax or hemothorax) can occur within days of discharge from the hospital, if other injuries (eg, rib fractures) permit.[47]

If blood enters the pleural cavity, the condition is called *hemothorax*. The presence of both blood and air in the thorax is a *hemopneumothorax* (Figure 7-17).[2] The signs and symptoms of hemothorax are similar to pneumothorax, but splashing can sometimes be auscultated in the lower lung lobes with changes in posture. Tension pneumothorax, hemopneumothorax, and pneumothorax with concomitant traumatic injuries require extensive medical care and a longer course of recovery.

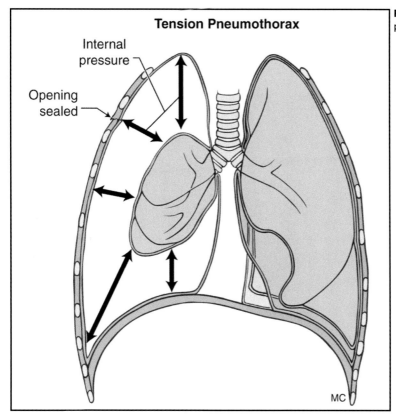

Figure 7-16. Tension pneumothorax.

Pneumomediastinum

Air can also spontaneously leak into the mediastinum, the anatomic space between pulmonary compartments, in a condition referred to as *pneumomediastinum*. Spontaneous pneumomediastinum occurs after a forceful effort that increases pressure in the thorax (eg, Valsalva maneuver, cough, or sneeze).[50,51] Asthma, diabetes, illicit drug use, anorexia nervosa, and pulmonary disorders are significant risk factors for this condition.[50]

Chest pain similar to pneumothorax appears but is localized to the sternum rather than the lateral thorax.[51] Neck pain or difficulty swallowing (*dysphagia*) may also be reported.[6,50] Pneumomediastinum is usually not an emergency, usually resolving within 10 days unless a more serious condition (eg, pulmonary embolism, pneumothorax) is also present. Physical activity can be gradually resumed once there are no symptoms and the condition does not recur.[50]

Lung Cancer

Lung cancer causes more cancer-related deaths in the United States among both sexes than any other type of cancer. In 2013, there were approximately 228,000 new cases of lung cancer diagnosed, and almost 160,000 deaths due to this disease. Lung cancer is associated with smoking; people who smoke are at a much larger risk for lung cancer. Up to 90% of lung cancer occurs in individuals who smoke. Smoking is thus the major risk factor for development of lung cancer.[52] Smoking and use of other tobacco products also greatly increase the risk of oral and throat cancers. Chronic exposure to other chemicals (eg, asbestos, hydrocarbons, polyethlenes) and radiation also increases the risk of lung cancer.[52]

Lung cancer is rarely diagnosed before age 35 years, most frequently occurring among people older than age 45 years. In early stages, pulmonary symptoms may be mild, such as a persistent productive cough, which is so common among people who smoke that it may be ignored.[52] As the

Figure 7-17. Hemopneumothorax.

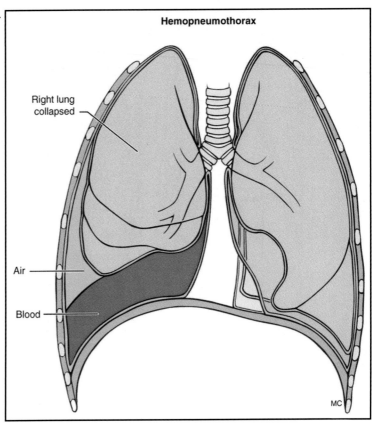

Hemopneumothorax

Right lung collapsed

Air

Blood

MC

lung cancer advances, loss of appetite, weight loss, and fatigue from impaired pulmonary function may occur.[52] Depending on the location of the tumor within the lung, dyspnea, stridor, pneumonia, pleurisy, and hemoptysis may appear. A tumor in the superior lung may grow large enough to impinge on the brachial plexus, causing shoulder and arm pain. Diagnosis is made with chest X-rays and laboratory tests.

Treatment is surgical resection of the affected portion of the lung, radiation therapy, chemotherapy, or a combination of these techniques. Treatment depends on the stage and extent of the tumor. Because of difficult early detection, prognosis is generally poor.[52] Less than 15% of patients survive 5 years after diagnosis. Bony metastases are very common and may cause chest (ribs), neck, or back (vertebrae) pain. The lungs also very commonly develop metastatic tumors from cancer of other organs.[52] Survival for lung cancer is poor. Five-year survival for early-stage lung cancer is less than 50%; for advanced lung cancer, 5-year survival is less than 2%. Certain types of lung cancer (small cell carcinoma) have 5-year survival rates less than 10% even when detected in the earliest stage.

PEDIATRIC CONCERNS

Asthma in Children

Asthma causes a large number of missed school days and is one of the most common chronic illnesses in children. Exposure to respiratory viruses in infancy or childhood has been suggested as a precipitating factor; the first asthma attack may at first appear to be a simple case of coryza (the common cold) before progressing to bronchospasm. Childhood attacks vary in severity but are similar in clinical presentation to adolescent or adult asthma attacks: wheezing, dyspnea, nonproductive cough, and use of accessory breathing muscles. If the attack progresses in severity, cyanosis and tachycardia appear; in extreme cases, wheezing is not heard because the airway is collapsing. A rapid progression may require emergency care. Asthma in children is treated by avoidance of known allergens and medication, similar to patients of other ages.

Cystic Fibrosis

Cystic fibrosis (CF) is the most inherited disorder among White Americans.[9,53] The genetic abnormality affects the exocrine glands, primarily those of the respiratory system, pancreas, and intestines.[53] Thick secretions from these glands block the airway, which tends to become infected.[9,46] Pneumonia, a bacterial pulmonary infection, is recurrent, progressively disabling, and eventually fatal. Blockage of glands also occurs in the pancreas and intestines, producing the respective effects of malnutrition from a lack of pancreatic enzymes to aid digestion and peritonitis from intestinal obstruction followed by rupture. Either effect may also cause death. Only half of those with CF will live to age 30 years.[9,46,53]

Treatment for CF includes nutritional support, regular pulmonary hygiene to clear secretions, and antibiotic medications.[9,46,53] Mild to moderate intensity exercise is recommended to improve aerobic fitness, survival time, and overall function.[9]

Neuromuscular Diseases

Respiratory disability accompanies chronic neuromuscular diseases (see Chapter 13) that affect the respiratory muscles or neural control of breathing.[9] In addition, chest wall deformities, either congenital or acquired, can restrict lung volumes and impair pulmonary function.[9] Deformities of the thorax, such as pectus excavatum, pectus carinatum, and scoliosis, should be referred for medical examination to rule out underlying cardiac or congenital disorders.[9]

Scoliosis

Severe scoliosis, an abnormal curvature in the spinal column, can impair the inflation of one or both lungs, thus decreasing vital capacity and overall pulmonary function. People with scoliosis are not restricted from sports participation unless the curve is progressing rapidly, prohibits trunk movement, or inhibits ventilation to a substantial degree.[9] Sports participation for individuals who have had surgical spinal fixation to correct scoliosis depends on residual pulmonary impairment and the limitations of the surgical hardware or trunk strength and motion.[9] The treating surgeon should provide a release specifying in which sports the person may participate.

Pertussis (Whooping Cough)

Infection with the bacteria *Bordetella pertussis* causes the respiratory infection known as pertussis, or whooping cough. The bacteria release a toxin that impairs the function of the cilia in the respiratory tree. The result is that secretions are not removed from the airway and the patient begins to cough violently in an effort to expel thickened mucus from the bronchial tree. The cough has a long inspiratory phase followed by a sudden violent cough; during inspiration, the narrowed airways produce the characteristic "whooping" sound. Pertussis is highly contagious, with 80% of people in contact with the infected patient themselves becoming infected. *B pertussis* is not carried by a vector but is strictly transmitted from person to person.

Following a relatively asymptomatic incubation phase of 7 to 21 days, the disease has 3 clinical stages. First, the catarrhal stage lasts 1 to 2 weeks and resembles a simple URI, with low-grade fever, sneezing, and coughing. It is during this first stage that the bacteria are most communicable to other people through aerosolization of respiratory secretions. Second, the paroxysmal stage is characterized by the whooping cough, gradually increasing in frequency and severity over 1 week and persisting for 6 to 10 weeks. Third, the convalescent stage heralds recovery, with gradual cessation of the cough over 2 to 3 weeks. Patients are susceptible to recurrence of the whooping-type cough with other respiratory infections for several months after pertussis infection. Fever remains low grade during the 3 clinical stages. Treatment is supportive to maintain hydration and facilitate mucus secretions and usually involves antibiotics. Other children in the patient's family should be isolated from the child who is ill, as should all individuals who have not completed the pertussis vaccination series.

Vaccination programs had decreased the prevalence of pertussis in the 1970s and 1980s in the United States, but since about the year 2000 the disease has again been on the rise. The reasons for this increase are unclear but may be related to inappropriate timing of vaccination. Approximately 12,000 cases per year are currently reported, most among children younger than 4 years of age, although older children and adolescents may also be affected. Older children typically have a less severe clinical presentation, but pose a risk to younger siblings and other children.

SUMMARY

The pulmonary system exchanges oxygen and carbon dioxide between the body and the environment, a process called respiration, by inspiring and expiring air, a process called ventilation. Dyspnea, cough, wheezing, cyanosis, thoracic chest pain, and abnormal breathing patterns are the most common signs and symptoms of pulmonary pathology. Percussion and auscultation are used to evaluate potential pulmonary disorders. Pulmonary pathology can occur as infections in the upper or lower respiratory tract, collapse of the interpleural space, or chronic obstructive conditions. The athletic trainer must be able to recognize, evaluate, and manage common acute and chronic pulmonary conditions in their patients.

CASE STUDY

Sarah, a 20-year-old basketball player who transferred to your school this year, is having difficulty with her in-season conditioning program. During the 3-mile outdoor runs that were added a few weeks ago, she reports that a few minutes into the runs she gets a tightness in her chest that takes her breath away, makes her cough, and keeps her from continuing. About 30 minutes later, she recovers fully and can complete the weight-lifting part of the workout. The conditioning coach thinks she just doesn't want to participate in the runs.

During your medical history, you discover that Sarah's condition is worse in colder weather, she has never been diagnosed with asthma or any other breathing problem, and that the shortness of breath has never caused her to feel like she was going to faint. She does not smoke.

Normal breath sounds are heard on auscultation of her lungs. Heart rate, respiration rate, and blood pressure are all normal (she came to see you before the workout).

Critical Thinking Questions

1. What conditions would you include in your differential diagnosis? Why?
2. What further tests might be needed to confirm or rule out a diagnosis?
3. How would the most likely diagnoses be managed?

REFERENCES

1. National Athletic Trainers' Association. *Athletic Training Education Competencies.* 5th ed. The Commission on Accreditation of Athletic Training Education; 2011.
2. Ganong WF. *Review of Medical Physiology.* 22nd ed. McGraw-Hill Medical; 2005.
3. Dantzker DR, Tobin MJ. Anatomical and physiological considerations. In: Andreoli TE, Carpenter CCJ, Plum F, Smith Jr LH, eds. *Cecil Essentials of Medicine.* 2nd ed. W.B. Saunders Company; 1990:126-135.
4. Loudon RG. Approach to the pulmonary patient. In: Beers MH, Berkow R, eds. *The Merck Manual of Diagnosis and Therapy.* 17th ed. Merck Research Laboratories; 1999:511-521.
5. Arnall D, Ryan M. Screening for pulmonary system disease. In: Boissonnault WG, ed. *Examination in Physical Therapy Practice: Screening for Medical Disease.* 2nd ed. Churchill-Livingstone; 1995:69-100.
6. Dantzker DR, Tobin MJ. Approach to the patient with respiratory disease. In: Andreoli TE, Carpenter CCJ, Plum F, Smith Jr LH, eds. *Cecil Essentials of Medicine.* 2nd ed. W.B. Saunders Company; 1990:124-126.
7. Stopka CB, Zambito KL. Referred visceral pain: what every sports medicine professional needs to know. *Athl Ther Today.* 1999;4:29-36.
8. Kizer KW, MacQuarrie MB. Pulmonary air leaks resulting from outdoor sports: a clinical series and literature review. *Am J Sports Med.* 1999;27(4):517-520.
9. Homnick DN, Marks JH. Exercise and sports in the adolescent with chronic pulmonary disease. *Adolesc Med.* 1998;9(3):467-481.
10. Mellman MF, Podesta L. Common medical problems in sports. *Clin Sports Med.* 1997;16:635-662.
11. Virant FS. Exercise-induced brochospasm: epidemilogy, pathophysiology, and therapy. *Med Sci Sports Exerc.* 1992;24:851-855.
12. Bickley LS, Szilagyi PG. *Bates' Pocket Guide to Physical Examination and History Taking.* 4th ed. Lippincott, Williams & Wilkins; 2004.
13. Bickley LS, Hoekelman RA. *Bates' Guide to Physical Examination and History Taking.* 7th ed. Lippincott, Williams & Wilkins; 1999.
14. Karnath B, Boyars MC. Pulmonary auscultation. *Hosp Physician.* 2002;38:22-26.
15. Kirton CA. Assessing breath sounds. *Nursing.* 1996;26(6):50-51.
16. Visich MA. Knowing what you hear: a guide to assessing breath sounds. *Nursing.* 1981;11:64-79.
17. Lechtzin N. Evaluation of the pulmonary patient. Merck & Co. Inc. The Merck Manual. Available at: http://www.merckmanuals.com/professional/pulmonary_disorders/approach_to_the_pulmonary_patient/evaluation_of_the_pulmonary_patient.html. Accessed May 20, 2013.
18. Ortega R HC, Elterman K, Woo A. Pulse oximetry. *N Engl J Med.* 2011;364:e33-e36.
19. Booker R. Pulse oximetry. *Nursing Stand.* 2008;22(30):39-41.
20. Dishuck J, Harrelson GL, Harrelson L. Educating the asthmatic athlete. *Athl Ther Today.* 2001;6:26-32.
21. Ellis EF. Asthma. In: Beers MH, Berkow R, eds. *The Merck Manual of Diagnosis and Therapy.* 17th ed. Merck Research Laboratories; 1999:556-568.
22. Miller MG, Weiler JM, Baker R, Collins J, D'Alonzo GD. National Athletic Trainers' Association position statement: management of asthma in athletes. *J Athl Train.* 2005;40(3):224-245.
23. Feld F. Airway management. In: Gorse K, Blanc R, Feld F, Radelet M, eds. *Emergency Care in Athletic Training.* F.A. Davis Company; 2010:36-39.
24. Gould BE. *Abnormal immune responses. Pathophysiology for the Health-Related Professions.* W.B. Saunders Company; 1997:22-40.
25. Houglum JE. The basics of asthma therapy for athletes. *Athl Ther Today.* 2001;6:16-21.
26. Spahn JD, Szefler SJ. The etiology and control of bronchial hyperresponsiveness in children. *Curr Opin Pediatr.* 1996;8(6):591-596.
27. Jain P, Golish JA. Clinical management of asthma in the 1990s: current therapy and new directions. *Drugs.* 1996;52(Suppl 6):1-11.
28. Casa DJ, Guskiewicz KM, Anderson SA, et al. National Athletic Trainers' Association position statement: preventing sudden death in sports. *J Athl Train.* 2012;47:96-118.
29. Kyle JM. Exercise-induced pulmonary syndromes. *Sports Med.* 1994;78:413-421.
30. Kovan JR, Mackowiak TJ. Exercise-induced asthma. *Athl Ther Today.* 2001;6:22-25.
31. Pope JS, Koenig SM. Pulmonary disorders in the training room. *Clin Sports Med.* 2005;24:541-564.
32. Nichols AW. Nonorthopedic problems in the aquatic athlete. *Clin Sports Med.* 1999;18:395-411.
33. Brenner IK, Shek PN, Shephard RJ. Infection in athletes. *Sports Med.* 1994;17(2):86-107.
34. Rubenstein CA. Respiratory infections in athletes. *Athl Ther Today.* 2004;9(3):38-39.
35. Sevier TL. Infectious disease in athletes. *Med Clin North Am.* 1994;78(2):389-412.
36. Weidner TG. Upper respiratory illness and sport and exercise. *Int J Sports Med.* 1994;15(1):1-9.
37. Weidner TG, Sevier TL. Sport, exercise, and the common cold. *J Athl Train.* 1996;31:154-159.
38. Hosey RG, Rodenberg RE. Training room management of medical conditions: infectious diseases. *Clin Sports Med.* 2005;24:477-506.

39. Koutures CG. Respiratory infections: practical advice for athletic trainers and therapists. *Athl Ther Today.* 2004;9(3):6-10.
40. DeGeorge KC, Ring DJ, Dalrymple SN. Treatment of the Common Cold. *American Family Physician.* 2019;100(5)281-289.
41. Roberts JA. Viral illnesses and sports performance. *Sports Med.* 1986;3:296-303.
42. Lorenc T, Kernan M. Lower respiratory infections and potential complications in athletes. *Curr Sports Med Rep.* 2006;5(2):80-86.
43. Bartlett JG. Acute bronchitis. Merck & Co. Inc. The Merck Manual. Available at: http://www.merckmanuals.com/professional/pulmonary_disorders/acute_bronchitis/acute_bronchitis.html. Accessed May 30, 2013.
44. Smoot MK, Hosey RG. Pulmonary infections in the athlete. *Curr Sports Med Rep.* 2009;8(2):71-75.
45. Bartlett JG. Community-acquired pneumonia. Merck & Co. Inc. The Merck Manual. Available at: http://www.merckmanuals.com/professional/pulmonary_disorders/pneumonia/community-acquired_pneumonia.html. Accessed May 30, 2013.
46. Dantzker DR, Tobin MJ. Obstructive lung disease. In: Andreoli TE, Carpenter CCJ, Plum F, Smith LH Jr, eds. *Cecil Essentials of Medicine.* 2nd ed. W.B. Saunders Company; 1990:140-147.
47. Amaral JF. Thoracoabdominal injuries in the athlete. *Clin Sports Med.* 1997;16:739-753.
48. Dean NL. Near drowning. In: Beers MH, Berkow R, eds. *The Merck Manual of Diagnosis and Therapy.* 17th ed. Merck Research Laboratories; 1999:2459-2460.
49. Cvengros RD, Lazor JA. Pneumothorax—a medical emergency. *J Athl Train.* 1996;31(2):167-168.
50. Ferro RT, McKeag DB. Neck pain and dyspnea in a swimmer: spontaneous pneumomediastinum presentation and return-to-play considerations. *Phys Sportsmed.* 1999;27(10):67-71.
51. Leiber JD, Phan NT. Pneumomediastinum and subcutaneous emphysema in a synchronized swimmer. *Phys Sportsmed.* 2005;33(8):40-43.
52. Gould BE. *Respiratory disorders. Pathophysiology for the Health-Related Professions.* W.B. Saunders Company; 1997:213-252.
53. Rosenstein BJ. Cystic fibrosis. In: Beers MH, Berkow R, eds. *The Merck Manual of Diagnosis and Therapy.* 17th ed. Merck Research Laboratories; 1999:2366-2371.

ONLINE RESOURCES

Auscultation

◊ **The Auscultation Assistant**
   ¤ www.med.ucla.edu/wilkes/intro.html
◊ **The RALE Repository**
   ¤ www.rale.ca

Pathology

◊ **American Academy of Asthma, Allergy, and Immunology**
   ¤ www.aaaai.org
◊ **American Lung Association**
   ¤ www.lung.org
◊ **National Heart, Lung, and Blood Institute**
   ¤ www.nhlbi.nih.gov

CHAPTER 8

Gastrointestinal and Hepatic-Biliary Systems

CHAPTER OUTLINE AND OBJECTIVES

Introduction

Review of Anatomy, Physiology, and Pathogenesis

◊ Describe basic gastrointestinal and hepatic-biliary anatomy and function.

◊ Review pathophysiological mechanisms of the gastrointestinal and hepatic-biliary systems.

◊ Describe the response of the gastrointestinal and hepatic-biliary systems to exercise.

Signs and Symptoms

◊ Discuss the general signs and symptoms of gastrointestinal and hepatic-biliary pathology.

Pain Patterns

◊ Describe the referred pain patterns associated with gastrointestinal and hepatic-biliary pathology.

Medical History and Physical Examination Procedures

◊ Discuss medical history findings relevant to gastrointestinal and hepatic-biliary pathology.

◊ Describe physical examination tasks relevant to the gastrointestinal and hepatic-biliary systems.

 ¤ Auscultation

 ¤ Percussion

 ¤ Palpation

Pathology and Pathogenesis

◊ Describe the etiology, signs, symptoms, interventions, medical referral guidelines, and, when appropriate, return-to-participation criteria for gastrointestinal infections.

 ¤ Viral Gastroenteritis

Bhojani RA, O'Connor DP, Fincher AL. *Clinical Pathology for Athletic Trainers: Recognizing Systemic Disease, Fourth Edition* (pp 199-233).
© 2022 Taylor & Francis Group.

- ¤ Food Poisoning
- ¤ Traveler's Diarrhea
- ◊ Describe the etiology, signs, symptoms, interventions, medical referral guidelines, and, when appropriate, return-to-participation criteria for criteria for upper gastrointestinal disorders.
  - ¤ Dyspepsia
  - ¤ Gastroesophageal Reflux Disease
  - ¤ Hiatal Hernia
  - ¤ Peptic Ulcer
  - ¤ Gastritis and Gastroenteritis
- ◊ Describe the etiology, signs, symptoms, interventions, medical referral guidelines, and, when appropriate, return-to-participation criteria for criteria for lower gastrointestinal disorders.
  - ¤ Inflammatory Bowel Diseases (Crohn's Disease and Ulcerative Colitis)
  - ¤ Irritable Bowel Syndrome
  - ¤ Appendicitis
  - ¤ Diverticulosis and Diverticulitis
  - ¤ Hernia
  - ¤ Colorectal Cancer
  - ¤ Hemorrhoids
- ◊ Describe the etiology, signs, symptoms, interventions, medical referral guidelines, and, when appropriate, return-to-participation criteria for abdominal trauma.
  - ¤ Spleen Trauma and Splenomegaly
  - ¤ Liver Trauma
- ◊ Describe the etiology, signs, symptoms, interventions, medical referral guidelines, and, when appropriate, return-to-participation criteria for hepatic-biliary diseases.
  - ¤ Hepatitis
  - ¤ Alcoholic Liver Disease and Cirrhosis
  - ¤ Gallstones and Gallbladder Disease
  - ¤ Pancreatitis

Summary

Case Study

- ◊ Develop critical-thinking and clinical decision-making skills.

Online Resources

This chapter addresses the following competencies from the *Athletic Training Education Competencies, Fifth Edition*[1]:

Content Area	Competency #
Prevention and Health Promotion (PHP)	3, 5
Clinical Examination and Diagnosis (CE)	1, 16, 17, 18, 20b, 20i, 21b, 21k, 22
Acute Care of Injury and Illness (AC)	7, 36g, 41
Therapeutic Interventions (TI)	30
Healthcare Administration (HA)	22
Clinical Integration Proficiencies (CIP)	5, 6

INTRODUCTION

Gastrointestinal (GI) symptoms, including nausea, vomiting, abdominal pain, diarrhea, and constipation, are common in athletes and the general population.[2,3] For instance, more than 10% of people are affected by irritable bowel syndrome (IBS) and experience GI symptoms almost daily.[3] Intense or long duration physical activity,[4,5] psychoemotional stress, and environmental factors can all alter the functions and digestive processes of the GI system. Pathological conditions of the liver and gallbladder (hepatic-biliary system), which are both intimately related to the GI system, are also included in this chapter.

Trauma, infection, and disease can affect the organs of the GI system, producing similar signs and symptoms regardless of etiology. Trauma to GI organs and the abdomen are relatively rare in sports but are also difficult to recognize and can have grave consequences.[6,7] Any athlete who sustains significant trauma to the abdomen should be examined and monitored closely.[7,8]

REVIEW OF ANATOMY, PHYSIOLOGY, AND PATHOGENESIS

The structures and organs of the GI system include the mouth, esophagus, stomach, small intestine (duodenum, jejunum, and ileum), large intestine, rectum, and anus (Figure 8-1). Figure 8-2 shows the relative position of the organs by abdominal quadrant. The functions of the upper GI system, from the mouth to the duodenum, are to take in and digest food. The functions of the lower GI system, from the jejunum to the rectum, are to absorb nutrients and water and, eventually, to expel the nondigestible waste products.[9]

Exercise and physical activity have several effects on the GI system.[5] Regular physical activity has been shown to be beneficial in both primary and secondary prevention of many GI disorders.[5] Gastric (stomach) emptying accelerates with the onset of exercise.[3,10] Once exercise intensity reaches about 75% of aerobic capacity, however, gastric emptying slows.[3,10] The general motility of the lower GI system (bowel) is higher in people who engage in regular exercise.[3] During exercise, small intestine motility slows as a result of decreased blood flow and exercise-induced hormone release.[5,10,11] Because gravity assists the passage of food through the GI system, upright physical activity increases bowel motility in persons who have been immobile. Jostling or other movement of the large bowel in the gut that may occur during exercise may cause diarrhea or mild abdominal cramping.[7,10] Proper hydration can prevent many exercise-associated GI symptoms.[3,5]

The liver, gallbladder, and exocrine pancreas each secrete various digestive enzymes into the duodenum at a common location, called the ampulla of Vater. The liver filters the blood on its way back to the heart from the intestines, colon, spleen, and pancreas, allowing the liver to absorb

Figure 8-1. Organs of the upper and lower gastrointestinal system and hepatic-biliary system.

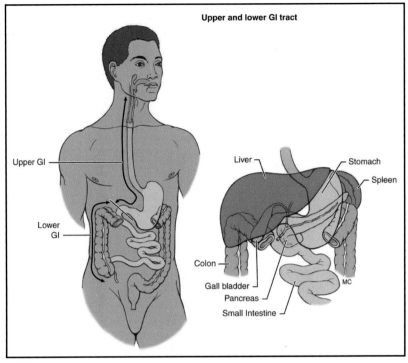

Figure 8-2. Abdominal quadrants and their contents.

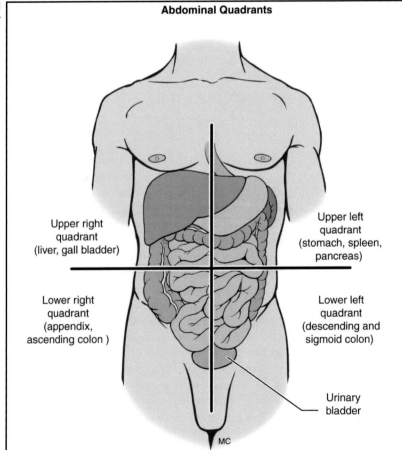

Table 8-1. Signs and Symptoms of Gastrointestinal and Hepatic-Biliary Pathology

Nausea and vomiting	Prandial or postprandial symptoms
Abdominal pain	Change in bowel habits
Abdominal rigidity	Change in stool quality
Loss of appetite	Rectal bleeding
Loss of body weight	Jaundice
Night pain	

nutrients and catabolize toxins. In addition, the liver regulates the metabolism of fats and cholesterol and stores large amounts of carbohydrate. It also forms bile, which contains pigments and salts that emulsify fat as part of the digestive process. Most of the bile salts are recycled through the GI-hepatic circulation, whereas the pigments are excreted in the stool.

Bile flows directly into the duodenum when food is present. Otherwise, it is stored in the gallbladder where it becomes concentrated. Disorders of the biliary (liver and gallbladder) system produce high levels of bilirubin, a yellow pigment, in the blood that leads to *jaundice*, a yellow discoloration of the skin, eyes, and mucosa. These disorders may also impair digestion and absorption of fats if the bile salts are lacking in the small intestine.

The pancreas consists of 2 functional segments. The endocrine pancreas, discussed in Chapter 10, secretes hormones (insulin, glucagon, and somatostatin) that regulate blood carbohydrate levels. The exocrine pancreas secretes several enzymes that are important to digestion of carbohydrates, proteins, and fats. Diseases affecting the exocrine pancreas thus affect digestion.

Signs and Symptoms

Table 8-1 summarizes the signs and symptoms of gastrointestinal and hepatic-biliary pathology.

Nausea and Vomiting

Nausea and vomiting (*emesis*) are hallmark symptoms of upper GI disorders. Nausea and vomiting occur when nerve endings in the upper GI are irritated by chemical, mechanical, or autonomic (vagus nerve) stimuli.[3] Stimulation of upper GI nerve endings reverses peristalsis, pushing partially digested contents back into the stomach. The associated contraction of the abdominal muscles increases intra-abdominal pressure and force the stomach contents up the esophagus and out of the mouth.

When blood appears in vomit, the condition is called *hematemesis*. A person with nose or mouth trauma may inadvertently swallow and then vomit bright red blood. If blood collects or pools for some time in the stomach before being vomited, as occurs with pathological upper GI bleeding, the vomitus has an appearance like coffee grounds. Gastric ulcers, excessive use of nonsteroidal anti-inflammatory drugs (NSAIDs), other drug use or abuse, alcohol abuse, or major systemic illness can produce upper GI bleeding. Rarely, extremely intense exercise can cause acute gastric hemorrhage and hematemesis.[10] See Algorithm 8-1 for clinical decision making related to nausea and vomiting.

Abdominal Pain

The location (ie, which abdominal quadrant; see Figure 8-2), severity, and quality of abdominal pain should be noted during the examination. Description of the pain may aid in discerning

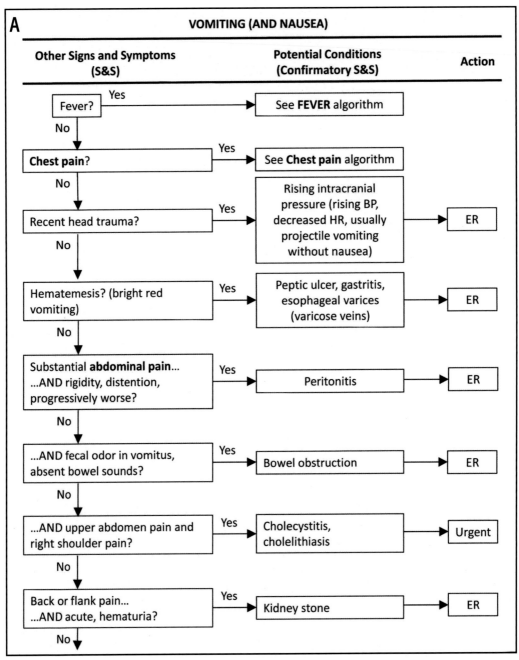

Algorithm 8-1. (A) *(continued)*

the affected structure or likely pathology. Severe, progressive cycles of intense cramping-type pain (called *colic*) are caused by acute inflammation or obstruction in an abdominal organ or duct; the intermittent cramping sensation results from the periodic contractions of these organs.[12] Acute, well-localized constant pain indicates inflammation of the parietal peritoneum (*peritonitis*), which is indicative of problems with the abdominal organs.[12] Mild abdominal cramps usually indicate lower GI disorders.[3] NSAIDs may temporarily eliminate pain of GI origin. See Algorithm 8-2 for clinical decision making related to abdominal pain.

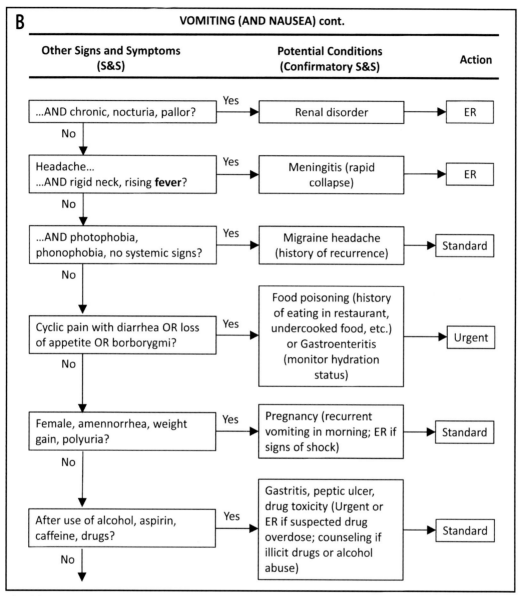

Algorithm 8-1. (B) *(continued)*

Abdominal Rigidity

Protective spasm of the muscles of the abdominal wall caused by pain from injury, internal bleeding, or disease in the organs is called abdominal *rigidity*. Rigidity is detected during palpation as a notable contrast to the normal supple compliance of the abdomen. Rigidity usually occurs in a specific quadrant or localized region rather than the whole abdomen. Significant abdominal pain and difficulty flexing the trunk accompanies rigidity. Abdominal rigidity indicates a significant injury or disease process and requires immediate medical attention.

Loss of Appetite and Significant Loss in Body Weight

Loss of appetite may indicate an upper GI problem.[3] A recent loss of significant body weight suggests poor nutritional absorption, dehydration from recurrent vomiting or diarrhea, or increased

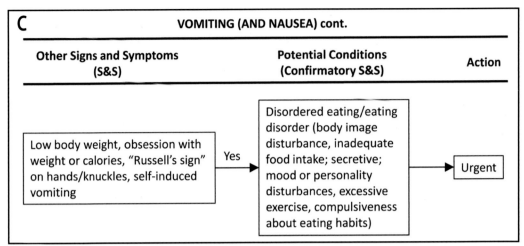

Algorithm 8-1. (C)

metabolic demand from a chronic disease. Infection and cancer also induce both loss of appetite by affecting the satiety center in the medulla oblongata and weight loss by increasing metabolism and creating an energy deficit.[3]

Night Pain

Abdominal pain that wakes a person at night is nearly always a symptom of serious pathology. Night pain is a result of the parasympathetic nervous system, which is more active at night, stimulating the GI organs and producing symptoms as function of the malfunctioning organ increases accordingly.

Prandial or Postprandial Symptoms

Prandial (while eating) and *postprandial* (after eating) symptoms suggest GI or biliary pathology. Stomach-associated pain typically begins about 1 hour after eating, as the food passes into the duodenum. Similarly, duodenal pain occurs 2 hours or more after a meal as food passes into the jejunum. Food usually irritates a gastric ulcer but may relieve a duodenal ulcer. In addition, caffeine, alcohol, and spicy foods may irritate a gastroesophageal reflux or peptic ulcer. Fatty foods may exacerbate gallbladder or pancreas pathology since fat increases demand on those organs.[9]

Change in Bowel Habits or Stool Quality

Changes in the frequency, regularity, or ease of defecation indicate lower GI pathology.[9] Changes in consistency, odor, or color of the stool (feces) are suggestive of disease in the lower GI or biliary systems.[9] Two types of disturbed bowel habits are diarrhea and constipation.

Diarrhea describes frequent or loose bowel movements caused by increased bowel motility, malabsorption syndromes, infection, or a combination of these factors.[13] Diarrhea typically means 3 or more loose stools within a 24-hour period. For example, an infectious agent or other irritant causes the cells in the small intestine and colon to release sodium, potassium, and water into the bowel. The result is a watery stool that moves quickly through the large intestine. Diarrhea can lead to dehydration, electrolyte imbalance, and, in severe cases, shock. Effective treatment involves hydration, electrolyte replacement (usually through sodium-glucose preparations), and medications (bismuth subsalicylate [Pepto Bismol] or loperamide [Imodium]) to reduce bowel output. The "BRAT" diet (bananas, rice, applesauce, and toast) is bland and easy to digest and can also be effective in managing diarrhea.

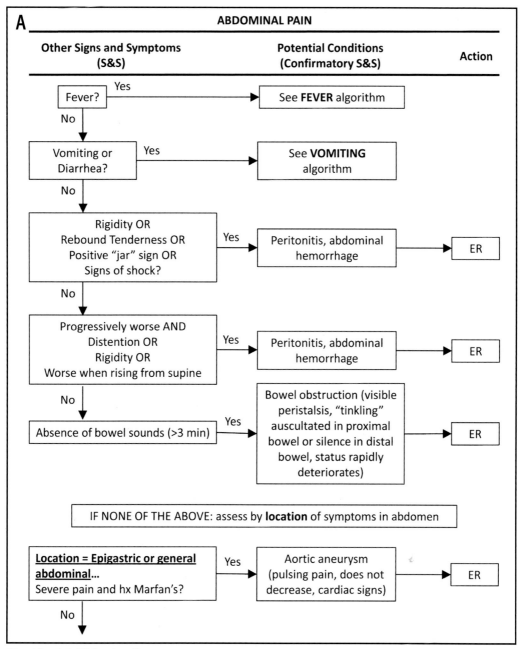

A ABDOMINAL PAIN

Other Signs and Symptoms (S&S)	Potential Conditions (Confirmatory S&S)	Action

Fever? — Yes → See **FEVER** algorithm
No ↓

Vomiting or Diarrhea? — Yes → See **VOMITING** algorithm
No ↓

Rigidity OR Rebound Tenderness OR Positive "jar" sign OR Signs of shock? — Yes → Peritonitis, abdominal hemorrhage → ER
No ↓

Progressively worse AND Distention OR Rigidity OR Worse when rising from supine — Yes → Peritonitis, abdominal hemorrhage → ER
No ↓

Absence of bowel sounds (>3 min) — Yes → Bowel obstruction (visible peristalsis, "tinkling" auscultated in proximal bowel or silence in distal bowel, status rapidly deteriorates) → ER

IF NONE OF THE ABOVE: assess by **location** of symptoms in abdomen

Location = Epigastric or general abdominal... Severe pain and hx Marfan's? — Yes → Aortic aneurysm (pulsing pain, does not decrease, cardiac signs) → ER
No ↓

Algorithm 8-2. (A) *(continued)*

Increased urgency or diarrhea occasionally occurs during or after bouts of vigorous exercise.[2,3,5] Some medications and drugs also can cause temporary diarrhea. Antibiotics, for instance, may allow overproduction of intestinal bacteria, causing colitis and increased intestinal motility. See Algorithm 8-3 for clinical decision making related to diarrhea.

Constipation is the abnormal retention of feces in the bowel as a result of hardened (dehydrated) stool or decreased bowel motility. Poor diet (high-sugar, low-fiber), dehydration, medications (eg, analgesics that decrease bowel motility), stress, inactivity, or GI disease can contribute to constipation. If chronically retained stool becomes impacted and cannot progress through the bowel, the

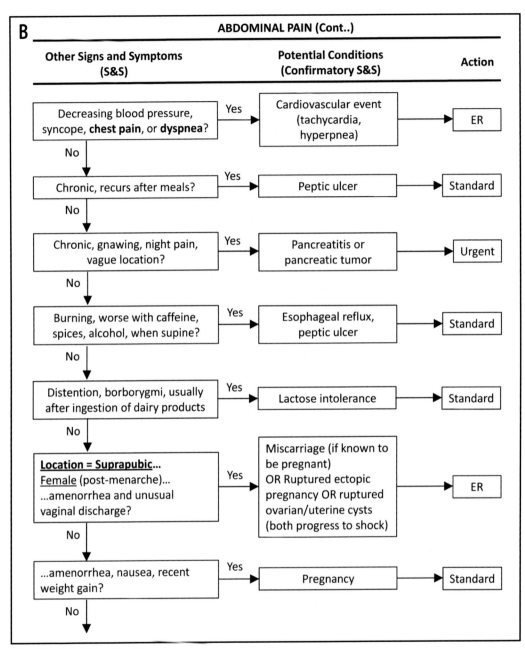

Algorithm 8-2. (B) *(continued)*

resulting bowel obstruction may require emergency surgery. Appropriate lifestyle changes relieve constipation due to a poor diet or inactivity, although laxatives may be needed in more resistant cases.

Rectal Blood

Bleeding from the rectum, either bright red or detected through testing in the feces (*hematochezia*), is a sign of lower GI pathology.[2] Most common causes include hemorrhoids or anal fissures, but a physician should examine the person to rule out IBS, cancer, or parasitic GI infection.[2,10] Black stools with a tar-like consistency, called *melena*, suggests upper GI bleeding. The

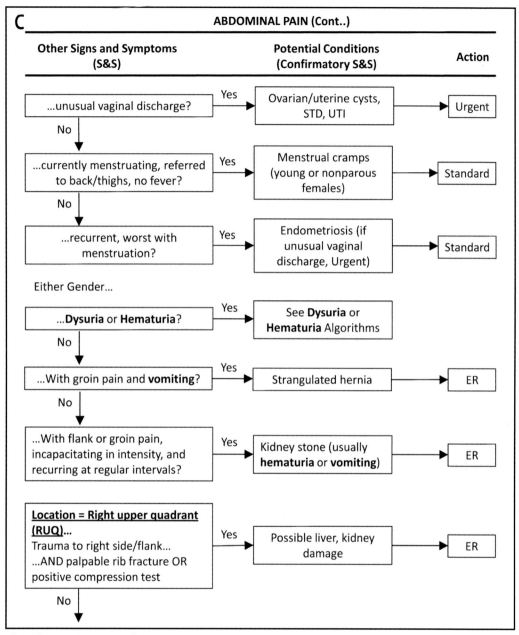

Algorithm 8-2. (C) *(continued)*

blood coagulates as it passes through the lower GI to produce this effect. Some medications can also cause melena, which may be ascertained during the medical history. Of note, other medications such as Pepto-Bismol, may discolor the stool and mimic melena. A high proportion of endurance athletes, particularly runners, have detectable hematochezia following an event or periods of heavy training.[5,11] This occult bleeding may be unnoticed by the athlete, but if it is severe enough it may be accompanied by fatigue, reduced performance, and mild anemia-like symptoms.[5]

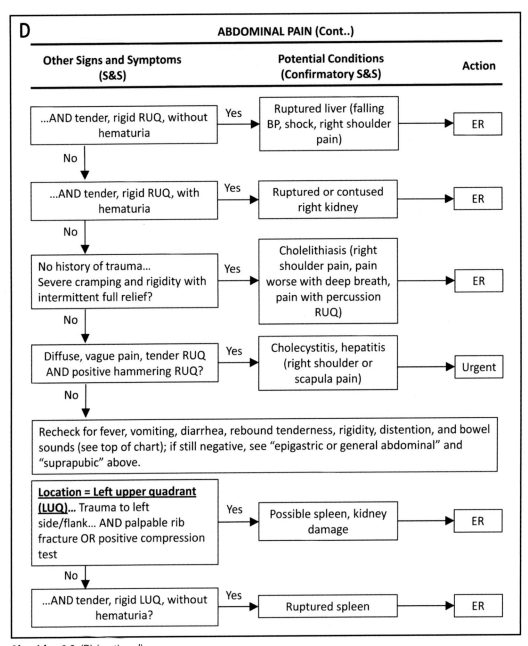

Algorithm 8-2. (D) *(continued)*

Jaundice

Jaundice, or *icterus*, is yellow discoloration of skin, eyes, and mucous membranes that occurs with high bilirubin levels in the blood. Pathology of the liver, gallbladder, exocrine pancreas, or the common bile duct that carries the secretions of these organs causes jaundice.[14] The urine progressively darkens and the stool progressively lightens in color as the kidneys filter the increased circulating bilirubin out of the blood and into the urine while bilirubin concentration decreases in the bowel.

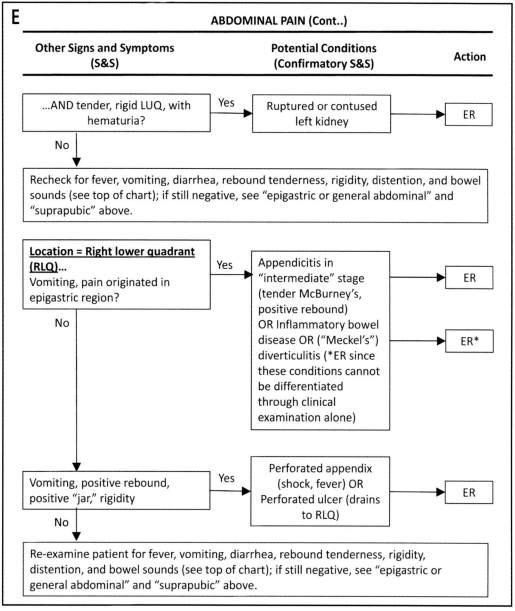

Algorithm 8-2. (E) *(continued)*

PAIN PATTERNS

Upper Gastrointestinal

Referred pain from the upper GI (Figure 8-3A) can be distributed similarly to referred cardiac pain (see Chapter 6), but history and accompanying signs and symptoms usually indicate the system of origin.[3,10] The esophagus causes substernal pain, although occasionally pain is also noted in the epigastric area or radiating to the back.[10] The stomach also produces epigastric pain, but may refer to the back or the left shoulder if the diaphragmatic pleura also becomes irritated.[15]

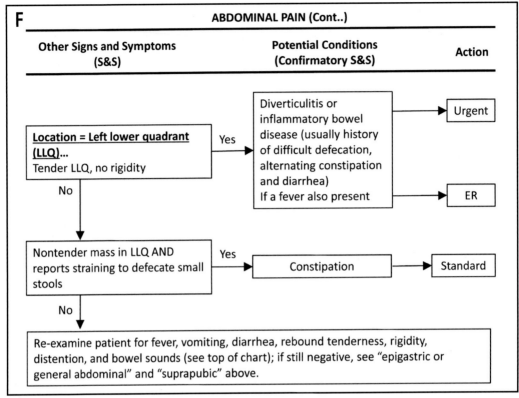

Algorithm 8-2. (F)

Lower Gastrointestinal

Pain from the small and large intestines present diffuse middle to lower abdominal pain (Figure 8-3B).[15] The visceral pain is accompanied by localized peritoneal pain and abdominal rigidity as the condition worsens.

The appendix classically produces midabdominal pain initially that gradually migrates to the right lower quadrant, one-third to one-half the distance from the anterior superior iliac spine toward the umbilicus (*McBurney's point*).[15] Pain from acute appendicitis may also refer to the central abdomen, hip, thigh, or lower back.

Liver

The liver refers pain to the epigastric region and right upper quadrant (RUQ) and can refer pain to the right shoulder, thoracic, or cervical spine if the diaphragm or diaphragmatic pleura become irritated.[15]

Gallbladder

The gallbladder produces a characteristic pattern along the right T8 dermatome, radiating to the right scapula as a sharp, stabbing sensation.[15] Gallbladder pain may be perceived initially as a sensation of "heartburn."

Pancreas

The pancreas produces epigastric pain referring to the middle or lower back. If the diaphragm becomes irritated, pain occurs in the left shoulder.

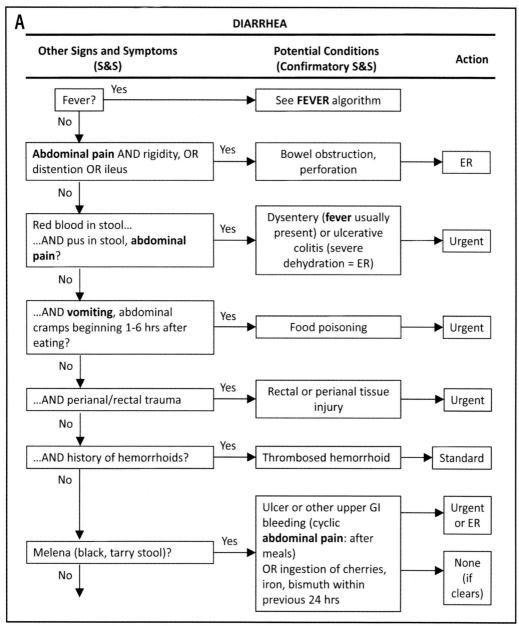

A

DIARRHEA

Other Signs and Symptoms (S&S)		Potential Conditions (Confirmatory S&S)	Action
Fever?	Yes	See **FEVER** algorithm	
Abdominal pain AND rigidity, OR distention OR ileus	Yes	Bowel obstruction, perforation	ER
Red blood in stool… …AND pus in stool, **abdominal pain**?	Yes	Dysentery (**fever** usually present) or ulcerative colitis (severe dehydration = ER)	Urgent
…AND **vomiting**, abdominal cramps beginning 1-6 hrs after eating?	Yes	Food poisoning	Urgent
…AND perianal/rectal trauma	Yes	Rectal or perianal tissue injury	Urgent
…AND history of hemorrhoids?	Yes	Thrombosed hemorrhoid	Standard
Melena (black, tarry stool)?	Yes	Ulcer or other upper GI bleeding (cyclic **abdominal pain**: after meals)	Urgent or ER
		OR ingestion of cherries, iron, bismuth within previous 24 hrs	None (if clears)

Algorithm 8-3. (A) *(continued)*

Spleen

The spleen, an abdominal organ that filters abnormal red blood cells and functions as part of the immune system, refers pain to the upper left quadrant and left shoulder. Referred pain from the spleen to the left shoulder is known as *Kehr's sign.*

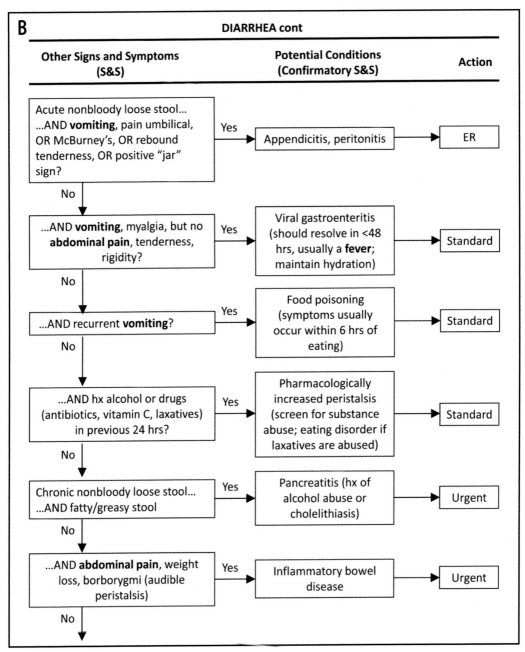

Algorithm 8-3. (B) *(continued)*

MEDICAL HISTORY AND
PHYSICAL EXAMINATION PROCEDURES

Family and Personal History

A complete GI history should be conducted for any person reporting nausea, vomiting, or abdominal pain as a primary complaint.[3] Recent GI illness, change in diet, current exercise or physical activity frequency and duration, and recent travel can be related to the etiology of GI pathology.[2]

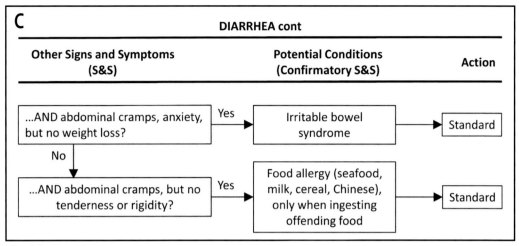

Algorithm 8-3. (C)

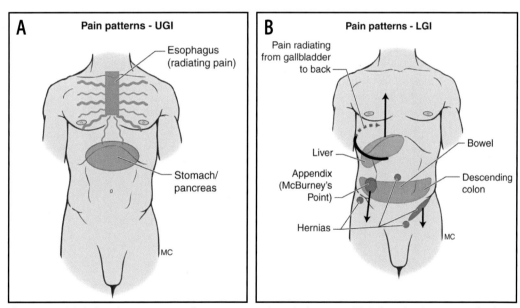

Figure 8-3. (A) Referred pain patterns for upper gastrointestinal system. (B) Referred pain patterns for lower gastrointestinal system.

Childhood diseases, recent surgery, current medications, and history of a similar condition should be ascertained.[12,16] Symptoms produced at night or while eating are usually more serious than postprandial heartburn or exercise-induced indigestion.[3] Regular use of caffeine, alcohol, nicotine, drugs, or medications should be noted.[9]

Direct trauma can damage the organs of the GI and hepatic-biliary systems.[7] Significant injuries to the liver, jejunum, or colon are rare in sports but do occur. Trauma from the end of a blunt instrument (bicycle handlebars, baseball bat) or that produces bruising or rib fractures should raise the index of suspicion for internal organ damage. A sudden deceleration of the thorax can cause the contents of the abdomen to collide with the rib cage and cause injury.[6]

Very recent trauma to the abdomen or thorax may not present signs or symptoms for several hours.[6] Signs and symptoms should be reevaluated at regular intervals for several hours following abdominal trauma.[7] Progressive deterioration of vital signs (shock) and persistent abdominal pain indicate serious injury and require emergency medical care.

Figure 8-4. Hook-lying position for abdominal examination.

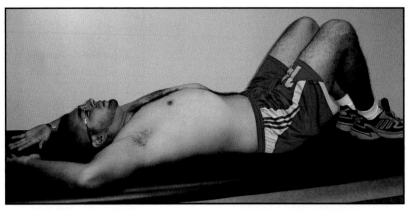

Inspection

An abnormally protruded abdomen indicates *ascites* (excess peritoneal fluid), distended bowels from an obstruction, or excessive gas in the bowels.[12] An asymmetric abdomen is a sign of ascites shifting with gravity, hepatomegaly (right-sided enlargement), or splenomegaly (left-sided enlargement).[9]

Other signs may be observable by close inspection. Small, bulging masses in the lower abdomen may be herniated bowel, particularly if tender or manually reducible. Pulsing in the abdomen may be observed with an aortic or iliac artery aneurysm (see Chapter 6).[12] Jaundice may be noted in the skin or sclera of the eyes. Acute pathology of the abdominal organs can cause severe spasms of the trunk muscles and cause a characteristic flexed or side lying *"fetal" posture*, with both arms wrapped around or crossing the belly.

Examination of the Abdomen

Physical examination of the abdomen should include auscultation, percussion, and palpation.[7,9,12,17] When examining the abdomen, the patient should be placed in a hook-lying position (supine with knees bent and feet flat on the table; Figure 8-4). This position relieves some of the stress on the abdomen that occurs when lying supine. Instructing the patient to raise the arms above the head will also improve examination of the upper abdominal quadrants because it causes the liver and spleen to extend slightly below the rib cage. Auscultation and percussion should be performed before palpation because palpation may disturb the contents of the GI and confound the other tests.

Auscultation should be performed within each quadrant to listen for bowel sounds. Bowel sounds will be heard as tinkling, clicking, or gurgling sounds, with a normal rate of 5 to 35 sounds per minute.[18] It may take up to 1 minute to begin hearing bowel sounds. Infrequent or completely absent bowel sounds may indicate a bowel obstruction or ileus. Other signs and symptoms of bowel obstruction are given in Table 8-2.

Percussion of the abdomen can be performed to identify the approximate borders of the liver and spleen if they extend abnormally below the rib cage. Also, percussion can be used to detect changes in resonance of the abdomen. Internal bleeding within the abdomen can produce a dull thud on percussion in place of the normal hollow sound. The technique for abdominal percussion is similar to that used for pulmonary percussion (see Chapter 7).

Superficial palpation should be performed using the palmar aspect of the fingers (the "finger pads") rather than poking with a single finger (Figure 8-5A). Deep palpation is performed similarly; however, the opposite hand is placed on top of the palpating hand (Figure 8-5B). When palpating the abdomen, the examiner should note any tenderness or palpated rigidity and abnormal masses. The liver and spleen should be palpated slightly below the rib cage in the RUQ and left upper quadrant (LUQ), respectively. Palpation of these structures can often be enhanced by placing one hand

Table 8-2. Signs and Symptoms of Bowel Obstruction

Vomiting	Inability to pass gas	Progressive cramping pain
Diminished bowel sounds	Distended abdomen	Tympanites
Foul breath odor	Systemic signs	

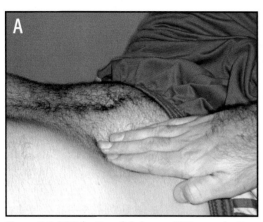 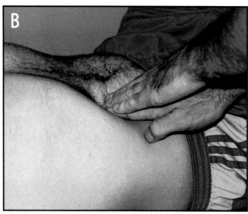

Figure 8-5. (A) Palpation of abdomen. (B) Deep palpation of abdomen.

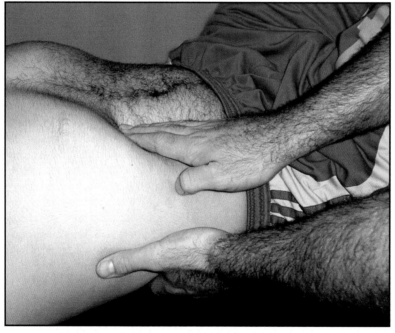

Figure 8-6. Enhancement of abdominal palpation.

underneath the appropriate quadrant and the other hand palpating the organ on top of the quadrant (Figure 8-6).

Differentiating musculoskeletal trauma, such as fractured ribs or strained abdominal muscles, from abdominal organ trauma or pathology can be difficult. If pain during abdominal palpation decreases significantly when the patient contracts their abdominal muscles (by raising the head in supine), injury to the internal organs is likely.[9] The contracted muscles provide a barrier between the organ and the palpating hand, such that the injured organ is not exacerbated by the palpation. In addition, placing the palm of the left hand flat on the quadrants or over specific abdominal organs and striking briskly with the ulnar edge of the right fist, an examination technique called *hammering*, sends a vibration through the abdomen that may increase the pain associated with injured organs.[17]

The test for rebound tenderness involves manually depressing the abdomen, on either the same or opposite side as the symptoms, and then quickly releasing the pressure. Pain produced by this maneuver suggests peritonitis, or inflammation of the peritoneum, the membrane that lines the abdominal cavity.[7,9] Another test for peritonitis is the *"jar" test*, also known as *Markle's sign*.[19] The person rises up on the toes then suddenly drops flatly onto the heels, jarring the body; a sharp increase in abdominal pain is positive for peritonitis.

Following trauma, initial physical examination may not suggest intra-abdominal injury, thus requiring repeated examinations.[7] Almost half of emergency room patients who have abdominal pain initially have a negative physical examination but actually end up having significant abdominal injuries.[3,7] Hence, emergency transportation should occur on the first sign that the condition is worsening after abdominal trauma.

Many GI disorders are associated with severe vomiting and diarrhea, which can lead to dehydration. The clinical detection of dehydration can be made by measuring the blood pressure and heart rate in both supine and standing positions (*orthostatic vital signs*).[18] When moving from a supine to a standing position, it is normal for the systolic blood pressure to decrease by 20 mm Hg and the pulse to increase by 20 bpm. If the systolic blood pressure decreases by more than 20 mm Hg, diastolic blood pressure decreases by more than 10 mm Hg, or the pulse increases by more than 20 bpm, these are signs that blood volume may be decreased and dehydration should be suspected.

PATHOLOGY AND PATHOGENESIS

Gastrointestinal Infections

GI infections include viral gastroenteritis, food poisoning, and so-called "traveler's diarrhea"[20] (Table 8-3). *Viral gastroenteritis* ("stomach flu") causes severe vomiting, diarrhea, and abdominal spasms and is accompanied by fever and myalgia.[20,21] The virus is contracted by ingesting food that has been contaminated. Most commonly, contamination is a result of infected food preparers improperly washing their hands after using the restroom. It can also be contracted by ingesting raw seafood or water that has been contaminated by sewage. This type of contamination, in which an infectious agent from the GI tract of an infected person is ingested by a healthy person, is known as the "fecal-oral" route of transmission. The illness, which lasts a few days, is usually self-limiting and rarely life threatening in healthy young people.[20] Primary treatment includes rest and hydration.[20,21] Occasionally, hydration by intravenous fluids is required if the person cannot tolerate oral ingestion of water or other fluids. Antidiarrheal and antiemetic (to inhibit vomiting) medications are not recommended because they delay elimination of the virus from the body.[20] Return to participation usually occurs within a week, depending on resolution of symptoms and restoration of hydration.

Food poisoning occurs with ingestion of food-borne bacteria, most commonly a species of *Salmonella* and *Campylobacter*.[20] The bacteria, usually passed into food from the hands or respiratory secretions of a food handler, produces a toxin as they reproduce and multiply on poorly refrigerated meat or dairy products.[20] Within 1 to 2 hours of bacterial ingestion, severe vomiting and diarrhea occur and persist for several hours. Rest and hydration are usually the only treatment needed. Antiemetic and antidiarrheal medications are not recommended since they delay elimination of the bacteria.[20]

Another type of food poisoning is caused by a strain of *Escherichia coli (E. coli)* that lives in the intestines of cattle. During slaughter or preparation, the E. coli contaminate the meat as it is being prepared for consumption. The bacterial contamination occurs when meat is not properly cooked, food preparers do not wash their hands after working with raw meat, or raw meat comes in contact

Table 8-3. Types of Gastrointestinal Infections

INFECTION TYPE	CAUSE	SIGNS AND SYMPTOMS
Viral gastroenteritis (stomach flu)	Improper hygiene by infected food handlers (fecal-oral route) or sewage-contaminated seafood	Fever Myalgia Severe vomiting Diarrhea Abdominal spasms
Food poisoning	Improper storage or cooking temperature allow bacteria (Staphylococcus) to replicate on food	Vomiting Diarrhea
	Improper food handling (eg, cross-contamination from raw meat) allows E. coli to replicate on food, and the ingested E. coli produces a toxin in the human GI system	Hematochezia/bloody diarrhea Severe abdominal cramping
Traveler's diarrhea	Improper hygiene by infected food handlers (fecal-oral route), improper food preparation or handling, or contaminated public water sources	Diarrhea Abdominal spasms

with other food. The E. coli strain produces a toxin in the human GI system, leading to bloody diarrhea and severe abdominal cramping. The bacteria can be communicated from an infected person to a healthy person through contact with infected feces. Most often this occurs when an infected person does not wash their hands properly after using the restroom. Treatment is generally supportive (hydration). Antidiarrheal medications should not be used because they allow the bacteria to remain in the body longer. There is no evidence that antibiotics lessen the duration or intensity of the infection. Occasionally, the toxins destroy red blood cells, which leads to kidney failure. This complication is a severe condition that results in a 5% rate of death even when intensive care is provided.

"Traveler's diarrhea" is so named because infectious diarrhea can occur in people while traveling to foreign countries, particularly from the United States to Asia or Latin American countries. Bacteria (Salmonella, etc) or viruses are transmitted through the fecal-oral route from improper hand washing, poor handling of uncooked food, improperly cooked food, and contamination of public water sources. Traveler's diarrhea may last up to 3 days and is similar to other GI infections, producing diarrhea, abdominal spasms, and fatigue from dehydration and decreased caloric intake.[20] Avoidance of potentially contaminated foods and water (ie, consume only bottled fluids and packaged foods) and the use of prophylactic bismuth subsalicylate (Pepto-Bismol) every 6 hours throughout travel can prevent infection while traveling. Treatment is similar to viral gastroenteritis and food poisoning, involving primarily rest and hydration. Antidiarrheal medications can be used to control traveler's diarrhea unless fever (indicating gastroenteritis) or bloody stool (hematochezia, indicating E. coli infection) occurs.[20]

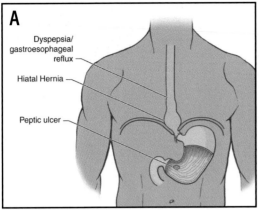
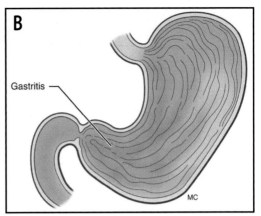

Figure 8-7. Upper gastrointestinal pathology. (A) Dyspepsia, gastroesophageal reflux, hiatal hernia, peptic ulcer. (B) Gastritis.

Upper Gastrointestinal Disorders

Burning pain in the chest, nausea, vomiting, and loss of appetite are hallmark signs and symptoms of upper GI pathology (Figure 8-7).[3]

Dyspepsia

The most common upper GI condition is dyspepsia, also known as indigestion or heartburn, which produces an uncomfortable burning sensation under the sternum and upper midabdominal discomfort or bloating.[13] Irritation of the mucosa in the upper GI from reflux of gastric acids, medications, drugs, alcohol, caffeine, pregnancy, or from certain states can cause dyspepsia.[13,22] Dyspepsia can usually be successfully managed with dietary changes and over-the-counter (OTC) antacids designed to reduce gastric acid.

Antacids are fast acting and generally provide relief within 15 minutes of dosing. They should be taken after meals and at bedtime. The duration of effect can be extended by taking them within 1 hour of meals. Antacids can interfere with the absorption of other medications, so they should not be taken with other medications. A general rule of thumb is to separate dosing of antacids and other drugs by at least 2 hours.[23] Other medications such as proton pump inhibitors (PPIs) or H_2 blockers can be more effective in treating heartburn, so individuals with chronic heartburn should consult their physician to discuss alternative medications.

The symptoms of dyspepsia are common to other, more serious GI disorders, including gastroesophageal reflux, peptic ulcer, and liver disease.[13] Other signs, such as weight loss, abnormal masses in the abdomen, hematochezia, or fever do not occur with benign dyspepsia and, therefore, warrant referral.

Gastroesophageal Reflux Disease

Gastroesophageal reflux disease (GERD) produces symptoms and impairment when the esophageal sphincter that controls flow of food from the esophagus into the stomach malfunctions, either because of an anatomical or functional abnormality and often after ingestion of certain types of foods, medications, high-carbohydrate fluids, or drugs (caffeine, alcohol). Presence of a hiatal hernia (described next) or obesity are also risk factors for GERD.[16,24] Symptoms are produced by acid from the stomach entering the esophagus, which has a thinner mucosal layer than the stomach and is irritated by the acid.[22,24] Exercise involving repeated vertical impact or intra-abdominal forces, such as running or power lifting, can also induce GERD by causing stomach acids to enter the esophagus.[5,10,16] Psychoemotional stress stimulates the vagus nerve, causing secretion of excess stomach acid and abnormal stomach contractions that may push acid into the esophagus.

GERD causes symptoms similar to those of dyspepsia but are usually more frequent, more intense, and of a longer duration. Most often, GERD can be controlled with dietary and lifestyle changes, such as avoidance of irritating foods or activities, stress management, and medications.[16] If the condition prevents participation in physical activity, persists for several weeks, or becomes significantly worse, the patient should be referred to a physician. Occasionally, prescribed medication is required and, in rare instances, surgery.[10]

PPIs and H_2 blockers inhibit acid production in the stomach and are effective in treating GERD.[16,24] Common PPIs include esomeprazole (Nexium), lansoprazole (Prevacid), omeprazole (Prilosec), and pantoprazole (Protonix). H_2 blockers include cimetidine (Tagamet), famotidine (Pepcid), and ranitidine (Zantac). The PPIs will often have an enteric coating to slow dissolution in the gut and should not be crushed, chewed, or split. For optimum use, they should be taken approximately 30 minutes before a meal. PPIs are generally more effective than H_2 blockers in treating GERD and are associated with a 30% greater rate of healing with the esophagus.[23,24]

Hiatal Hernia

A herniation is the abnormal protrusion of an organ through the surrounding tissue. A hiatal hernia is the protrusion of part of the proximal stomach through the diaphragm and into the thorax. This displacement impairs the function of the lower esophageal sphincter, which regulates the flow of food from the esophagus into the stomach. The effect is an increased risk of gastroesophageal reflux, although many people who have small hiatal hernias have no symptoms and no apparent effects. Symptoms are worse when lying down because the stomach acids flow more easily into the esophagus, and they are relieved by sitting because gravity pulls the acid back into the stomach. Diagnosis is made using barium fluoroscopy to image the upper GI system. Treatment involves medication to reduce stomach acid and surgery in recalcitrant cases.

Peptic Ulcer

A peptic ulcer occurs when the gastric juices digest the submucosal layers of the stomach or duodenum.[9] The mucosal layer of the stomach is normally protected from stomach acid by the mucosal barrier, which consists of secreted mucus and bicarbonate. Anything that disrupts this protective barrier increases the risk of peptic ulcer. Chronic infection by *Helicobacter pylori* has been strongly associated with the development of peptic ulcers; this bacteria interferes with the protective mucosal barrier of mucus and bicarbonate.[25] Chronic use of NSAIDs, such as aspirin and ibuprofen, which are often used by athletes during training, also increases the risk of peptic ulcers because they inhibit prostaglandins, which are necessary for the secretion of mucus and bicarbonate in the stomach.[16] Some diseases that increase acid secretion in the stomach can also lead to ulcers by overwhelming the mechanisms in the protective barrier. Ulceration into the muscular layer produces scarring, and erosion beyond the muscular layer can perforate blood vessels, causing severe gastric hemorrhage and shock.[25]

Risk of peptic ulcer increases with advancing age, chronic use of NSAIDs (eg, for arthritis), and regular heavy use of nicotine and alcohol. Ulcers can occur in physically active individuals who are under psychological and physiological stress.[9]

A peptic ulcer produces intermittent pain in the upper or middle abdomen that radiates to the thoracic spine, chest, and neck.[9] The symptoms may improve or worsen after eating and may disappear and recur over several weeks or months. Abdominal pain at night is very common. If the condition persists, recurrent vomiting and loss of appetite may cause weight loss.[9] A perforated ulcer may produce bloody vomitus (*hematemesis*), coffee-grounds vomitus, or melena.[9]

Avoidance of foods that irritate the condition and the use of antacids usually provide symptomatic relief.[25] Prescription antibiotics for *H. pylori* (after testing and confirmation of the bacteria either by urea breath test, stool antigen, and/or blood antibody) and acid-reducing medications, such as PPIs (with the exception of Nexium) and H_2 blockers, often succeed in healing peptic ulcers, with a 5% to 10% recurrence rate. Relatively few patients with ulcers require surgery, which is performed to stop excessive gastric bleeding or to biopsy for a suspected malignancy.[25]

Gastritis and Gastroenteritis

Gastritis describes stomach inflammation resulting from a disease causing erosion of the entire mucosa, chronic use of NSAIDs, H. pylori infection, or autoimmune diseases.[9] Gastritis can be acute or chronic, erosive or nonerosive.

Acute erosive gastritis occurs in patients who have severe chronic illnesses, such as severe burns, head or spinal trauma, shock, and hepatic or renal failure or who require mechanical ventilation. These conditions cause severe gastric stress by impairing the mucosal barrier mechanism, leading to the erosion of the mucosa. Treatment of the causative medical condition takes precedence.

Chronic erosive gastritis is most commonly attributed to long-term use of NSAIDs, alcohol abuse, irritable bowel disease, or viral infection.[25] Nausea, vomiting, and vague upper abdominal pain may be present in such cases. Dietary restrictions and symptomatic treatment with antacids are used as treatment, although recurrences are frequent, particularly if the causative condition persists.

Acute and chronic nonerosive gastritis is frequently a result of H. pylori infection, potentially causing gastric irritation, mucosa breakdown, peptic ulcers, and stomach cancer.[25] Symptoms, when present, are similar to erosive gastritis and peptic ulcer. A course of antibiotics along with a PPI eliminates the bacteria and the gastritis.

Lower Gastrointestinal Disorders

The cardinal signs of lower GI (includes the jejunum, colon, and rectum) pathology are persistent diarrhea or hematochezia. Table 8-4 compares the signs and symptoms of common lower GI conditions. Diarrhea is a symptom, not a disease. Most commonly, a lower GI infection causes diarrhea that resolves within 5 days with simple supportive interventions, such as hydration and electrolyte replacement.[13] A pattern of similar GI signs and symptoms at the same time among family or teammates suggests an infectious origin. In such cases, the affected individuals should be temporarily isolated from others to prevent cross-contamination.

Bismuth subsalicylate (Pepto-Bismol) and loperamide (Imodium) are both OTC medications that are effective in treating diarrhea. As mentioned previously, bismuth subsalicylate is especially effective in preventing and treating traveler's diarrhea. People with a known allergy to aspirin should not take bismuth subsalicylate.[23]

Radical changes in diet, excessive alcohol consumption, mechanical vibration of the bowels such as may occur with running long distances, and psychoemotional stress can also cause a bout of diarrhea. An athlete with diarrhea should be withdrawn from participation until the syndrome resolves to prevent dehydration. Return to play is allowed once normal, fully hydrated body weight is restored.

Occasionally, diarrhea is the chief compliant in a person with more serious pathology, particularly if it is notably unusual in color or odor, or accompanied by fever, vomiting, or severe abdominal cramps. Recurrent or persistent diarrhea, particularly leading to weight loss or accompanied by other systemic signs and symptoms (eg, fever, fatigue) requires urgent referral to a physician.[2]

Inflammatory Bowel Diseases (Crohn's Disease and Ulcerative Colitis)

The inflammatory bowel diseases are *Crohn's disease* and *ulcerative colitis*. Both are genetic autoimmune disorders in which the small intestine and colon initiate an immune reaction against their own cells. This reaction causes widespread ulceration, fibrosis, and necrosis in the small and large intestines.[26] Onset of the disease is usually in adolescence or early adulthood, and the condition often coexists with other immune disorders.

Inflammatory bowel diseases can cause a variety of signs and symptoms, including abdominal pain, chronic diarrhea, hematochezia, weight loss, a palpable abdominal mass (particularly in the

Table 8-4. Comparison of Lower Gastrointestinal Conditions

	INFLAMMATORY BOWEL DISEASE	IRRITABLE BOWEL SYNDROME	APPENDICITIS	DIVERTICULITIS	COLORECTAL CANCER
ABDOMINAL PAIN AND CRAMPING	Chronic, recurrent	Chronic, recurrent	Acute, severe	Acute, severe	Little to none
PAIN LOCATION	General lower abdominal	General lower abdominal	Epigastric progressing to LRQ	LLQ	Rectal, lower abdomen, if any
SYSTEMIC SIGNS AND SYMPTOMS	Chronic diarrhea Hematochezia Palpable LRQ mass Skin rash	Intermittent diarrhea or constipation, or alternating both	Nausea Rebound tenderness LRQ May have fever	Alternating diarrhea and constipation Fever Rectal bleeding	Rectal bleeding Intermittent diarrhea and constipation

LLQ, lower left quadrant; LRQ, lower right quadrant.

right lower quadrant), loss of appetite, skin rash, and intermittent joint pain.[26] A key to recognition is the chronic recurrence of whichever signs and symptoms are present. Inflammatory bowel diseases cannot be cured, but they are usually not disabling and can be medically managed with diet, lifestyle changes, medication, and surgery as needed. Treatment with medication often involves a combination of drugs depending on the symptoms. Combination therapies include the use of corticosteroids, NSAIDs, antibiotics, and immunosuppressants.[23] Approximately 30% of patients with ulcerative colitis and 70% of patients with Crohn's disease will require surgery.[26]

People with inflammatory bowel disease should be monitored during physical activity to ensure adequate hydration. Exacerbation of symptoms is common with heavy exercise or physical activity, but inflammatory bowel disease is not necessarily a contraindication to sports; the treating physician should make this determination.

Irritable Bowel Syndrome

A less severe and far more common condition is IBS, thought to be a reaction to psychophysical stress and poor diet.[27] IBS produces intermittent abdominal pain and cramping and is most prevalent among young women.[22,27] This disorder affects the motility of the intestines, causing either diarrhea or constipation, or alternating episodes of both. Bloating or abdominal distention may also appear as gas builds up in the colon. Relief of abdominal pain usually occurs after defecation.[27]

IBS does not cause inflammation in the bowels, which distinguishes it from other disorders. In addition, IBS rarely interrupts sleep.[27] Stress reduction, dietary changes, and reasonable amounts of physical activity are the usual course of treatment.[22] Alcohol, nicotine, and caffeine use should be curtailed, and a physician should review any medication use. Medication may be prescribed to assist with decreasing stress or relieving symptoms.[27] OTC antidiarrheals and laxatives, depending on the predominant symptom, are the primary medications used to treat IBS. Bulk-forming laxatives (psyllium [Metamucil] or methylcellulose [Citrucel]) are usually preferred over stool softeners (docusate [Colace]) or osmotic laxatives (magnesium hydroxide [Milk of Magnesia]).[23] With appropriate treatment, IBS only very rarely affects function or ability.

Appendicitis

The appendix lies in the lower right quadrant of the abdomen, at the junction where the terminal ileum becomes the cecum and then the ascending colon. When the appendix becomes acutely inflamed by physical irritants or infection, a general, progressively increasing epigastric abdominal pain appears. The abdominal pain eventually migrates to the lower right quadrant (the right iliac region). McBurney's point, about one-third of the distance from the anterior superior iliac spine toward the umbilicus, becomes exquisitely sensitive to palpation, and rebound tenderness or a positive "jar sign" is present. Passive extension (*iliopsoas sign*) or active flexion (*obturator sign*) of the right hip may be painful because the inflammation sometimes affects the psoas muscle.[17] Loss of appetite and nausea are usually present, although vomiting is rare.[6] Other signs of infection may be present, such as fever and malaise.

The traditional treatment is surgical removal of the appendix, although nonsurgical medical treatment is becoming increasing successful (ie, intravenous antibiotics, percutaneous drainage of abscess) in adults as compared to children. Return to activity after surgery occurs in 1 to 2 weeks in children and 3 to 4 weeks in adults depending on type of surgery.[6] If the condition goes untreated, the appendix may inflame to the point that it ruptures and spills its infected contents into the peritoneal cavity. A ruptured appendix is a medical emergency and requires prompt surgical treatment. Early recognition and proper management of appendicitis are key to preventing rupture.

911

Diverticulosis and Diverticulitis

Multiple herniations of the mucosa and submucosa of the intestine through the muscular layer of the intestinal wall is a condition called *diverticulosis*. Ten percent of Americans, and as many as

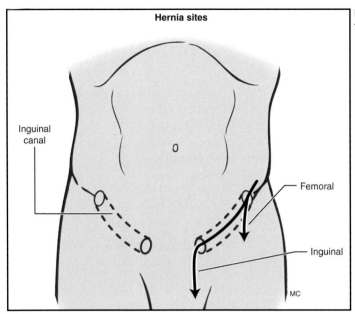

Figure 8-8. Location of inguinal and femoral hernias.

half of the older adult population, have this anatomical disorder. In most cases, diverticulosis is asymptomatic.

If feces or food items such as nuts or seeds become trapped in a herniated section or such a section becomes obstructed, an inflammation of the herniated section, called *diverticulitis*, results. Symptoms include severe abdominal cramping and constant pain in the lower left quadrant; this pain may radiate to the back.[9] Additional signs include alternating constipation and diarrhea, fever, and rectal bleeding. The pain and cramping usually worsen a few hours after eating and may briefly resolve after defecation. Typically, antibiotics are used to treat and may warrant surgical intervention depending on severity, response to conservative treatment, and recurrence.

Treatment with a high-fiber diet and light exercise to encourage bowel motility is common. In more severe cases involving infection or a complete bowel obstruction (causing an ischemic bowel segment), antibiotics and emergency surgery may be required.

Colorectal Cancer

Cancer of the colon and rectum causes the second most cancer deaths in the United States annually. Age over 50 years, a family history of colorectal cancer, history of other colon disorders, presence of polyps in the colon, and a high-fat, high-sugar, low-fiber diet are risk factors for colorectal cancer. Colorectal cancer can exist for a long time before symptoms are noticed. Bleeding from the rectum or bloody stools is usually the first sign. Change in bowel habits, including intermittent diarrhea and constipation, and a continuing sense of bowel fullness even after a bowel movement are other potential symptoms of colorectal cancer. Depending on the stage of the cancer, treatment will usually involve surgery, chemotherapy, radiation, or a combination of these. Prognosis depends on the stage of the disease when diagnosed. Early detection is associated with a 5-year survival rate of nearly 100%; the survival rate in advanced disease is very low.

Hernia

Herniation occurs when an organ or part of an organ protrudes through a defect in the tissue surrounding that organ.[9,17] A segment of small intestine can herniate into the inguinal canal, under the inguinal ligament and into the femoral canal (which contains the neurovascular bundle), or through the linea alba near the umbilicus (Figure 8-8). Inguinal, femoral, and umbilical hernias often cause a palpable bulge at the herniation.[6,9] With an indirect inguinal hernia, the herniated segment travels down the inguinal canal and into the scrotum, where the bowel loop may be palpated by the patient during showering or self-examination. History may include a sudden tearing sensation that occurred during a specific physical exertion, although many persons with hernias do not remember a particular episode. Many hernias are detectable only by medical imaging and may be completely asymptomatic.[6,9]

The primary symptom of a hernia is a burning pain in the groin. This pain worsens with activity, an increase in abdominal pressure (Valsalva maneuver), or body position.[9] Pain from an inguinal or femoral hernia may radiate into the anterior thigh if it irritates the femoral nerve. An umbilical hernia produces pain in the abdominal wall near the point of herniation. The intestinal segment may herniate only intermittently, and thus cause only intermittent symptoms. Herniation of a large bowel segment that does not retract, a condition called *strangulation* of the bowel, requires surgical repair to prevent bowel ischemia or obstruction.[9] Most hernias requiring surgery can be operated on laparoscopically. Gradual return to physical activity can be expected in about 1 week after laparoscopic surgery, whereas open surgical repair requires an additional 1 to 2 weeks of recovery.[6]

The so-called *"sports hernia"* is not a true hernia but describes otherwise unexplained chronic groin pain often following vigorous pivoting, cutting, or kicking activity.[28] The pathophysiology is unclear, with several conditions potentially being classified as sports hernia, including tear of the external oblique aponeurosis with injury to the ilioinguinal nerve, adductor strain, osteitis pubis, hip joint syndromes, and inguinal wall disorders.[28] The distinguishing characteristic between sports hernia and a true inguinal or femoral hernia is the absence of the intestines protruding under or through a defect in the inguinal ligament.

Hemorrhoids

Hemorrhoids, also called "piles," are veins in the rectum or anus that become dilated. The reason for the dilation is poorly understood but is thought to be related to genetic predisposition, frequent constipation, liver disease, or any other condition that increases pressure in the anorectal veins. *Internal hemorrhoids* occur inside the rectum; *external hemorrhoids* protrude through the anal border. In either case, bright red blood may appear with defecation, although no pain occurs unless the rectum or anus is fissured (split) or the veins become strangulated (ischemic). Pain and itching accompany external hemorrhoids, particularly during sitting.

Very common and bothersome but usually not medically serious (unless they are a sign of other pathology), hemorrhoids are treated with changes in diet to soften the stool and reduce constipation and topical medications to relieve symptoms. Topical medications are available in a variety of dosage forms, including creams, suppositories, ointments, and pads. Although minimal, some systemic absorption may occur with medications, depending on the dosage form. Occasionally surgery is needed to provide relief. Examination of the rectum provides clues to this diagnosis. Prompt referral to a physician should be made for uncontrolled bleeding from a hemorrhoid, failure to respond to OTC medications and lifestyle changes, or thrombosed hemorrhoid.

Abdominal Trauma

911 Persistent abdominal pain, localized tenderness, abdominal rigidity, or upper GI signs (eg, nausea, vomiting) after a blow to the ribs or abdomen requires emergency referral. If an athlete sustains a blow that fractures ribs, causes bruising in the abdomen, causes abdominal cramping, or produces rigidity, a physician should examine them as soon as possible.[6] In sports, the spleen and liver are the abdominal organs most susceptible to injury.

Spleen Trauma and Splenomegaly

The spleen stores platelets and other types of blood cells and filters the blood to remove small particles and deformed or old red blood cells. In adults, the spleen lies on the left side of the abdomen between the ninth to the eleventh ribs. In younger children, the inferior aspect of the spleen extends slightly below the rib cage. A direct blow to the LUQ is the most common mechanism of

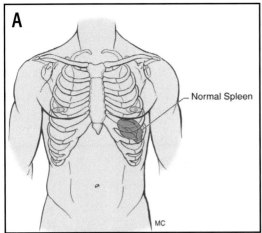 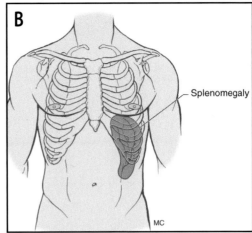

Figure 8-9. (A) Normal spleen size and location. (B) Splenomegaly.

injury.[6,8] Eliciting an accurate and careful history is important. Any blow to the LUQ or abdomen should be noted, because apparently benign contact may damage the spleen (eg, falling on a football).[8] History of a recent infectious disease or fever may also be relevant, because these conditions may result in splenomegaly (see next) and increase the risk of injury.

Signs and symptoms of splenic injury include shock, nausea, vomiting, rigidity in the LUQ, abdominal pain, and pain referred to the left shoulder (known as Kehr's sign).[3,6] The pain in the left shoulder is a result of left-side diaphragmatic irritation caused by inflammation and bleeding of the spleen. Occasionally, signs of serious injury to the spleen appear gradually and are difficult to recognize. The spleen's ability to splint itself through clotting may cause a delay in the presentation of symptoms. Later disruption of the clot or "splint" will cause symptoms to develop hours or days after the original injury, leading to severe shock and death. Consequently, more severe splenic injury may result in several days of hospitalization for close medical monitoring.[8] Any suspicion of splenic injury, by history, symptoms, or signs, requires immediate withdrawal from participation and urgent medical referral and testing, which often includes computed tomography and ultrasound imaging to assess and grade the injury.[8] In cases of severe injury or bleeding, the spleen may be surgically removed (*splenectomy*). Return to play following nonoperative treatment is gradual and is often restricted to light activity for at least 3 months to ensure full healing and decrease the risk of re-rupture. Return to activity following surgical removal is dictated primarily by healing of the surgical wounds because no risk of re-rupture exists.[8] Of note, patients who have had splenectomy for any causes need to consult with physicians to be updated on their immunizations against certain bacteria along with management plan for infections as they are at higher risk for certain pathogens.

People with *splenomegaly* (Figure 8-9), a pathological enlargement of the spleen resulting from medical conditions such as mononucleosis (see Chapter 4), require at least 3 weeks of rest before resuming physical activity and may require up to an additional 1 month or more before returning to strenuous athletic activity.[3,13] Splenomegaly greatly increases the risk of splenic rupture, so physician clearance is required before return to contact or collision sports.[3,6]

Liver Trauma

Trauma to the liver is more subtle in its clinical presentation than trauma to the spleen,[3,6,29] and liver injury is less common than splenic injury. The mechanism of liver injury is a direct blow to the RUQ. Persistent abdominal pain, RUQ tenderness, and upper GI signs (eg, nausea, vomiting) are signs of liver injury that warrant an emergency medical examination.[6,29] Many liver injuries recover naturally and do not require surgery, but all such injuries should be monitored in a hospital and followed by a physician on discharge.[6,7,29] Recovery, from either surgical or nonsurgical treatment, can

Table 8-5. Types of Hepatitis by Cause

TYPE	CAUSE	SIGNS AND SYMPTOMS	CLINICAL COURSE
Viral	Infection with hepatitis virus (types A, B, C, D)		
Initial stage		Fatigue, loss of appetite, nausea, diarrhea, weight loss, joint pain, dark urine, light stools, hepatomegaly	3 to 4 weeks
Icteric stage		Jaundice, splenomegaly, lymph node swelling	6 to 8 weeks
Recovery stage		Fatigue	4 or more months (hepatitis B can be fatal)
Toxic	Exposure to hepatotoxic chemical or drug (antibiotics, oral contraceptives, acetaminophen, psycho-tropics, cytotoxins)	Jaundice, fatigue, loss of appetite, dark urine, light stools, fever, joint pain, and pain in right upper quadrant	Progressive until toxin is removed; severity depends on extent of tissue damage
Chronic	Viral infection, chronic toxic exposure, idiopathic	Jaundice, arthritis, signs of kidney impairment, anemia	Poor; often progressing to cirrhosis and liver failure
Alcoholic	Chronic alcohol consumption	Fever, abdominal pain, jaundice, elevated white blood cell count	Varies widely, depends on extent of tissue damage; poor prognosis if drinking continues

take weeks or months.[29] A liver injury severe enough to require surgery often results in a permanent exclusion from sports.[6]

Hepatic-Biliary Diseases

Hepatitis

Hepatitis, meaning literally "inflammation of the liver," occurs primarily with viral infection or liver toxicity; the inflammation response affects liver function, which causes the signs and symptoms. Viral infection is the leading cause of hepatitis in the United States, but there are numerous other causes (Table 8-5).

Viral hepatitis types (A, B, C, D, E) refer to the different viruses that infect the liver.[30] Hepatitis A virus is transmitted through close personal contact (oral-oral route) or by contamination when food preparers do not wash their hands appropriately (fecal-oral route). Hepatitis B, C, and D require direct exposure to body fluids, including blood, urine, feces, saliva, mucous, tears, vomit, semen, or vaginal secretions.[30,31] Children and adolescents usually acquire hepatitis A, whereas young adults are more likely to contract hepatitis B or C. Hepatitis D occurs primarily as a complication of type B. Hepatitis B and C cause more damage to the liver than the other types.

Health care workers are at increased risk for contracting viral hepatitis because they are exposed to many people who have chronic illnesses.[9] Vaccines are available for hepatitis viruses A and B, and vaccination is recommended for all health care workers. There are newer guidelines for screening for certain viral hepatitis strains (such as hepatitis C) by multiple organizations due to risk of transmission from blood transfusions. Frequent hand-washing and strict adherence to standard precautions (eg, gloves; mask and gown as needed) also offer protection against exposure and spread of hepatitis.[30,31]

Three stages of hepatitis infection are described: initial, icteric, and recovery. The *initial stage* may be asymptomatic, although the hepatitis virus is highly communicable during this time.[30] During this stage, general systemic signs and symptoms may appear, including fatigue, loss of appetite, nausea, diarrhea, weight loss, and joint pain.[9] As hepatitis progresses, urine darkens and stool lightens in color as a result of the pigment bilirubin increasing in concentration in the blood.[9,30] During this stage, the liver swells and becomes tender to palpation.

The *icteric stage* begins 3 or 4 weeks later, producing jaundice that lasts 6 to 8 weeks as the systemic signs slowly resolve. Near the end of this stage, the liver begins to return to normal size, but the spleen enlarges and cervical lymph nodes may swell. The virus is no longer communicable at this point. The *recovery stage*, when it occurs, can last 4 months or longer. Fatigue is the most prominent symptom as liver function normalizes.[30]

Specific medical treatments do not exist for hepatitis, although antiviral agents and supportive measures are usually administered. Practicing infection control measures, such as rigorous hand-washing when working with food or between patient contacts, and inoculating health care workers are prudent preventative measures. Most people infected with hepatitis A recover fully. Recovery from the other hepatitis types depends on the aggressiveness of infection and the timing of medical intervention. Hepatitis B can be fatal.

Toxic hepatitis is an inflammation of the liver that occurs after exposure to certain chemicals or drugs, including antibiotics, oral contraceptives, acetaminophen, psychotropics, and cytotoxic drugs used to treat cancer. The chemicals damage liver cells, which become necrotic and cause an inflammatory response. The symptoms and signs depend on the extent of the necrosis. Clinical presentation resembles viral hepatitis, including jaundice, fatigue, loss of appetite, dark urine, light stools, fever, joint pain, and RUQ pain. Treatment is removal of the offending agent and strict avoidance of the toxin.

Chronic hepatitis can develop from viral infection, chronic exposure to toxins, or idiopathic (unknown) etiology.[30] Chronic hepatitis often progresses to liver necrosis and irreparable scarring, a condition called cirrhosis. Many secondary syndromes develop, such as arthritis, kidney disorders, and anemia, as waste products that go unprocessed by the diseased liver flood the bloodstream. Chronic hepatitis is treated with steroids to reduce the inflammation; unfortunately, the steroids themselves cause many complications and side effects. The prognosis for chronic hepatitis is poor.

Alcoholic Liver Disease and Cirrhosis

Alcohol abuse is the leading cause of liver disease in the United States.[9] Prolonged consumption of large amounts of alcohol leads to hepatitis, cirrhosis, hepatic failure, and death. To stop drinking alcohol in such cases is critical but difficult both physically and psychologically. Chapter 14 discusses the psychological aspects of alcohol abuse.

Alcohol causes several types of pathological changes in the liver. Alcohol consumption changes the liver structure and function by affecting its enzymatic and cellular actions.[32,33] *Alcoholic fatty liver disease*, an abnormal accumulation of fat in the liver as a result of chronically altered enzymes and cell function, occurs proportionately to the dose of alcohol consumed. Virtually all heavy drinkers have enlarged, fatty livers. Alcoholic fatty liver by itself is essentially asymptomatic and appears to have no serious effects on liver function but indicates recurrent, heavy drinking that increases the risk of other health problems. If the person stops drinking alcohol, these fatty changes will resolve and the liver will return to its normal structure.

Some heavy drinkers who have fatty liver disease will develop *alcoholic hepatitis*, an inflammation that occurs when there is necrosis (death) of liver cells. Alcoholic hepatitis produces fever, abdominal pain, jaundice, and laboratory signs of inflammation, such as an increased white blood cell count.[32] The severity of alcoholic hepatitis varies from relatively mild, with less cellular damage that has potential to heal, to severe, with permanent liver damage, liver failure, and potentially death.

Cirrhosis is the result of the combined effects of any chronic liver disease (eg, fatty liver, hepatitis, infectious or toxic damage) and malnutrition that results in irreversible damage to the liver cells.[33] Alcohol abuse is a leading cause of cirrhosis, although there are a number of other common causes such as chronic (nonalcoholic) hepatitis and acetaminophen overdose.

Cirrhosis produces extensive cellular damage and necrosis, which lead to fibrotic changes in the liver. The fibrous tissue eventually interferes with the liver's vascular supply and function, leading to ascites, splenomegaly, central and peripheral neurological effects, and various GI system signs and symptoms.[32,33] Cirrhosis is incurable; the fibrous scarring cannot return to normal liver tissue. Medical treatment includes addressing the underlying cause (eg, alcohol abuse or chronic hepatitis) to prevent further necrosis and supportive measures. Extensive cirrhosis often requires a liver transplant because the host liver becomes increasingly unable to function effectively (liver failure).

Gallstones and Gallbladder Disease

Gallstones (cholelithiasis) and *gallbladder disease (cholecystitis)* both produce intermittent RUQ pain that worsens after meals that include fatty foods. Secretion of bile increases when fatty foods are eaten. The increased activity of the gallbladder after such a meal produces the pain when disease or gallstones are present.

Gallstones are composed primarily of cholesterol and bilirubin and account for nearly 20% of all hospital admissions among adults. An increased risk of gallstones is associated with older than age 40 years, obesity, a high-cholesterol diet, and diabetes. Females are at higher risk, most likely because of elevated estrogen levels, oral contraceptive use, or multiple births. Increased estrogen levels inhibit the production of bile acid, which leads to collection of cholesterol and bilirubin in the gallbladder.

Cholecystitis results when gallstones block the cystic duct, which is the gallbladder's attachment to the common bile duct. Fever, jaundice, vomiting, RUQ tenderness, and referred right shoulder or right scapular pain suggest an acute gallbladder attack.[9] Right shoulder pain is the result of irritation of the diaphragm by the inflamed gallbladder. Chronic cholecystitis may present severe RUQ pain, accompanied by intolerance for spicy or fatty foods, heartburn, burping, constipation, or diarrhea. Biliary dyskinesia is a functional gallbladder disorder that is a result of decreased gallbladder motility that may be in the differential diagnosis for gallbladder pathology. Laparoscopic surgery can remove the gallstones or gallbladder to relieve symptoms. Recovery depends on the size and extent of the gallstones.

Pancreatitis

Acute pancreatitis occurs when the pancreatic enzymes become active within the pancreas rather than in the duodenum. The activated enzymes self-digest the pancreatic cells, causing an inflammatory response.[34] The inflammation cascades into severe peritonitis, sudden and excruciating epigastric and LUQ pain, left shoulder pain, LUQ rigidity, and possibly shock. Infection can lead quickly to septicemia (bacteria in the bloodstream) and death. Acute pancreatitis is a medical emergency that has a clear and dramatic clinical presentation of severe illness.[34]

SUMMARY

Many GI disorders can be attributed to lifestyle, including diet, nicotine and alcohol use, and physical inactivity. Other serious disorders are caused by infection, chronic disease processes, or obstruction of the GI tract or its organs' ducts. Common signs and symptoms of GI disorders include nausea, vomiting, diarrhea, constipation, and abdominal pain. The liver, gallbladder, spleen, and exocrine pancreas produce upper abdominal pain that may refer to the shoulders as inflammation of those organs irritates the diaphragm. Pathology in these organs usually disturbs digestion. Medical emergencies of the abdomen, containing the GI system, hepatic-biliary system, and spleen, often produce peritonitis, recognizable by abdominal pain, tenderness, localized rigidity, and positive rebound or jar signs. Peritonitis causes fever or shock as it progresses, thereby demanding immediate medical care.

CASE STUDY

One of the football coaches runs into your office and states that he thinks Bill, the offensive line coach, is having a heart attack. Bill is a 45-year-old male who is obese and has high cholesterol.

On your way to Bill's office, the assistant coach tells you that he and Bill had gone for chili cheeseburgers and french fries a couple of hours ago for lunch. Immediately after lunch Bill had complained of an upset stomach but did not think much of it since he usually gets an upset stomach after a big meal. It usually goes away in a couple of hours.

When you get to Bill's office, you find him bent over in obvious pain. His skin appears to be a very pale green, and he is leaning over and vomiting into his wastebasket. He is fully alert and oriented. He describes having a severe aching pain in the right shoulder and shoulder blade. He denies having any chest pain.

Bill's heart rate is strong and regular at 90 beats per minute. His respirations also appear strong and regular, and he denies having any problems breathing. You notice while taking his pulse that he feels warm to the touch, and he is sweating profusely. You palpate his abdomen and find that he is acutely tender in the RUQ.

Critical Thinking Questions

1. Based on Bill's clinical presentation, do you think he is having a heart attack? What other conditions might be causing his signs and symptoms?

2. What tests might you conduct to determine whether Bill is having a heart attack or experiencing a different condition?

3. What other steps might you take to manage Bill's condition?

REFERENCES

1. National Athletic Trainers' Association. *Athletic Training Education Competencies.* 5th ed. The Commission on Accreditation of Athletic Training Education; 2011.
2. Butcher JD. Runners' diarrhea and other intestinal problems of athletes. *Am Fam Physician.* 1993;48:623-627.
3. Green GA. Gastrointestinal disorders in the athlete. *Clin Sports Med.* 1992;11:453-470.
4. Martin D. Physical activity benefits and risks on the gastrointestinal system. *South Med J.* 2011;104:831-837.
5. de Oliveira EP, Burini RC. The impact of physical exercise on the gastrointestinal tract. *Curr Opin Clin Nutr Metab Care.* 2009;12:533-538.
6. Amaral JF. Thoracoabdominal injuries in the athlete. *Clin Sports Med.* 1997;16:739-753.
7. Ryan JM. Abdominal injuries and sport. *Br J Sports Med.* 1999;33:155-160.
8. Gannon EH, Howard T. Splenic injuries in athletes: a review. *Curr Sports Med Rep.* 2010;9:111-114.

9. Koopmeiners MB. Screening for gastrointestinal system disease. In: Boissonnault WG, ed. *Examination in Physical Therapy Practice: Screening for Medical Disease.* 2nd ed. Churchill-Livingstone Inc; 1995:101-116.

10. Moses FM. The effect of exercise on the gastrointestinal tract. *Sports Med.* 1990;9:159-172.

11. Perlowski AA, Jaff MR. Vascular disorders in athletes. *Vasc Med.* 2010;15:469-479.

12. Stone R. Primary care diagnosis of acute abdominal pain. *Nurse Pract.* 1996;21:19-20,23-26,28-30,35-41.

13. Mellman MF, Podesta L. Common medical problems in sports. *Clin Sports Med.* 1997;16:635-662.

14. Barrett KE, Barman SM, Boitano S, Brooks H. *Ganong's Review of Medical Physiology.* 24th ed. McGraw-Hill Medical; 2012.

15. Stopka CB, Zambito KL. Referred visceral pain: what every sports medicine professional needs to know. *Athl Ther Today.* 1999;4:29-36.

16. Waterman JJ, Kapur R. Upper gastrointestinal issues in athletes. *Curr Sports Med Rep.* 2012;11:99-104.

17. Bickley LS, Szilagyi PG. *Bates' Guide to Physical Examination and History Taking.* 10th ed. Lippincott, Williams & Wilkins; 2009.

18. Putukian M. Assessment of abdominal conditions in athletes. *Athl Ther Today.* 2000;5(6):20-29.

19. George B, Markle IV. A simple test for intraperitoneal inflammation. *Am J Surg.* 1973;125:721-722.

20. Marder EP, Cieslak PR, Cronquist AB, et al. Incidence and Trends of Infections with Pathogen Transmitted Commonly Through Food and the Effect of Increasing Use of Culture-Independent Diagnostic Tests on Surveillance – Foodborne Diseases Active Surveillance Network, 10 U.S. Sites, 2013-2016. *MMWR Morb Mortal Wkly Rep.* 2017;66(15):397.

21. Boyce TG. Gastroenteritis. In: Beers MH, Berkow R, eds. *The Merck Manual of Diagnosis and Therapy.* 17th ed. Merck Research Laboratories; 1999:283-292.

22. Casey E, Mistry DJ, MacKnight JM. Training room management of medical conditions: sports gastroenterology. *Clin Sports Med.* 2005;24:525-540.

23. Houglum JE, Harrelson GL. *Principles of Pharmacology for Athletic Trainers.* 2nd ed. Slack Incorporated; 2011.

24. Leggit JC. Evaluation and treatment of GERD and upper GI complaints in athletes. *Curr Sports Med Rep.* 2011;10:109-114.

25. Finn S, Hirschowitz BI. Gastritis and peptic ulcer disease. In: Beers MH, Berkow R, eds. *The Merck Manual of Diagnosis and Therapy.* 17th ed. Merck Research Laboratories; 1999:245-255.

26. Sachar DB, Walfish J. Inflammatory bowel diseases. In: Beers MH, Berkow R, eds. *The Merck Manual of Diagnosis and Therapy.* 17th ed. Merck Research Laboratories; 1999:302-311.

27. Olden K. Functional bowel disorders. In: Beers MH, Berkow R, eds. *The Merck Manual of Diagnosis and Therapy.* 17th ed. Merck Research Laboratories; 1999:312-317.

28. Caudill P, Nyland J, Smith C, Yerasimides J, Lach J. Sports hernias: a systematic literature review. *Br J Sports Med.* 2008;42:954-964.

29. Ray R, Lernire JE. Liver laceration in an intercollegiate football player. *J Athl Train.* 1995;30:324-326.

30. Simon JB. Hepatitis. In: Beers MH, Berkow R, eds. *The Merck Manual of Diagnosis and Therapy.* 17th ed. Merck Research Laboratories; 1999:377-385.

31. Buxton BP, Daniell JE, Buxton BHJ, Okasaki EM, Ho KW. Prevention of hepatitis B virus in athletic training. *J Athl Train.* 1994;29:107-112.

32. Damjanov I. *The liver and biliary tract. Pathology for the Health-Related Professions.* 2nd ed. W.B. Saunders; 2000:277-305.

33. Porth CM. *Alterations in hepatobiliary function. Essentials of Pathophysiology.* Lippincott Williams & Wilkins; 2004:494-516.

34. Freedman SD. Pancreatitis. In: Beers MH, Berkow R, eds. *The Merck Manual of Diagnosis and Therapy.* 17th ed. Merck Research Laboratories; 1999:269-274.

ONLINE RESOURCES

Case Examples Including Auscultation Samples

◊ http://www.practicalclinicalskills.com/abdominal-course-contents.aspx?courseid=120

Gastrointestinal

◊ **American College of Gastroenterology**

¤ www.acg.gi.org/patients

◊ **Colorectal Cancer Network**

¤ http://www.cancernetwork.com/colorectal-cancer

◊ **Medscape's collection of online gastroenterology articles**
  ¤ http://emedicine.medscape.com/gastroenterology
◊ **National Digestive Diseases Information Clearinghouse**
  ¤ https://www.niddk.nih.gov/health-information/community-health-outreach/information-clearinghouses

Hepatic-Biliary

◊ **American Liver Foundation**
  ¤ www.liverfoundation.org
◊ **Gallstones (National Institute of Diabetes and Digestive and Kidney Diseases)**
  ¤ https://www.niddk.nih.gov/health-information/digestive-diseases
◊ **Hepatitis Foundation International**
  ¤ https://hepatitisfoundation.org/

CHAPTER 9

Renal and Urogenital Systems

CHAPTER OUTLINE AND OBJECTIVES

Introduction

Review of Anatomy, Physiology, and Pathogenesis

◊ Describe the basic renal and urogenital structures and their functions.
◊ Describe the pathophysiological mechanisms of the renal and urogenital systems.
◊ Describe the response of the renal and urogenital systems to exercise.

Signs and Symptoms

◊ Identify the general signs and symptoms of renal pathology.
◊ Identify the general signs and symptoms of urogenital pathology.

Pain Patterns

◊ Identify the referred pain patterns associated with pathology of the renal and urogenital systems.

Medical History and Physical Examination Procedures

◊ Discuss medical history findings relevant to renal and urogenital pathology.
◊ Describe the physical examination procedures associated with renal and urogenital pathology.
  ¤ Inspection
  ¤ Palpation
  ¤ Urinalysis
  ¤ Refractometry

Bhojani RA, O'Connor DP, Fincher AL. *Clinical Pathology for Athletic Trainers: Recognizing Systemic Disease, Fourth Edition* (pp 235-262).
© 2022 Taylor & Francis Group.

Pathology and Pathogenesis

◊ Discuss the signs, symptoms, management, medical referral guidelines, and, when appropriate, return-to-participation criteria for pathology involving the renal system.

  ¤ Renal and Bladder Trauma

  ¤ Renal, Bladder, and Genital Infections

   • Urinary Tract Infection

  ¤ Sexually Transmitted Infections

  ¤ Renal Disorders

   • Urolithiasis

   • Renal Failure

◊ Discuss the signs, symptoms, management, medical referral guidelines, and, when appropriate, return-to-participation criteria for pathology involving the urogenital system.

  ¤ Male Urogenital Disorders

   • Monorchidism

   • Prostate Disorders

   • Prostate Cancer

   • Scrotum and Testicular Trauma

   • Testicular Torsion

   • Varicoceles

   • Testicular Cancer

  ¤ Female Urogenital Disorders

   • Endometriosis

   • Pregnancy

   • Ruptured Ectopic Pregnancy

   • Female Athlete Triad

   • Breast Disorders

   • Breast Cancer

   • Ovarian Cysts

   • Cervical, Ovarian, and Uterine Cancers

Pediatric Concerns

◊ Primary Amenorrhea

◊ Kidney Trauma

◊ Cryptorchidism

Summary

Case Study

◊ Develop critical-thinking and clinical decision-making skills.

Online Resources

This chapter addresses the following knowledge and skills from the *Athletic Training Education Competencies, Fifth Edition*[1]:

Content Area	Knowledge and Skills
Prevention and Health Promotion (PHP)	5
Clinical Examination and Diagnosis (CE)	1-3; 13; 17-19; 20 a-c, j; 21 l; 22-23
Therapeutic Interventions (TI)	30-31

INTRODUCTION

The renal system is responsible for regulating body fluid levels and removing waste products from the blood. The urinary system functions to excrete these waste products from the body. The genital system contains the organs of reproduction that are specific to each gender. Trauma, infection, tumors, hormonal imbalances, and congenital conditions can cause pathology in the renal and urogenital systems. In addition to disorders of the renal and urogenital systems, this chapter includes discussions of other gender-specific medical conditions that affect physical activity.

REVIEW OF ANATOMY, PHYSIOLOGY, AND PATHOGENESIS

Renal-Urinary System

The renal-urinary system, which consists of the kidneys, ureters, bladder, and urethra (Figure 9-1), filters the blood, regulates body fluids, and eliminates metabolic waste from the blood. The kidneys remove waste products and excess water from the blood and regulate electrolyte levels in the body. These substances are collected and sent through the ureters to the bladder, exiting the body through the urethra as urine. The kidneys contribute to homeostasis by providing hormonal and osmotic (fluid balance) control of blood pressure (BP), regulating red blood cell production, and regulating calcium levels.[2,3]

Urine normally contains water, salt, and the by-products of protein metabolism, namely urea, creatine, and various acids. Urine may also normally contain small amounts of glucose, dead cells, crystallized salts, and mucus. Blood cells and whole proteins should not be present in urine because they are too large to be normally absorbed through the renal system.[3] The detection of protein during urinalysis is thus by definition pathological.

The kidneys have a dual role in the control of BP. First, the kidneys secrete the hormone renin, an enzyme that converts angiotensinogen, a protein that circulates in the blood, to angiotensin I. In the presence of angiotensin-converting enzyme, angiotensin I becomes angiotensin II. Angiotensin II increases vascular resistance by causing vasoconstriction, which in turn increases BP. Thus, the secretion of renin by the kidneys leads to an increase in BP. Angiotensin II also increases the reabsorption of sodium by the renal tubules. Renin secretion is stimulated by decreasing BP detected by receptors in the kidneys and by increasing catecholamines and norepinephrine released by sympathetic nervous system activity. Renin secretion is inhibited by angiotensin II and by increases in electrolyte (sodium, chlorine, and potassium) levels that are detected by receptors in the kidneys. The second function of the kidneys in regulating BP is to eliminate excess fluid, thus maintaining a consistent fluid level in the body and the blood.[2,4] The regulation of fluid level directly affects BP.

If the overall fluid level drops, as occurs with severe bleeding or dehydration, BP decreases. When BP decreases for any reason, the kidneys release renin to restore BP. Conversely, if the kidneys are unable to remove excess fluid from the body or if the blood retains excess fluid (*hypervolemia*),

Figure 9-1. Organs of the renal system and urogenital tract.

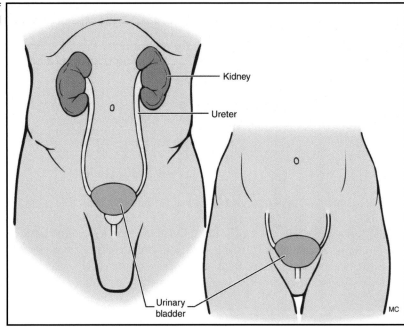

BP increases as the increased volume of fluid in the vascular system exerts more pressure on the vascular walls.[2] With chronic secretion of renin or hypervolemia, systemic hypertension results. Chronic hypertension, whether caused by hormonal or fluid imbalances, damages the nephrons of the kidney, which accentuates and perpetuates the problem.

During resistance exercise, systolic and diastolic BP increases in proportion to exercise load. People with cardiovascular or kidney problems are thus advised to avoid resistance training. During endurance exercise, systolic BP first increases moderately, then levels off, and gradually decreases back to normal as exercise continues. Diastolic BP changes very little during endurance exercise. Moderate intensity endurance exercise is thus usually recommended for persons who have pathology of the cardiovascular or renal systems or those who have hypertension.

The kidneys can be damaged by trauma, toxins, chronic disease, obstruction of urine collection or flow, and chronically high concentrations of glucose (as occurs in diabetes mellitus), urea, or creatine in the blood.[3] Regardless of the etiology, kidney pathology affects the function of the nephrons; nephrons are the basic unit of the kidney and consist of a glomerulus (the vascular component) and the tubular system for collecting and concentrating urine.[3] Simply stated, pathology changes the kidney's filtering process. The kidney either extracts elements from the blood that it should not, fails to extract elements it should, or both. The osmotic pressure in the kidney capillaries (glomeruli) becomes closer to the osmotic pressure in the blood. The nephron then begins to absorb a large amount of fluid to restore proper osmotic tension. The increased fluid in turn affects the ability of the kidney to draw solutes (waste products) into the urine, so the waste products accumulate in the blood.

Over time, the buildup of metabolic by-products in the blood damages other organ-systems. The most notable effects occur in the cardiovascular and neurological systems. Chronic kidney disorders often result in hypertension as they impair the kidneys' role in regulation of BP. Disturbance of acid-base balance produces metabolic imbalances (acidosis or alkalosis) that either depress or excite the central nervous system.

Reproductive System

The male genital system includes the prostate gland, spermatic cord, testes, epididymis, vas deferens, seminal vesicles, urethra, and penis (Figure 9-2). The female genital system includes the

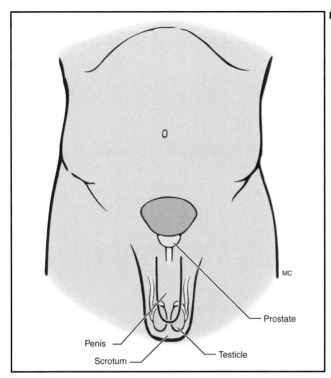

Figure 9-2. Organs of the male genital system.

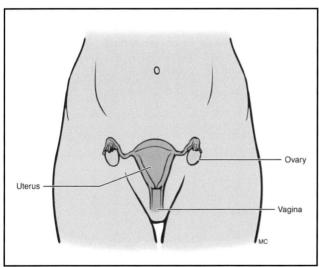

Figure 9-3. Organs of the female genital system.

ovaries, fallopian tubes, uterus, cervix, and vagina (Figure 9-3). Some organs of the genital system are stimulated by hormones of the hypothalamus (gonadotropin-releasing hormone, prolactin-releasing hormone, and prolactin-inhibiting hormone) and pituitary (prolactin, follicle-stimulating hormone, and luteinizing hormone) to release gender specific hormones. The testes produce testosterone, and the ovaries produce estrogen, although both sexes have small circulating amounts of the opposite sex's hormones. The "sex hormones" induce puberty, the development of sexual maturation and secondary sex characteristics, and regulate sexual health and function. Testosterone stimulates development of the penis, prostate, and seminal vesicles during puberty, and causes enlargement of the larynx and thickening of the vocal cords, producing the characteristic deeper voice of males. Testosterone also influences the growth of face and body (axilla, chest) hair, aggressive behaviors,

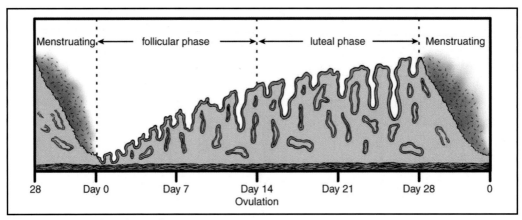

Figure 9-4. Hormonal regulation of menstruation.

muscular development, and sebaceous gland activity. Estrogen stimulates uterine and ovarian blood flow and growth, as well as enlargement of the breasts, breast ducts, and vagina—although many of the secondary female characteristics (narrow shoulders, broader hips, higher-pitched voice, less body hair) depend at least as much on the absence of testosterone and other androgens as on the presence of estrogen. Estrogen also increases libido (sexual motivation) in both sexes.

Several hormones produced by the hypothalamus regulate menstruation. The hypothalamus hormones also stimulate the pituitary gland to release hormones that affect estrogen and progesterone production in the ovaries (Figure 9-4).[5,6] Estrogen and progesterone interact to produce endometrial development in the presence of *ovulation*, the release of an ovum from the ovaries that occurs approximately 2 weeks before menses. Thickening of the endometrium is needed to nurture a fertilized ovum in the event of pregnancy. When estrogen and progesterone levels decrease, the thick, blood-rich endometrium is expelled (menses) to prepare the uterus for the next cycle. The menstrual cycle is very sensitive to hormonal levels and nutrition. *Amenorrhea*, the absence of menses, occurs with pregnancy, endocrine disorders, and malnutrition.

Finally, the urogenital system also has a musculoskeletal component. The organs of the pelvis are supported by a horizontal sling of muscles within the pelvic ring. These muscles suspend the organs within the pelvic cavity and assist in urinary and sexual function. Impairment of these muscles can cause urinary or sexual disability.

Signs and Symptoms

Hematuria

Blood in the urine is a sign of kidney or bladder pathology. Gross hematuria after a blow to the back or abdomen suggests kidney, ureter, or bladder injury and is therefore a medical emergency. Infection of the kidney or bladder produces subtle hematuria.

Exertional or "sports" hematuria develops from either exercise-induced renal ischemia during long duration, high intensity exercise, or repetitive microtrauma of the kidney or bladder during running or other vigorous activity ("heel strike hemolysis").[7] Treatment is rest, medical referral, and gradual return to activity. Activities can resume 24 hours after urine returns to normal.[7] See Algorithm 9-1 for clinical decision making related to hematuria or dysuria.

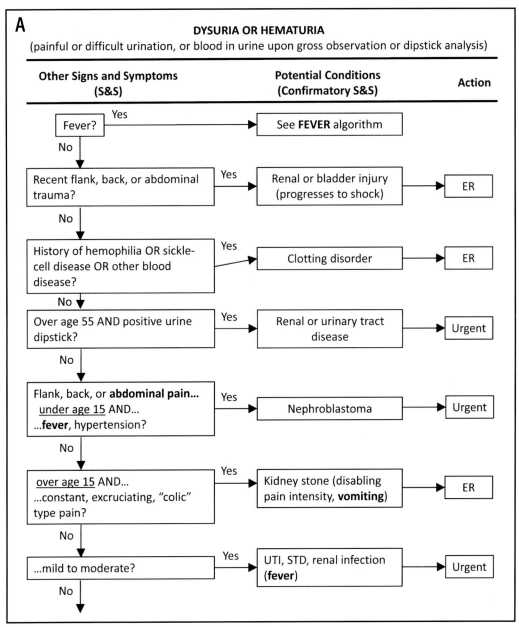

A

DYSURIA OR HEMATURIA
(painful or difficult urination, or blood in urine upon gross observation or dipstick analysis)

Other Signs and Symptoms (S&S)	Potential Conditions (Confirmatory S&S)	Action
Fever? — Yes →	See **FEVER** algorithm	
No ↓		
Recent flank, back, or abdominal trauma? — Yes →	Renal or bladder injury (progresses to shock)	ER
No ↓		
History of hemophilia OR sickle-cell disease OR other blood disease? — Yes →	Clotting disorder	ER
No ↓		
Over age 55 AND positive urine dipstick? — Yes →	Renal or urinary tract disease	Urgent
No ↓		
Flank, back, or **abdominal pain...** under age 15 AND... ...**fever**, hypertension? — Yes →	Nephroblastoma	Urgent
No ↓		
over age 15 AND... ...constant, excruciating, "colic" type pain? — Yes →	Kidney stone (disabling pain intensity, **vomiting**)	ER
No ↓		
...mild to moderate? — Yes →	UTI, STD, renal infection (**fever**)	Urgent
No ↓		

Algorithm 9-1. (A) *(continued)*

Change in Urinary Habit

Changes in an individual's urinary frequency, particularly if sudden or progressive, can indicate a urogenital disorder. *Dysuria* (difficult urination), *nocturia* (frequent waking from sleep to urinate), unusual urgency, and *incontinence* (inability to control urinary excretions) are symptoms of urogenital pathology. *Oliguria* (very infrequent urination) and *anuria* (absence of urination) result from serious renal, urinary, or metabolic disorders and warrant referral.

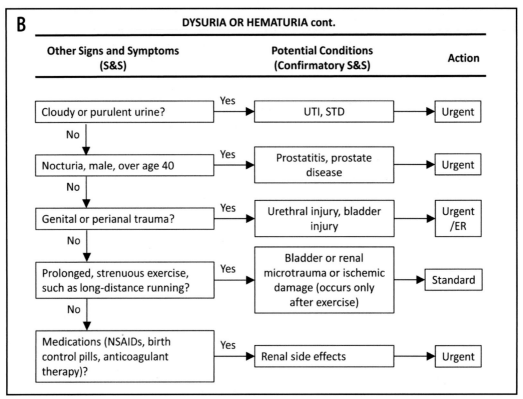

Algorithm 9-1. (B)

Nipple Discharge

Serous (watery), sanguineous (bloody), or serosanguineous (mixed) discharge may occur with breast cancer and other more benign breast conditions, such as gland infection and hormonal imbalances.[8] Patients who present with nipple discharge should be referred to a physician for evaluation.

Hypertension

High BP may be a sign of kidney pathology because of the kidneys' role in regulating BP.

Anemia

Kidney pathology may affect the production of erythropoietin, a hormone that regulates red blood cell production. The decrease in erythropoietin decreases the number of red blood cells, leading to anemia.

Sexual Dysfunction

Impotence, painful intercourse, blood in the semen (*hematospermia*), unusual vaginal bleeding during intercourse, or loss of *libido* (psychoemotional sex drive) are symptoms of urogenital pathology. Individuals reporting these symptoms should see a physician.

Menstrual Irregularities

The *menstrual cycle* is defined as the number of days between the first day of bleeding with one menstrual episode to the first day of bleeding with the next menstrual episode. Menstrual irregularities, such as increased menstrual bleeding (*menorrhagia*), changes in time between episodes of

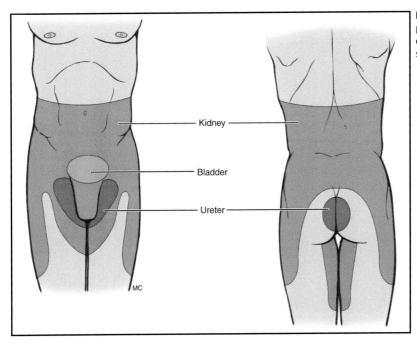

Figure 9-5. Referred pain patterns for the organs of the urogenital system.

menstruation (*metrorrhagia*), or frequency changes between episodes of menstruation (*oligomenorrhea*), can occur with pathology of the female urogenital system.

PAIN PATTERNS

Kidneys, Ureters, and Bladder

The kidneys refer pain to the ipsilateral lower back at the costovertebral angle or to the abdomen or can cause general lower abdominal pain (Figure 9-5).[9] The ureters usually cause severe pain in the groin, thigh, and abdomen.[9] Bladder pain occurs in the suprapubic region with referral to the lower back or thighs.[9]

An obstruction in a kidney or ureter, as occurs with kidney stones, produces acute intermittent pain in the abdomen and unilateral lower back that radiates to the ipsilateral lower abdominal quadrant, groin, or perineum. An obstruction in the bladder or urethra produces an aching pain in the lower abdomen.

Male Urogenital System

Testicular trauma produces a distinct, temporarily incapacitating pain. Pain persisting longer than 10 minutes suggests more serious urogenital injury. Testicular disease may refer a deep, aching pain to the lower abdomen or sacrum.[9] The prostate gland refers pain to the lower back, scrotum, or perineum.[9]

Female Urogenital System

The uterus refers pain to the middle and lower back, whereas the ovaries and fallopian tubes refer pain to the lower abdomen (suprapubic) and sacrum. Breast pain is usually localized to the affected breast but may refer symptoms into the ipsilateral axilla and upper arm.

MEDICAL HISTORY AND PHYSICAL EXAMINATION PROCEDURES

Family and Personal History

A history of an untreated urinary infection or sexually transmitted disease can cause significant long-term health problems. A family history of renal disease, such as kidney stones or personal history, of systemic disorders, such as diabetes, hypertension, or sickle cell anemia, increases the risk of urogenital system pathology. Exposure to certain toxins may also affect renal function, including heavy metals, radioactive substances, and medications such as nonsteroidal anti-inflammatory drugs, antibiotics, and narcotics.[2] The use of contraceptives, including birth control pills, should also be ascertained.

For young females, age of *menarche* (first menses) and menstrual history (pain, difficulty, regularity, etc), including the date of the last period, should be obtained if a urogenital condition is suspected.[5] A history of a family member with breast cancer, particularly with onset at an early age, is important with complaints of breast pain, mass, or discharge.[8]

Males and females should be asked whether they perform regular self-examinations when they have symptoms related to the urogenital systems. Sexual dysfunction, urethral discharge, or abnormal menses, as discussed above, are symptoms requiring medical referral.

Inspection

Edema in the extremities usually occurs in the late stages of kidney disease. Other urogenital conditions present few signs that would be noticeable on gross inspection.

Palpation

The kidneys, particularly the right kidney, can sometimes be palpated in the posterior thorax, near the vertebral column just below the costal border of the twelfth rib, at the costovertebral angle. Tenderness to palpation at this location is abnormal. Pain reproduced by percussion (or "hammering") directly over the kidney indicates inflammation, infection, or injury.

The athletic trainer relies on history, symptoms, and other signs to raise suspicion of pathology in the genital system. If necessary, the person can be instructed to perform a self-examination and report the findings.

Urinalysis

Hematuria (blood in urine), *proteinuria* (protein in urine), and *glucosuria* (glucose in urine) can be detected through a urinalysis performed microscopically in a laboratory or clinically using chemical test strips. Although athletic trainers are not trained in performing laboratory urinalyses, they can use urine test strips to perform screening urinalyses to identify persons with possible pathology, such as during preparticipation physical examinations. A screening urinalysis can also be used to check for ketones or glucose in an athlete with diabetes who is having difficulty regulating the disease. Specific gravity can be assessed through urinalysis to determine levels of hydration.

Urinalysis test kits can be purchased to test urine concentration levels in a variety of substances. Table 9-1 provides a summary of the more common substances tested and their associated pathology. The test strips are thin plastic strips that contain square pads impregnated with specific chemicals that are designed to react with specific substances in urine (Figure 9-6). Although these test strips are not as accurate as microscopic tests or refractometer assessment, they are convenient and easy to use in screening patients for pathology such as dehydration, urinary tract infections, kidney injuries, and complications associated with diabetes (eg, ketoacidosis). A *clean catch (midstream) urine sample* provides the most accurate test results as it avoids the collection of contaminants or bacteria that might be present on the skin and be carried into the initial urine flow. To obtain a clean

Table 9-1. Urinalysis Test Substances and Associated Pathology

TEST	POSSIBLE PATHOLOGY
Specific gravity	Normal levels range from 01.002 to 01.029. Increased specific gravity is associated with increased concentration of solutes and dehydration. Decreased levels are associated with excessive fluid intake.
pH	Urine pH ranges from 4.5 to 8 with 7 being considered neutral. pH > 7 is considered alkaline, pH < 7 considered acidic. Alkaline urine is associated with the following: • Urinary tract obstruction • Hyperventilation • Chronic renal failure • Salicylate (aspirin) intoxication Acidic urine is associated with the following: • Acidosis • Uncontrolled diabetes • Dehydration • Vomiting • Diarrhea
Leukocytes	Presence of leukocytes in the urine suggests possible infection.
Protein	The presence of greater than trace amounts of protein in the urine is associated with kidney disease. Presence of protein in the urine warrants referral to a physician.
Glucose	Associated with excessive levels of glucose in the blood (hyperglycemia).

(continued)

catch urine sample, male patients should wipe the head of the penis and female patients should wipe between the labia (front to back) with a prepackaged sterile wipe. Patients should be instructed to urinate a small amount into the toilet and then place the sterile urine cup into the urine stream. After collecting 1 to 2 ounces of urine, the cup is removed from the stream without stopping the flow. The patient then secures the lid on the urine cup.

The athletic trainer should apply gloves prior to handling the urine specimen. The cup should be placed on a flat, firm surface to prevent spilling. The chemically treated end of the reagent test strip is inserted fully into the urine specimen for 1 second and then promptly removed. The test strip should be tapped on the edge of the urine cup to remove any extra drops of urine and then blotted with a paper towel or other absorbent material to further remove excess urine. Excess urine on the test strip can cause mixing of the reagent chemicals from the different test pads, affecting the accuracy of the test. After 60 seconds, the color of the pads on the test strip should be compared to the color indicator chart on the bottle (see Figure 9-6, color indicator posters are also available). Leukocytes require a wait of 120 seconds (depending on the kit used) before color comparison. Minor traces of blood in the urine are normal in females during their menstruation cycles.

In addition to the urinalysis test values, changes in the color, odor, or volume of urine may also indicate a urinary disorder. Urine is normally a pale yellow, but will darken considerably as fluid content decreases or relative concentration of solute increases. Red or brownish urine usually

Table 9-1 (continued). Urinalysis Test Substances and Associated Pathology

TEST	POSSIBLE PATHOLOGY
Glucose	Associated with excessive levels of glucose in the blood (hyperglycemia).
Ketones	Ketones are by-products of fat metabolism and can be present in urine as a result of the following: • Diabetic ketoacidosis • Anorexia (or other form of starvation) • Excessive vomiting • High-protein/low-carbohydrate diets The presence of ketones in a patient with diabetes warrants an injection of insulin.
Blood (hemoglobin)	The presence of greater than trace amounts of blood is associated with kidney or bladder injury. This warrants a referral to a physician.
Nitrite	Positive test for nitrite indicates the presence of bacteria.
Urobilinogen	Normal values range from 0 to 8 mg/dL. Increased values suggest liver pathology (eg, infection, cirrhosis). Decreased values suggest blockage of bile passage or decreased bile production.
Bilirubin	Bilirubin is a yellowish pigment found in bile. Positive test indicates possible liver or gallbladder pathology such as: • Gallstones • Cirrhosis of the liver • Hepatitis • Liver tumor

indicates the presence of blood, hemoglobin, myoglobin, bilirubin, or other metabolic proteins and is therefore never normal.[2] Of note, over-the-counter medications to help with urinary symptoms such as Azo can also change the urine color red and interfere with a urinalysis. A clouded or milky appearance indicates infection, which is usually accompanied by a foul or strong odor.[2] Any abnormal test values or discoloration should be followed up by a physician.

Refractometry

A handheld refractometer is easy to use and provides a more accurate and objective measure of urine specific gravity for determining an individual's hydration status (Figure 9-7).[10] *Urine specific gravity* is a measure of urine density, or the kidneys' ability to concentrate or dilute urine. Normal urine specific gravity values in healthy adults range from 1.013 to 1.029.[11,12] Urine specific gravity values greater than 1.030 indicate dehydration, whereas values between 1.001 and 1.012 indicate hyperhydration.

Using a refractometer to measure urine specific gravity requires the collection of a urine sample (following the same procedures as those described above for performing a urinalysis). The refractometer can be calibrated by placing a few drops of distilled water on the stage of the device and then pointing the view piece toward a light source. The scale should be adjusted to 1.000. Once

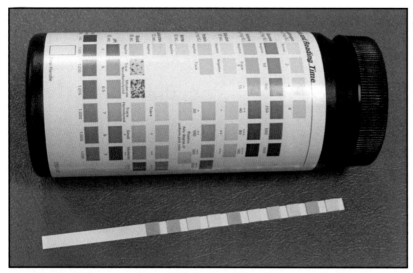

Figure 9-6. Urinalysis test strips and color indicator chart.

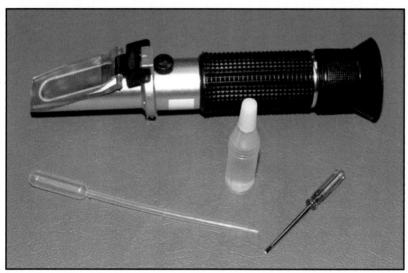

Figure 9-7. Refractometer for measuring urine specific gravity.

calibrated and the glass plate has been wiped with a clean cloth, 1 to 2 drops of urine can be placed on the glass plate and covered with the flap. The refractometer is again pointed to the light source while the examiner looks through the view piece and reads the scale for specific gravity. Currently, there are no standardized protocols for using urine specific gravity for hydration replenishment.

PATHOLOGY AND PATHOGENESIS

Renal and Bladder Trauma

A direct blow to the middle or lower back, a sudden deceleration of the trunk, or a fractured rib can injure the kidney. The hallmark of renal injury is hematuria, as bleeding in the kidney passes into the urine.[13] Tenderness or swelling may appear in the back, over ribs 10 through 12. Grossly observable blood in the urine after a blow to the back or other abdominal trauma requires emergency medical imaging and diagnostic studies.

Most kidney trauma can be treated without surgery but needs close medical monitoring. Return to sports is slow, usually taking at least 6 to 8 weeks before evidence of healing is observable on

Table 9-2. Signs and Symptoms of Urinary Tract Infection by Site of Colonization

SITE	SIGNS AND SYMPTOMS
Urethra	Dysuria, discharge
Bladder	Dysuria, urgency, decreased urine volume, nocturia, back pain, pyuria or hematuria
Prostate	Fever, urgency, back pain, dysuria, nocturia, hematuria
Kidney	Fever, back pain, vomiting, costovertebral tenderness

medical imaging.[13] Collision and contact sports may be contraindicated for persons who have only a single kidney.[14] This decision should be made by either the athlete's physician or the team physician.

The urethra and bladder may also sustain trauma during physical activity; however, significant bladder injuries are rare in athletics. The bladder is more commonly injured in high-energy trauma, such as a car accident. Hematuria and pain in the lower abdomen usually occur with bladder injuries.

Urethral bleeding happens with traumatic impact of the genitals or perineum. If inflammation obstructs the urethra, surgery to drain urine and hospitalization until healed are indicated.[13] The immediate course of action includes application of ice packs and physician referral.

Renal and Bladder Infections

Urinary Tract Infections

Urinary tract infections (UTIs) are very common and can be caused by bacteria, fungi, or parasites. Bacterial infection is by far the most prevalent type of UTI. Regardless of the type of invading organism, possible consequences include urethritis (inflamed urethra), cystitis (inflamed bladder), prostatitis (inflamed prostate), and pyelonephritis (inflamed kidney) as the organism progresses up the urinary tract. Symptomatic infection with yeast (*Candida albicans*), which causes vulvar irritation, is very common in women. Men can carry and transmit yeast infections while remaining asymptomatic, so sexual partners may need to be treated to prevent repeat infections. Signs and symptoms of UTIs depend on the primary site of colonization in the urinary tract (Table 9-2). Treatment consists of antibiotics or antifungal medications, as well as analgesics or antipruritics (itch inhibitors) to control symptoms.

Renal Disorders

Nephrolithiasis

Nephrolithiasis, commonly known as kidney stones, results when excess insoluble salts, calcium, or uric acid enter the kidney filtrate. Because these substances cannot be excreted in the urine, they collect in the kidney and form solid masses. When these stones grow large enough to block the flow of urine or irritate the urinary tract, sudden severe pain appears as the renal tubules or capsule becomes distended with urine.

History will be negative for trauma. The characteristic clinical presentation is severe, with unilateral pain in the lower back and abdomen that radiates around the flank and into the anterior thigh.[4] Vomiting, pallor, and tachycardia may also be noted. Signs of shock (decreased BP and rapid, weak pulse) will not be present since no internal hemorrhaging occurs.

Small kidney stones (< 5 mm) are treated with pain medication and hydration; the hydration increases urine output, which helps to pass the stones out of the body. In addition, there are new medications such as tamsulosin (Flomax) which may be given to expedite the excretion of the small stone. Large stones (>5 mm) or stones that are accompanied with infectious symptoms may need to be fragmented by sound, shock (lithotripsy), or light (laser) treatments. Recovery is usually complete, although recurrences are not uncommon. Risk of kidney stones decreases with proper diet and hydration.[4] Risk factors may include high animal protein diet, excessive vitamin C/D, low fluids, sugar-sweetened beverages, alcoholic beverages.

Renal Failure

Acute renal failure occurs as a result of toxins or acute obstruction of the ureter.[4] Signs include sudden weight gain, generalized edema, hypertension, and signs of left-sided heart failure (see Chapter 6).[2] These signs are the result of the kidneys failing to remove water and waste products from the bloodstream. Water and waste products accumulate in the blood, producing hypertension and left-sided heart failure, and eventually must be moved from the blood into the interstitial tissues, producing edema and weight gain. Causes of acute renal failure in the athletic population may include rhabdomyolysis, dehydration, and nonsteroidal anti-inflammatory drug overuse.

Chronic renal failure is unlikely among physically active persons. As a complication of diabetes, hypertension, or other kidney disease, however, chronic renal failure is not uncommon among the American population. Diabetes and hypertension irreparably damage the nephrons, as does chronic kidney disease. Once the nephrons are damaged, the function of the kidney is permanently impaired and chronic renal failure results. In early stages, chronic renal failure may be asymptomatic. As the disease progresses, nocturia, hypertension, gastrointestinal symptoms, impaired cognitive function, neurological changes (decreased reflexes, paresthesias), bone degeneration, muscle dysfunction, and cardiovascular complications gradually occur as waste products normally filtered out by the kidney accumulate and damage other organs.[4] Chronic renal failure is not curable because damaged kidney cells cannot regenerate.

Male Urogenital Disorders

Monorchidism

Monorchidism, or the absence of one testicle, congenitally occurs in 0.02% (1 in 5000) of males, but can also be traumatically acquired.[15] Monorchidism should not exclude a male from contact sports; however, it does necessitate the need for wearing a protective cup.[14] More rarely, complete absence of both testicles or the presence of more than 2 testicles occurs.[15] Decisions regarding sports participation in these conditions should be deferred to a urologist or endocrinologist.

Prostate Disorders

Prostate disorders often gradually produce symptoms that are related to chronic or acute inflammation (*prostatitis*). The prevalence of prostate disorders increases with age. The most frequent cause of prostatitis is infection, although it can occur with cancer or other urogenital disease.[4] Dysuria, painful urination, an increase in urinary urgency and frequency, and nocturia are common symptoms.[4] In addition, a dull ache may develop in the lower back or sacrum. The gland also enlarges with age (benign prostatic hypertrophy), causing the signs and symptoms to recur chronically.[4] Acute bacterial prostatitis can occur with cystitis, urethritis, and other infections and is more common in the younger male population. The bacterial most commonly associated with this include *E. Coli*, *Proteus* species, and sexually-transmitted infections such as *Neisseria gonorrhoeae* and *Chlamydia trachomatis*. These patients are typically ill and require extended duration of antibiotic therapy. Return to play decisions are based on symptoms.[16]

Prostate Cancer

Prostate cancer is primarily a disease of aging males and becomes progressively more prevalent each decade after age 40 years. Prostate cancer is the most common cancer among men (after skin cancer).[17] Prostate cancer causes the second most cancer deaths among men, after lung cancer; the lifetime risk of prostate cancer is 1 in 6 men, and 1 in 36 men will die of the disease. More than 230,000 cases are diagnosed each year, and prostate cancer causes almost 30,000 deaths per year.[17] As of 2013, there were more than 2 million prostate cancer survivors living in the United States.[17] Although the etiology is unknown, prostate cancer is more prevalent in the Black race than in any other races. Also, males with a history of a first-degree relative (father or brother) with prostate cancer are twice as likely to develop the disease. Other risk factors include smoking, obesity, and a diet high in red meat or dairy fat.

Metastases to the spine, pelvis, hips, lung, and liver are very common and are often the first indication of prostate cancer. As tumor size increases, the urethra becomes progressively obstructed and urinary function becomes impaired. Pain in the low back, hips, and upper thighs, along with dysuria and nocturia, suggest prostate enlargement in middle-aged men, which may be a result of prostate cancer or benign prostate changes with age (benign prostatic hypertrophy). The American Cancer Society recommends annual prostate screening tests via *prostate-specific antigen* in males aged 50 years and older or aged 45 years for men at high risk. A digital rectal examination has been shown in recent studies to have low sensitivity and low specificity in detecting abnormalities in the prostate gland. A history of diagnosed prostate cancer increases the probability of vertebral metas- tasis. If history is suspicious for prostate involvement, the person should be referred to his physician for X-rays and medical testing. A diagnosis of prostate cancer is made through biopsy. Depending on the stage of the disease, treatment may include surgery, radiation, chemotherapy, or hormone therapy. The 5-year survival rate for prostate cancer that has not metastasized is nearly 100%; the 5-year survival rate drops to 34% once the cancer has metastasized.

Scrotum and Testicular Trauma

The scrotum is vulnerable to trauma in sports, necessitating the use of a protective cup. Unfortunately, male athletes often refuse to use a cup consistently. Most scrotum trauma is relatively benign, even though the initial trauma may produce excruciating testicular pain. Scrotal or testicu- lar pain that does not improve in 10 minutes is highly suspicious of a more serious injury, such as testicular torsion which requires a referral to an emergent medical setting.

Testicular Torsion

Testicular torsion occurs primarily during late childhood or adolescence because the still- developing scrotum may allow rotation of the testicle and its connective tissue capsule.[15] When this rotation occurs, the spermatic cord twists, compressing arteries and veins and causing ischemia of the affected testicle.[4]

A history of trauma or previous torsion may or may not be present.[13] Table 9-3 compares benign scrotum trauma with the clinical presentation of testicular torsion. Nausea and vomiting are also common.[15] The twisted spermatic cord elevates the affected testicle from its normal position; the athlete can perform a self-examination to detect this change. Emergency surgery is necessary to save the testicle, even if spontaneous or manual "derotation" occurs.[15]

Varicoceles

Varicose veins in the scrotum (*varicoceles*) occur most commonly in adolescents and cause a sensation of heaviness or tenderness.[4,15] Varicoceles are caused by faulty valves in the veins that run alongside the spermatic cord. The faulty valves allow blood flow to back up in the veins, causing them to increase in diameter. Varicoceles range in diameter from 1 to 2 cm, are more prominent when standing, and may be described as a "bag of worms."[15] Surgical correction may be necessary because varicoceles do not spontaneously regress and may lead to fertility problems.[15] Trauma may produce a testicular *hydrocele*, or a fluid-filled sac, which produces similar signs and symptoms to varicocele, but with sudden onset after trauma. Medical referral is warranted both for varicoceles and hydroceles.

Table 9-3. Simple Scrotum Trauma Versus Testicular Torsion

	SCROTUM TRAUMA	TESTICULAR TORSION
PAIN	Bilateral, lasting less than 10 minutes	Unilateral, lasting longer than 10 minutes
SCROTUM SWELLING	None	Progressive
NAUSEA/VOMITING	None or very brief nausea	Increasing nausea and eventual vomiting
TESTICULAR POSITION	Normal	Unilateral elevation

Testicular Cancer

Testicular cancer is the most common cancer among males aged 15 to 35 years; approximately 8000 new cases are diagnosed each year. Although primarily genetic in nature, a history of cryptorchidism (undescended testicle) is a risk factor for developing testicular cancer. White males are 5 times more likely to develop testicular cancer than Black males. Although usually detectable on regular self-exam as a progressive, unilateral testicular swelling or nodule, the disease may go unrecognized until metastases to the spine cause back pain or other symptoms such as abdominal pain, fatigue, weight loss, or nausea. The American Cancer Society recommends that males perform monthly testicular self-examinations (TSEs) starting at age 15 years (Figure 9-8) for high risk males. Other societies now do not recommend for testicular cancer screening. Table 9-4 summarizes the steps for correctly performing a TSE.

Testicular cancer is curable. Treatment is based on the stage of the disease and usually includes surgery, radiation, and chemotherapy. Early detection is critical for long-term survival; the 5-year survival rate for non-metastatic testicular cancer is greater than 99%. Metastases to the spine have a worse prognosis, with survival rates dropping below 75%.

Female Urogenital Disorders

Menstrual Dysfunction

Amenorrhea is defined as the absence of menstruation[18] and can be classified as primary or secondary. Primary amenorrhea is when *menarche* (first menses) fails to occur by age 16 years. The most common causes are hormonal imbalance, genetic disorders, and reproductive organ diseases.[19,20] If the patient is not already receiving medical care, referral to a pediatrician or gynecologist is appropriate. *Secondary amenorrhea* is defined as fewer than 3 cycles per year or lack of menstruation for 3 consecutive months.[5,6,18] Possible causes of secondary amenorrhea include pregnancy, severe dietary restriction, hormonal imbalance, and excessive exercise. Adolescents display a wide variation in regularity and intensity of menses, but amenorrhea (primary or secondary) in young, healthy females is not normal and requires a medical evaluation.[21]

Oligomenorrhea refers to infrequent menstruation and is defined by cycles in excess of 35 days.[22] *Dysmenorrhea* is disabling pain or discomfort that occurs with menstruation. *Premenstrual syndrome* is a complex of physical and psychological signs and symptoms that occurs several days before menstruation. In premenstrual syndrome, the specific signs and symptoms, as well as their intensity and duration, varies from woman to woman. Treatment focuses on identifying the underlying etiology in addition to diet and lifestyle changes.

Figure 9-8. Testicular self-examination.

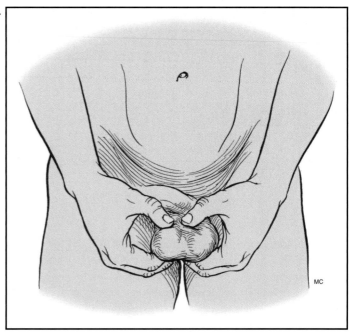

Endometriosis

Endometriosis occurs when endometrial tissue grows outside of the uterus and is most common between age 30 and 40 years.[4] The etiology is unknown. Menstruation becomes painful and the volume of menstrual discharge increases. Painful intercourse and pain in the lower back are also usually reported. Fibrosis and infertility can result, so prompt referral is important. Treatment consists of hormone therapy or surgery.[4] Recognition of disproportionate or refractory pain with menstruation or unusual pain patterns with menstruation should warrant referrals to a physician.

Pregnancy

Pregnancy involves significant anatomical and physiological changes that occur over time. This time period is divided into 2 distinct phases: prenatal and postpartum. The prenatal phase includes the time period between conception and birth and typically lasts a little more than 9 months. The prenatal period is further divided into 3 fairly equal trimesters. The postpartum phase begins immediately after birth and lasts approximately 6 weeks.[23]

Early signs and symptoms, which are caused by higher-than-normal levels of estrogen and progesterone in the bloodstream, are often the first indication of pregnancy. Initial symptoms include amenorrhea; recurrent nausea and vomiting, referred to as "morning sickness"; fatigue; and abdominal bloating. Other signs and symptoms appear as pregnancy advances and the size of the fetus increases, including frequent urination, hypotension in the supine position, peripheral neurovascular occlusion syndromes (from fluid retention and edema), and breast enlargement and tenderness. A weight gain of 25 to 30 pounds during the course of a pregnancy is normal but may cause increased fatigue and musculoskeletal strain syndromes.[24]

Resting heart rate (HR) increases early in pregnancy and increases to as much as 15 beats per minute (bpm) over normal throughout the pregnancy.[24] BP, however, progressively decreases and is lower by 8 to 10 mm Hg by the 20th week. The decrease in BP is exacerbated in the supine position, so exercise in this position should be avoided after the fourth month.[24] As a precaution, pregnant women should be taught the symptoms of rapidly decreasing BP, including dizziness, syncope, and nausea, so they can change positions to restore BP.

Table 9-4. Testicular Self-Examination

1. The TSE should be performed right after a hot bath or shower when the skin of the scrotum is relaxed and soft.
2. Become familiar with the normal size, shape, and feel of each testicle.
3. Standing in front of a mirror, check for swelling of the scrotum.
4. Using both hands, cup the index and middle fingers under each testicle with the thumbs on top.
5. Gently roll each testicle between the thumb and fingers. (One testicle may be larger than the other; however, this is normal.)
6. Identify the epididymis, which will feel like a rope-like or tube-like structure on the top and back of each testicle. (This structure is normal and should not be mistaken for a lump.)
7. Feel for any abnormal lumps. This tissue will feel like a piece of uncooked rice or small peanut.
8. Any lump or swelling detected during TSE should be reported to a physician.

The physician managing the woman's prenatal care should be consulted before recommending any type of exercise or rehabilitation program. Regular physical activity has been shown to be beneficial both to the mother and developing fetus. Exercise regimen changes should not be altered during pregnancy other than for medical indications. However, exercise may be contraindicated for pregnant women who have diabetes, hypertension, a history of miscarriage, or the presence of multiple fetuses.[19,25]

The American College of Obstetrics and Gynecology recommends that women with low-risk pregnancies exercise 30 minutes or more per day, up to 7 days a week.[26] For women who were active prior to becoming pregnant, aerobic intensity can be set at 50% to 75% of the age-predicted maximum HR.[27] However, it should be noted that during the second and third trimesters, resting HR can increase by 15 bpm, making HR a potentially unreliable indicator for determining exercise intensity. For this reason, the American College of Sports Medicine (ACSM) recommends that healthy pregnant women use the Rating of Perceived Exertion scale to establish their level of intensity rather than HR. Women with low-risk pregnancies are recommended to exercise at a moderate intensity level, which would be 12 to 14 (somewhat hard) on the 6 to 20 perceived exertion scale.[28] In general, women should not exceed the intensity levels that they used prior to their pregnancy. Pregnancy is not the time to seek significant increases in fitness levels but rather is a time to maintain an active lifestyle. To prevent complications, the duration and intensity of exercise sessions should be adjusted to avoid injury (due to increased strain from weight gain and change in center of gravity), elevation of core body temperature, energy deficits (ie, depletion of blood glucose), or dehydration.[19,25,28] Ideally, women should exercise in a thermo-neutral environment (ie, air conditioning) during pregnancy. If exercising outdoors in the heat, the duration should be reduced to 15-minute sessions. Sedentary women need an additional 300 kcal per day to meet the energy needs associated with pregnancy. Therefore, pregnant women who are exercising regularly will need to increase their caloric intake by more than 300 kcal per day.[28] To ensure that adequate hydration is maintained when exercising during pregnancy, women should weigh themselves before and after their workout. For every 1 pound lost, 1 pint (16 ounces or 500 mL) of fluid should be consumed.

The NCAA has a published guideline that recommends avoidance of contact and collision sports and urges the pregnant athlete in noncontact sports to continue at sub-competitive intensities; it also recommends that if a pregnant athlete chooses to compete, she should sign an informed consent about the risks and her institution should obtain approval from her personal physician, the team physician, and an institutional official.[29] Athletic trainers working in a university or high

Table 9-5. Signs and Symptoms Warranting the Cessation of Exercise During Pregnancy

Vaginal bleeding	Calf pain or swelling
Shortness of breath before exercise	Preterm labor
Dizziness	Decreased fetal movement
Headache	Amniotic fluid leakage
Chest pain	Muscle weakness

Adapted from Klossner D, ed. NCAA guideline 2q: pregnancy in the student-athlete. *NCAA Sports Medicine Handbook.* National Collegiate Athletic Association; 2012-2013. © National Collegiate Athletic Association. 2013. All rights reserved.

school setting should be familiar with their institutions' policies regarding pregnant athletes. Table 9-5 provides a list of signs and symptoms that warrant the termination of exercise in a pregnant athlete.[30]

The circulating concentration of the hormone *relaxin* increases substantially during pregnancy. Relaxin increases the extensibility of connective tissues, such as ligaments, which will allow for expansion of the pelvic girdle during labor and delivery. Relaxin also makes skeletal joints susceptible to injury during physical activity and thereby prohibits vigorous sports participation. Precaution is also needed during manual therapy techniques, such as joint mobilization.

Returning to a "regular" exercise regimen may take several months after delivery. Physical changes of pregnancy often persist up to 6 weeks postpartum.[19] Activities to avoid in the immediate postpartum stage include: exercise in hot, humid weather (dehydration); high-impact or high-intensity exercise; excessive stretching or joint motions (due to relaxin); and sudden changes in posture (orthostatic hypotension).[24] An additional 400 to 600 kcal per day may be required for women who are breastfeeding to meet their basic metabolic demands.[24] This caloric intake increases with additional physical activity.

Ruptured Ectopic Pregnancy

An ectopic pregnancy occurs when a fertilized ovum attaches outside of the uterus, usually in a fallopian tube. The usual signs of pregnancy may or may not occur. When the embryo grows large enough, it ruptures the tube and causes severe internal hemorrhaging. The first indication of the pregnancy may not occur until the embryo ruptures. Ruptured ectopic pregnancy produces acute, lacerating lower abdominal pain with lower quadrant tenderness, vaginal bleeding, syncope, and shock.[31] Syncope associated with abdominal pain in a female of childbearing age always requires prompt medical attention.[31] An embryo implanted ectopically has no chance of surviving. The condition may be life threatening for the mother unless emergency surgery is performed.[31] Recognition of systemic signs and symptoms of acute abdominal pain warrants prompt referral to a physician or an emergency room setting.

Female Athlete Triad

The *female athlete triad* was originally described as the simultaneous presence of disordered eating, amenorrhea, and osteoporosis in an otherwise healthy woman.[5,6] With their 2007 position statement, the ACSM redefined this triad to be a syndrome composed of 3 interrelated spectra that can range in severity along a continuum: energy availability, menstrual function, and bone mineral density (BMD).[22] Energy availability can be defined as caloric balance, or the difference between caloric intake and caloric expenditure. Low energy availability can occur intentionally through severe calorie restriction or unintentionally by honestly failing to take in enough calories to offset the energy demands of a high-intensity workout session. Intentional efforts to produce a negative caloric balance can range from occasional fasting to binge eating and purging to anorexia. The spectrum of menstrual function can range from eumenorrhea (normal menses) to amenorrhea. The spectrum of BMD can range from normal to osteopenia to osteoporosis.

The ACSM recommends that athletes be screened for female athlete triad during their preparticipation examination.[22,32] Also, BMD should be assessed in any female athlete who experiences a stress fracture or with any woman who is known to be 6 months post-diagnosis of an eating disorder.[22] Treatment of the triad requires a multidisciplinary team composed of a physician or other health care provider (ie, physician assistant or nurse practitioner), a registered dietician, and a mental health professional (for those with an eating disorder).[22,32] Treatment should focus on increasing caloric intake and reducing the caloric expenditure by reducing the intensity and duration of the individual's exercise.

Breast Disorders

In an adult woman, breast masses, changes in breast shape or resiliency, tenderness, or discharge warrant referral to a physician, particularly if the woman has a positive family history of breast cancer. However, most cases of breast cancer have no history. In adolescents, however, some breast changes, including tender lumps detected during self-examination, are often benign.[8] The proper term for these benign breast changes is *proliferative breast changes*, formerly called *fibrocystic breast disease*. Small multiple lumps accompanied by cyclic pain (pain associated with the menstrual cycle) are common with proliferative breast changes. Genetic and hormonal factors are linked to the development of these changes.[8] Most cases of proliferative breast changes have no adverse long-term health consequences; however, any new lump found on self-examination should be evaluated by a physician. Treatment of benign breast lesions is usually observation, aspiration or core biopsy, or surgical excision.[8]

Breast pain may be a result of direct trauma or repetitive strain from activities such as running with poor support.[13] Ice is recommended following a painful blow to the breast. Anti-inflammatories should be avoided because they may increase bleeding and subsequent scarring. Use of a sports bra can prevent repetitive strain injuries caused by sprain of the suspensory (Cooper's) ligaments of the breast.[13]

Breast Cancer

Breast cancer is the most common malignancy among women. One in 8 women will be diagnosed with breast cancer at some point in their lifetime. Approximately 268,600 cases are diagnosed each year, nearly 2600 of which are among men, and around 40,000 deaths a year are attributable to breast cancer. As of 2019, it was estimated that there were approximately 3.1 million breast cancer survivors living in the United States.[33] A positive family history increases risk and is associated with an earlier age of onset.[34] Hormonal factors are also involved because women who experienced an early onset of menarche, have never been pregnant, have a first child after age 35 years, or did not breast-feed their children, all of which affect estrogen and progesterone levels, are at increased risk.[34] Other risk factors for developing breast cancer include having the *BRCA1* or *BRCA2* gene mutation, being overweight, smoking, excessive alcohol consumption (2 to 5 drinks daily), and physical inactivity. Breast cancer typically occurs in women over age 40 years, but appearance at an earlier age usually indicates greater severity of the disease.

The first physical sign of breast cancer is a palpable lump in the breast tissue.[34,35] In addition, the breast may be unusually tender, display dimpling, or produce discharge from the nipple.[35] Common sites of metastasis from breast cancer include the bones of the ribs, vertebrae, or hips.[34] The American Cancer Society previously recommended monthly breast self-examinations (BSEs) beginning by age 20 years (Figure 9-9) but currently does not recommend this screening modality. Table 9-6 summarizes the proper steps for performing a BSE. Approximately 90% of breast lesions are discovered in this manner. Women between 40 and 44 should be given the option to start

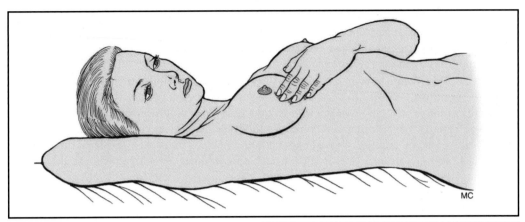

Figure 9-9. Breast self-examination. (A) Supine. (B) Standing.

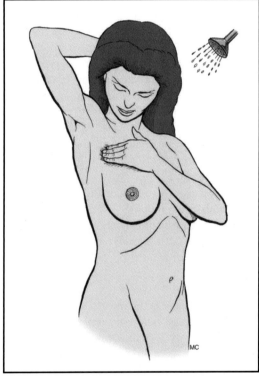

screening with mammography ever year and becomes standard between age 45 to 54. After the age 55, mammography should be utilized every other year until life expectancy decreases to under 10 years.[33] Mammography and other imaging tests may be able to identify breast cancer before it becomes a palpable tumor. Definitive diagnosis of breast cancer requires a biopsy to obtain sample tissue.

Depending on the stage of the disease, breast cancer is generally treated with either a lumpectomy (removal of the tumor) or a mastectomy (removal of the entire breast and underlying muscle tissue). Also, depending on the stage of the cancer, chemotherapy and radiation therapy are often part of the overall treatment plan. If the tumor is estrogen and progesterone positive (ER/PR+; meaning the tumor's growth was stimulated by estrogen and progesterone hormones), breast cancer patients will also be treated with estrogen suppressants such as tamoxifen. Unfortunately, for these patients, maintaining low levels of estrogen can lead to other health complications, such as decreased BMD and osteoporosis.

Table 9-6. Breast Self-Examination

1. Lie supine with a pillow under the right shoulder and the right arm behind the head.
2. Use the finger pads of the 3 middle fingers on the left hand to feel for lumps in the right breast.
3. Press firmly enough to feel the tissue below the skin.
4. Check the entire breast area following either a vertical or circular pattern (be consistent with each evaluation).
5. Repeat the evaluation on the left breast, using the finger pads of the right hand.
6. Repeat the evaluation of both breasts while standing, with one arm again placed behind the head. The upright position makes it easier to check the upper outer part of the breasts (toward the axilla). Approximately 50% of breast cancers are found in this area. The standing examination can be performed in the shower. Soapy hands allow the hands to glide over the wet skin, making it easier to detect abnormal lumps.
7. After completing the BSE, inspect the breasts by standing in front of a mirror looking for any changes in appearance, such as dimpling of the skin, changes in the nipple, changes in contour, redness, or swelling.

Breast cancer in early stages is curable, with 5-year survival rate of 99% for localized breast cancer. For invasive breast cancer, the 5-year and 10-year survival rates are 90% and 83%, respectively.

Ovarian Cysts

Fibrous cysts (vascularized, fluid-filled sacs) can form within the female urogenital system, including the ovaries.[4] Although usually asymptomatic and benign, occasionally they cause significant health problems. *Ovarian cysts* may cause unusual bleeding or interfere with the menstrual cycle. If ovarian cysts are large or numerous (polycystic ovary syndrome), they may interfere with normal estrogen production, causing coarse hair to grow on the chest and face (*hirsutism*).[4] Although many ovarian cysts will resolve on their own, others may require surgical removal. Furthermore, ovarian cysts can also rupture, producing sudden and severe internal hemorrhaging. Ruptured ovarian cysts lead to acute lower quadrant abdominal pain, peritonitis, shock, and, occasionally, death.[4,36,37] Recognition of abrupt onset of lower abdominal pain often following sexual intercourse warrants referral to a physician depending om systemic symptoms.[38]

911

Cervical, Ovarian, and Uterine Cancers

Cancers of the female reproductive system occur primarily in women older than age 45 years and are typically asymptomatic until metastases exist. These cancers vary with respect to prevalence and survival rates. *Cervical cancer* is diagnosed in about 10,000 women and causes more than 3700 deaths each year. The 5-year survival rates for the early stages range from 80% to 90%; the rate decreases to below 20% for advanced disease. *Ovarian cancer* is diagnosed in about 22,000 women and causes 16,000 deaths each year. The 5-year survival early in the disease is 90%, but decreases to 20% in the most advanced stage. *Uterine cancer* is diagnosed in 40,000 women and causes more than 7000 deaths each year. The 5-year survival rate is 50% in the earliest stage and decreases below 10% for advanced uterine cancers.

Unusual vaginal bleeding or discharge may be the only indication of cancer in these organs. Early pre-cancerous changes of the cervix can be detected during routine medical examination with a medical test called a Pap smear, which resulted in much higher survival rates than were observed in the mid-20th century. Risk factors for these cancers include a history of numerous sexual partners, postmenopausal estrogen supplementation, endocrine disorders, never becoming pregnant, family history, and an age of 40 years or older.[35,39] Presence of the human papillomavirus (HPV) is also associated with cervical cancer, and HPV vaccination in preadolescent girls before they become sexually active has been recommended for prevention.

Sexually Transmitted Infections

Sexually transmitted infections (STIs) are communicated to sexual partners by direct contact with genital wounds or body fluids. These diseases can infect the rectum, eyes, and mouth in addition to the genitals. Use of condoms reduces the risk of contracting an STI, although they do not guarantee prevention. Contact of any mucous membrane with contaminated fluids or lesions greatly increases the probability of infection. There are several common STIs: gonorrhea, chlamydia, syphilis, genital warts, herpes, and pelvic inflammatory disease. Each condition is discussed next.

Gonorrhea

Bacteria (*Neisseria gonorrhoeae*) that cause gonorrhea incubate for 1 to 3 weeks, then induce purulent urethral discharge and painful dysuria. Other mucous membranes (mouth, throat, eyes, rectum) may be infected, producing pain, erythema, edema, or purulent exudate in those areas. A significant portion of infected people experience no symptoms themselves but are contagious and can transmit the organism to others. Gonorrhea often coexists with other STIs, such as chlamydia and syphilis. Vigorous and meticulous medical care is necessary to address gonorrhea and all comorbid infections. Sexual contact with others must be strictly avoided until the infection is eliminated. Recent (previous 3 to 6 months) sexual partners must be contacted and reported to the state health department in order to get them examined and/or treated.

Chlamydia

Chlamydia (*Chlamydia trachomatis*), estimated to be the most common STI, is a bacterial infection with an incubation period of 1 to 4 weeks in men. Infected women, although usually asymptomatic, transmit the bacteria to their sexual partners. Symptoms include painful dysuria and clear or purulent urethral discharge. Similar to gonorrhea, other mucous membranes may be affected. Treatment is by antibiotics and screening for comorbid STI. Abstention from sexual activity is required until infection resolves. Recent (3 to 6 months) sexual partners must be contacted, examined, and treated.

Syphilis

Syphilis is caused by yet another bacterium (*Treponema pallidum*) that invades the urogenital system during sexual contact, although the organism ultimately infects other systems, such as nervous and cardiovascular. Symptoms may not occur for up to 3 months after initial exposure. A painless epithelial lesion on the region exposed to the bacteria, called a *chancre*, appears and spontaneously resolves within 2 months. Inguinal lymphadenitis may occur, but the nodes are usually not tender and may not be noticed. A skin rash erupts within 2 months and may persist for 2 to 3 additional months. Low-grade fever, fatigue, headache, loss of appetite, and myalgia may also appear during this stage.

If untreated, the disease goes into remission, becoming asymptomatic sometimes for decades. Invasion of bone, skin, myocardium, or the central nervous system eventually occurs, leading to serious and irreversible changes to those systems. Cardiac and central nervous system complications are the most severe, disabling, and ultimately fatal. Treatment begins with early recognition and consists of appropriate antibiotic therapy and identification of coexisting STIs.

Genital Warts

Various papillomaviruses (HPV 6 and 11 mostly) cause *genital warts*. External warts, cauliflower-like in appearance, appear on the genitals after 1 to 6 months. Internal warts may appear on the rectum, vagina, or cervix but require physical examination by a physician to identify them.

Treatment is by surgical removal and topical medications, although recurrences are common and, in some cases, total resolution may not be possible. During exacerbation, sexual abstinence is required to prevent communicating the virus. Two papillomavirus (*human papillomavirus*) has been implicated as a cause of cervical cancer (16 and 18).

Herpes

Genital herpes, caused by herpes simplex viruses types 1 and 2, occurs after contact with the genital lesions of an infected person. These viruses can infect any mucous membrane. Once infected, the virus remains in the ganglia of the associated nerves for the remainder of the host's lifetime. Periodically, the virus reactivates and causes recurrence of the characteristic lesions.

Small vesicles appear within 1 week of the initial infection. These lesions are circular and painful, appear in clusters, and generally heal in 1 to 2 weeks. Dysuria, paresthesia, and other neurological signs may appear. General systemic signs, including fever, malaise, and inguinal lymphadenitis, may be present after initial infection. Subsequent recurrences usually have shorter duration and are less symptomatic. Diagnosis requires medical laboratory tests. Treatment involves medications to control symptoms during outbreaks and to limit recurrent episodes. Abstention from sexual activity when lesions are present is essential to prevent spreading the virus.

Pelvic Inflammatory Disease

Pelvic inflammatory disease (PID) results from infection of the cervix, uterus, or fallopian tubes. Chlamydia and gonorrhea, usually contracted during sexual intercourse, are the most common organisms that infect these organs in PID. Signs and symptoms include abdominal pain, high-grade fever, nausea, and purulent or bloody vaginal discharge. PID can cause infertility, ectopic pregnancy, chronic pelvic pain, or death. Once the organism is identified, immediate antibiotic treatment begins. Clinically, the signs and symptoms of acute PID are difficult to discern from ectopic pregnancy, thus requiring an emergency medical examination.

911

PEDIATRIC CONCERNS

Kidney Trauma

Among children, kidney injuries resulting from traumatic blows to the abdomen or trunk are more frequent than spleen or liver injuries.[13] The kidneys are exposed below the costovertebral angle until adolescence. Hence, a child who has received trauma to the trunk or back should be screened for signs (hematuria, shock) and symptoms (flank pain) of renal damage.

Cryptorchidism

Cryptorchidism, which describes an undescended testicle, is the most common congenital abnormality of the male genitalia.[15] Normally, both testicles descend from the abdomen into the scrotum just before birth or during the first year of life.[4] Usually detected in infancy during regular pediatric care, cryptorchidism occasionally persists into early childhood. The undescended testicle has a high rate of malignancy and infertility if uncorrected.[4,15] There is also a high rate of inguinal hernia that is associated with cryptorchidism.[15] Although such hernias are usually surgically corrected before age 2 years, a history of cryptorchidism may be an indication of a recurrent hernia when assessing groin pain.

SUMMARY

The renal and urinary systems remove metabolic wastes from the blood and have a major role in regulation of body fluid levels, electrolyte levels, and BP. The signs of renal damage include hematuria, an abnormal dipstick test (proteinuria, glucosuria), and hypertension. Symptoms include pain in the back and abdomen, tenderness to percussion at the costovertebral angle, and change in urinary habit (frequency, urgency, volume). The genital or reproductive system contains the organs of procreation specific to each gender. The male genitals are prone to traumatic injury, most of which is temporary and benign. Unilateral scrotum pain or swelling, however, may indicate an emergency condition. The menstrual cycle is an indication of female reproductive system function. If menses is unusually heavy or painful or very infrequent or absent, pathology may exist in the uterus or ovaries. Pregnancy produces certain characteristic signs and symptoms and requires precautions both during and after pregnancy to prevent injury to the mother or fetus. Female athlete triad involves 3 interrelated spectra of conditions (energy availability, menstrual function, and BMD), with the severity of each ranging along a continuum from normal to severe. Early recognition and intervention are necessary to prevent long-term complications. Any sign of renal or genital pathology accompanied by shock indicates internal bleeding and is an emergency. Cancers commonly involve both male and female genital structures. Self-examinations and regular physician examinations are important in the prevention and early detection of these diseases.

CASE STUDY

You are asked by the women's athletic director to develop an education and prevention program for the female athlete triad. The goals of the program are to educate the female athletes on the causes and the short- and long-term consequences of the triad and to provide the coaches with a simple way to screen athletes for signs of potential female athlete triad.

Critical Thinking Questions

1. What are the important points to include in your presentation to the athletes?
2. What advice are you going to provide to the coaches to help them screen for the female athlete triad among their athletes?

REFERENCES

1. National Athletic Trainers' Association. *Athletic Training Education Competencies.* 5th ed. The Commission on Accreditation of Athletic Training Education; 2011.
2. Andreoli TE, Culpepper RM, Thompson CS, Weinman EJ. Section III-Renal disease. In: Andreoli TE, Carpenter CCJ, Plum F, Smith LH Jr, eds. *Cecil Essentials of Medicine.* 2nd ed. W.B. Saunders Company; 1990:176-252.
3. Ganong WF. *Review of Medical Physiology.* 22nd ed. McGraw-Hill Medical; 2005.
4. Gould BE. *Urinary system disorders. Pathophysiology for the Health-Related Professions.* W.B. Saunders Company; 1997:299-319.
5. Putukian M. The female athlete triad. *Clin Sports Med.* 1998;17:675-696.
6. West RV. The female athlete: the triad of disordered eating, amennorrhea, and osteoporosis. *Sports Med.* 1998;26:63-71.
7. Abarbanel J, Benet AE, Lask D, Kimche D. Sports hematuria. *J Urol.* 1990;143:887-890.
8. Neinstein LS. Breast disease in adolescents and young women. *Pediatr Clin North Am.* 1999;46:607-629.
9. Stopka CB, Zambito KL. Referred visceral pain: what every sports medicine professional needs to know. *Athl Ther Today.* 1999;4:29-36.
10. Stuempfle KJ, Drury DG. Comparison of 3 methods to assess urine specific gravity in collegiate wrestlers. *J Athl Train.* 2003;38:315-319.
11. Armstrong LE, Maresh CM, Castellani JW, et al. Urinary indices of hydration status. *Int J Sport Nutr.* 1994;4:265-279.

12. Armstrong LE, Soto JA, Hacker FT Jr, Casa DJ, Kavouras SA, Maresh CM. Urinary indices during dehydration, exercise, and rehydration. *Int J Sport Nutr.* 1998;8:345-355.
13. Amaral JF. Thoracoabdominal injuries in the athlete. *Clin Sports Med.* 1997;16:739-753.
14. Stricker PR. Preparticipation physical examination. In: Garrett WE Jr, Kirkendall DT, Squire DL, eds. *Principles and Practice of Primary Care Sports Medicine.* Lippincott Williams & Wilkins; 2001:19-20.
15. Pillai SB, Besner GE. Pediatric testicular problems. *Pediatr Clin North Am.* 1998;45:813-830.
16. Coker TJ, Dierfeldt DM. Acute Bacterial Prostatitis: Diagnosis and Management. *Am Fam Physician.* 2016;93;114.
17. American Cancer Society. What are the key statistics about prostate cancer? Available at: http://www.cancer.org/cancer/skincancer-melanoma/detailedguide/melanoma-skin-cancer-survival-rates. Accessed June 12, 2013.
18. Pinkerton JV. Amenorrhea. The Merck Manual for Health Care Professionals. Available at: http://www.merckmanuals.com/professional/gynecology_and_obstetrics/menstrual_abnormalities/amenorrhea.html. Accessed June 13, 2013.
19. Teitz CC, Hu SS, Arendt EA. The female athlete: evaluation and treatment of sports-related problems. *J Am Acad Orthopaedic Surg.* 1997;5:87-96.
20. Worthington G. Athletic amenorrhea: updated review. *Athl Train.* 1991;26:270-273.
21. Wilson CA, Abdenour TE, Keye WR. Menstrual disorders among intercollegiate athletes and non-athletes: perceived impact on performance, preventative medical care for the female athlete. *Athl Train.* 1991;26:170-177.
22. Nattiv A, Loucks AB, Manore MM, et al. American College of Sports Medicine position stand. The female athlete triad. *Med Sci Sports Exerc.* 2007;39:1867-1882.
23. Blackburn S. Maternal, Fetal, & Neonatal Physiology: A Clinical Perspective. St. Louis, MO: Saunders; 2003.
24. Artal R. Exercise and pregnancy. *Clin Sports Med.* 1992;11:363-377.
25. Weiss Kelly AK. Practical exercise advice during pregnancy: guidelines for active and inactive women. *Phys Sportsmed.* 2005;33(6):24-30.
26. American College of Obstetrics and Gynecology. *Exercise during pregnancy and the postpartum period.* American College of Obstetrics and Gynecology; 2002.
27. Prather H, Spitznagle T, Hunt D. Benefits of exercise during pregnancy. *PMR.* 2012;4:845-850.
28. Artal R, O'Toole M. Guidelines of the American College of Obstetricians and Gynecologists for exercise during pregnancy and the postpartum period. *Br J Sports Med.* 2003;37:6-12.
29. NCAA Committee on Competitive Safeguards and Medical Aspects of Sport. *Guideline 3B: Participation by the Pregnant Student-Athlete.* National Collegiate Athletic Association; 2002.
30. National Collegiate Athletic Association. Guideline 2q: pregnancy in the student-athlete. In: Klossner D, ed. *2012-2013 NCAA Sports Medicine Handbook.* National Collegiate Athletic Association; 2012:86-87.
31. Stone R. Primary care diagnosis of acute abdominal pain. *Nurse Pract.* 1996;21:19-20,23-26,28-30,35-41.
32. Deimel JF, Dunlap BJ. The female athlete triad. *Clin Sports Med.* 2012;31:247-254.
33. Cancer Facts and Figures. American Cancer Society; 2019.
34. Randall T, McMahon K. Screening for musculoskeletal system disease. In: Boissonnault WG, ed. *Examination in Physical Therapy Practice: Screening for Medical Disease.* 2nd ed. Churchill-Livingstone Inc; 1995:223-255.
35. Gould BE. Reproductive system disorders. *Pathophysiology for the Health-Related Professions.* W.B. Saunders Company; 1997:428-452.
36. Giudice L. Menstrual abnormalities and abnormal uterine bleeding. In: Beers MH, Berkow R, eds. *The Merck Manual of Diagnosis and Therapy.* 17th ed. Merck Research Laboratories; 1999:1932-1942.
37. Hendrix S. Pelvic pain. In: Beers MH, Berkow R, eds. *The Merck Manual of Diagnosis and Therapy.* 17th ed. Merck Research Laboratories; 1999:1944-1948.
38. Kim JH, Lee SM, Lee JH, et al. Successive conservative management of ruptured ovarian cysts with hemoperitoneum in healthy women. *PLoS One.* 2014;9(3):e91171.
39. Gould BE. Neoplasms. *Pathophysiology for the Health-Related Professions.* W.B. Saunders Company; 1997:54-69.

ONLINE RESOURCES

◊ **American Cancer Society**

   ¤ www.cancer.org

◊ **American College of Sports Medicine**

   ¤ www.acsm.org

◊ **The American Congress of Obstetricians and Gynecologists**

   ¤ www.acog.org

◊ **Breastcancer.org**

   ¤ www.breastcancer.org

◊ **National Cancer Institute**

  ¤ www.cancer.gov

◊ **National Collegiate Athletic Association**

  ¤ www.ncaa.org

◊ **National Institute of Diabetes and Digestive and Kidney Diseases**

  ¤ https://www.niddk.nih.gov/health-information/digestive-diseases

◊ **Prostate Cancer Foundation**

  ¤ www.prostatecancerfoundation.org

◊ **Susan G. Komen Breast Cancer Foundation**

  ¤ www.komen.org

CHAPTER 10

Endocrine and
Metabolic Systems

CHAPTER OUTLINE AND OBJECTIVES

Introduction

Review of Anatomy, Physiology, and Pathogenesis

◊ Describe basic endocrine system structures and their functions.
◊ Review pathophysiological mechanisms of the endocrine system, including contributions to homeostasis and metabolism.
◊ Explain how the endocrine system contributes to the regulation of body energy.
◊ Explain how the endocrine system contributes to the regulation of body temperature.
◊ Explain how the endocrine system contributes to the regulation of body fluid.
◊ Describe the response of the endocrine system to exercise.
◊ Describe basic metabolic responses to exercise.

Signs and Symptoms

◊ Identify the general signs and symptoms of pathology involving the endocrine and metabolic systems.

Pain Patterns

◊ Identify the referred pain patterns associated with illnesses and diseases involving the endocrine and metabolic systems.

Bhojani RA, O'Connor DP, Fincher AL. *Clinical Pathology for Athletic Trainers: Recognizing Systemic Disease, Fourth Edition* (pp 263-294).
© 2022 Taylor & Francis Group.

Medical History and Physical Examination Procedures

◊ Discuss medical history findings relevant to endocrine and metabolic pathology.

◊ Perform physical examination tasks and interpret findings relevant to the endocrine system and metabolic systems.

¤ Urinalysis

¤ Glucometer

¤ Rectal Temperature

Pathology and Pathogenesis

◊ Describe the pathophysiology associated with type I and type II diabetes.

◊ Discuss the etiology, signs, symptoms, interventions, medical referral guidelines, and, when appropriate, return-to-participation guidelines for diabetic emergencies (hypoglycemia and ketoacidosis).

◊ Explain the therapeutic strategies used for treating diabetes mellitus.

◊ Discuss the etiology, signs, symptoms, interventions, medical referral guidelines, and, when appropriate, return-to-participation guidelines for disorders of the pituitary gland.

◊ Discuss the etiology, signs, symptoms, interventions, medical referral guidelines, and, when appropriate, return-to-participation guidelines for disorders of the thyroid and parathyroid.

◊ Discuss the etiology, signs, symptoms, interventions, medical referral guidelines, and, when appropriate, return-to-participation guidelines for disorders of the adrenals.

◊ Discuss the etiology, signs, symptoms, management, medical referral guidelines, and, when appropriate, return-to-participation guidelines for exertional heat illnesses (heat cramps, heat exhaustion, heat stroke, and hyponatremia).

◊ Discuss the etiology, signs, symptoms, interventions, medical referral guidelines, and, when appropriate, return-to-participation guidelines for hypothermia.

◊ Describe the relationship between obesity and the development of chronic diseases.

◊ Describe the methods used to identify obesity in individuals and populations.

◊ Describe the contributing factors that lead to the development of obesity.

◊ Discuss the etiology, signs, symptoms and interventions for gout.

◊ Discuss the etiology, signs, symptoms, interventions, medical referral guidelines, and, when appropriate, return-to-participation guidelines for metabolic bone diseases.

Pediatric Concerns

◊ Discuss the etiology, signs, symptoms, interventions, and medical referral associated with osteogenesis imperfecta.

Summary

Case Study

◊ Develop critical-thinking and clinical decision-making skills.

Online Resources

This chapter addresses the following competencies from the *Athletic Training Education Competencies, Fifth Edition*[1]:

Content Area	Competency #
Prevention and Health Promotion (PHP)	3, 5, 10, 11, 12, 17d, 17e, 36
Clinical Examination and Diagnosis (CE)	1, 16, 17, 18, 20j, 21p, 22
Acute Care of Injury and Illness (AC)	6, 7, 27, 28, 29, 30, 36d, 36h, 36m, 41
Therapeutic Interventions (TI)	28, 30
Healthcare Administration (HA)	22
Clinical Integration Proficiencies (CIP)	1, 5, 6

INTRODUCTION

The endocrine system works with the nervous system to maintain homeostasis. The endocrine system releases many different hormones that regulate the functions of many other organ systems, including reproduction, growth and development, mobilization of defenses against stressors, blood glucose levels, and core body temperature, as well as water, electrolyte, and nutrient levels. One of the primary functions of the endocrine system is the regulation of the metabolism.

Metabolism describes the biochemical functions and interactions of the organ systems of the body. Metabolic processes respond to the normal cyclic increases and decreases in organ activity, internal energy demands, environmental factors, and nutrition. Metabolic activity is affected internally by hormones and organs and externally by environmental factors and intake of calories, carbohydrates (CHOs), protein, fat, water, minerals, and vitamins. Thus, metabolism is a primary manifestation of the endocrine system's attempt to maintain homeostasis. Acute and chronic diseases can develop involving one or more of the glands within the endocrine system, which disrupts homeostasis and affects many other systems and bodily functions.

REVIEW OF ANATOMY, PHYSIOLOGY, AND PATHOGENESIS

The endocrine system consists of several small glands located throughout the body (Figure 10-1). These glands secrete chemicals called *hormones* into the blood to stimulate or repress activity in the organ systems of the body, including inhibition or stimulation of other glands and hormones. The endocrine system also interacts with and receives input from the nervous, gastrointestinal (GI), cardiovascular, hepatic, and renal systems.

Almost all of the hormones produced by the endocrine system can be categorized as amino acid derivatives, peptides, or steroids, although most are amino acid derivatives. Hormones circulate throughout the body but will only produce a response in their specific target cells. For a certain hormone to affect a cell, that cell must have a specific protein receptor to receive the hormone. Table 10-1 lists the endocrine glands, their primary hormones, and the targets of their hormones.[2-4]

The *hypothalamus* serves as a communication link between the nervous system and the endocrine system. It is stimulated by a number of hormones and direct neural connections from the brain stem. The responses of the hypothalamus regulate the endocrine system in 3 key ways. First, the hypothalamus stimulates the adrenal medullae to release epinephrine and norepinephrine in response to sympathetic activation. Second, the hypothalamus produces 2 hormones, antidiuretic hormone (ADH, also called vasopressin) and oxytocin (OT), which are transported to the posterior pituitary to be released into the bloodstream. Third, the hypothalamus secretes a number of

Figure 10-1. Glands of the endocrine system.

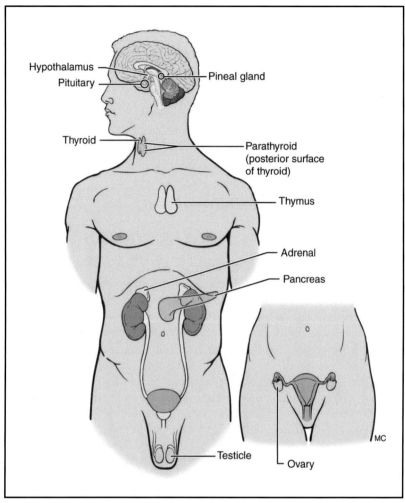

hormones that stimulate the anterior pituitary to release its own hormones that in turn regulate all of the other endocrine glands.

The *pituitary gland* is divided into an anterior lobe and a posterior lobe. The *anterior lobe* produces a number of hormones that are responsible for regulating other endocrine glands. As the name implies, thyroid-stimulating hormone (TSH) stimulates the thyroid gland to produce thyroid hormones. Adrenocorticotropic hormone (ACTH) stimulates the adrenal cortex to release glucocorticoids and androgens. Follicle-stimulating hormone (FSH) and luteinizing hormone (LH) both regulate the secretion of hormones from the ovaries and testicles. The anterior lobe also secretes growth hormone (GH), an anabolic hormone, that stimulates protein synthesis and tissue growth. GH also promotes the use of fats for fuel, providing a glucose-sparing effect. The *posterior pituitary* releases ADH and OT from the hypothalamus into the bloodstream.

The *thyroid*, the largest of the endocrine glands, is a butterfly-shaped gland located on the trachea along the anterior aspect of the neck. This gland secretes 2 hormones, thyroxine (T4) and triiodothyronine (T3). These hormones regulate the basal metabolic rate and are considered to be the body's major metabolism-regulating hormones. These 2 hormones also work together to affect the normal functioning of almost every system in the body, including the nervous, cardiovascular, muscular, skeletal, GI, reproductive, and integumentary systems. For this reason, as will be discussed later, dysfunction or pathology of the thyroid leads to dysfunction in many other systems.

Table 10-1. Endocrine Glands, Selected Associated Hormones, and Hormone Functions

GLAND	HORMONE(S)	TARGETS	HORMONE FUNCTION
Hypothalamus	Antidiuretic hormone (ADH)	Posterior pituitary	Stimulate release of hormones by posterior pituitary
	Oxytocin (OT)		
Anterior pituitary	Growth hormone (GH)	All cells	Growth and development; protein synthesis; breakdown of fats for energy
	Adrenocorticotropic hormone (ACTH)	Adrenal cortex	Cause adrenals to release cortisol
	Thyroid-stimulating hormone (TSH)	Thyroid gland	Increase thyroid function; stimulate release of thyroid hormones (T3 and T4)
	Follicle-stimulating hormone (FSH)	Ovaries	Increase estrogen release
		Testes	Increase sperm production
	Luteinizing hormone (LH)	Ovaries	Stimulate ovulation
		Testes	Increase testosterone release
	Prolactin (PRL)	Mammary glands in females	Production of milk
Posterior pituitary	Antidiuretic hormone (ADH)	Kidneys	Reabsorption of water; increased blood volume; increased blood pressure
	Oxytocin (OT)	Uterus, mammary glands (females)	Labor contractions, milk secretion
		Ductus deferens, prostate glands (males)	Contractions of ductus deferens and prostate; ejection of secretions
Thyroid	Thyroxine (T4)	Most cells	Increase metabolism, protein synthesis, growth and development
	Triiodothyronine (T3)	Most cells	Increase metabolism, protein synthesis, growth and development
	Calcitonin (CT)	Bones, kidneys	Decrease demineralization of bone
Parathyroid	Parathyroid hormone (PTH)	Bones, kidneys	Increase calcium in blood by demineralizing bone
Thymus	Thymosins	Lymphocytes	Increase effectiveness of immune system

(continued)

Table 10-1 (continued). Endocrine Glands, Selected Associated Hormones, and Hormone Functions

GLAND	HORMONE(S)	TARGETS	HORMONE FUNCTION
Adrenal	Aldosterone	Kidneys	Increase reabsorption of water and sodium ions in kidneys
	Cortisol	Most cells	Anti-inflammatory effects, tissue catabolism, respond to stress, increases synthesis of glucose and glycogen formation
	Epinephrine	Most cells	Respond to stress (increase heart rate, increase blood flow to muscle, decrease blood flow to internal organs), increases glycogen breakdown and release of lipids from adipose tissue
	Norepinephrine	Most cells	Vasoconstriction
Pancreas (endocrine)	Insulin	All cells (except those of brain, kidneys, gastrointestinal, epithelium, and red blood cells)	Increase glucose transport out of blood and into cells
	Glucagon	Liver, adipose tissues	Breakdown of glycogen in liver, release glucose from liver into blood, release of fat stores
Testes	Testosterone	Most cells	Produce secondary male sex characteristics, increase protein synthesis, increase sperm production, inhibit luteinizing hormone release
Ovaries	Estrogen	Most cells	Produce secondary female sex characteristics, regulate menstrual cycle, inhibit luteinizing hormone release
	Progesterone	Uterus, mammary glands	Prepares uterus for egg implantation, secretory function of mammary glands
	Relaxin	Pubic symphysis, uterus, mammary glands	Relaxes uterine muscles and pubic symphysis
Pineal	Melatonin	All cells	Inhibits release of FSH and LH, slows maturation of reproductive organs, assists in regulation of circadian rhythms, works as antioxidant to protect the central nervous system (CNS) and boost immune system

The *parathyroid* secretes parathyroid hormone (PTH), which functions primarily to regulate the level of calcium in the blood. Calcium blood levels are important for the conduction of nerve impulses, normal muscle contraction, and blood clotting.

The *adrenal glands* are actually a set of paired glands located just above the kidneys. The adrenal *medulla*, or inner part of each adrenal gland, secretes epinephrine and norepinephrine and is associated with the sympathetic nervous system. The outer portion of the adrenals, or adrenal *cortex*, secretes many corticosteroid hormones, including aldosterone and cortisol, and androgens (testosterone and related molecules). Aldosterone increases blood levels of sodium while decreasing levels of potassium. The regulation of these and other electrolytes in the blood affects blood volume and blood pressure. Cortisol has many functions, including raising blood glucose levels by stimulating gluconeogenesis, which is the production of glucose from noncarbohydrate sources (ie, fats and proteins). Cortisol also suppresses the immune system and produces anti-inflammatory effects, and chronic high levels can decrease cartilage and bone formation. Dysfunction of the adrenals is associated with 2 disorders: Addison's disease and Cushing's syndrome.

The *pancreas* is located posterior to the stomach and is composed of both endocrine and exocrine cells. Injuries and illnesses involving the exocrine pancreas were discussed in Chapter 8. The endocrine portion of the pancreas secretes glucagon and insulin. Glucagon is considered a hyperglycemic hormone and increases blood glucose levels. Glucagon stimulates the breakdown of glycogen to glucose in the liver and facilitates gluconeogenesis. Insulin is a hypoglycemic hormone that works to lower blood glucose levels by promoting the transport of glucose from the bloodstream into tissue cells.

Women and men have sex-specific endocrine glands. Women have *ovaries* that secrete estrogen and progesterone. These hormones are responsible for the development of the female reproductive organs, secondary sex characteristics, and the menstrual cycle. Men have *testicles* that secrete testosterone, which promotes the maturation of the male reproductive organs, secondary sex characteristics, sperm production, and sex drive. Pathological conditions involving the ovaries and testicles were addressed in Chapter 9.

Regulation of Body Energy

Glucose is the body's primary energy source. The endocrine system maintains normal blood glucose levels to meet the body's constantly changing energy needs. This complex balance is achieved through the functions of multiple hormones including insulin and glucagon from the pancreas; epinephrine, norepinephrine, and cortisol from the adrenal glands; and GH from the pituitary gland.

As mentioned previously, insulin lowers blood glucose levels by transporting glucose from the blood into the cells for energy. When glucose levels exceed the body's need for fuel, insulin removes the excess glucose from the blood to be stored as either glycogen in the liver and the muscles or as fat in the adipose tissues. Glucagon, epinephrine, norepinephrine, cortisol, and GH all function as insulin antagonists that counter the activity of insulin and thereby increase blood glucose levels. These hormones stimulate the release of glucose from glycogen stores and promote gluconeogenesis, both of which increase blood glucose levels.

During exercise, insulin levels decrease as metabolic demand for glucose increases. Glucose is released in response to this increased fuel demand, primarily through the function of glucagon.[5,6] Simultaneously, insulin receptors on muscle cells become more sensitive; this change increases the muscular uptake of glucose despite decreases in blood insulin level.[5] Epinephrine and norepinephrine are released as exercise begins, and GH and cortisol are released during extended exercise. All of these hormones inhibit insulin production, thereby further aiding release of glucose from the liver.[5]

Regulation of Body Temperature

Normal metabolic processes produce energy while the body is at rest. Most of this energy is released as heat, which maintains the body's resting temperature. The body can also regulate heat loss or heat production in response to environmental conditions.[7]

With the onset of exercise or physical exertion, core body temperature increases slightly and the physiological heat-dissipating mechanisms begin to function, primarily sweating and evaporation of water from the skin and increased radiation of heat from the head and neck. Ideally, a steady state is reached where heat production and heat dissipation stabilizes body temperature.[7] In very humid environments, the capacity for evaporation is reduced, which decreases the effectiveness of sweating for cooling the body.[8] This impairment of one of the body's major thermoregulation responses is related to the development of the exertional heat illnesses discussed later in this chapter.

The hypothalamus responds to changes in blood temperature by increasing or decreasing TSH in the pituitary gland. In response to decreases in body temperature, increased TSH increases thyroid hormone, which causes the metabolism to increase. A higher metabolism requires more energy-producing biochemical reactions, which increases body temperature. Through the opposite set of reactions, increased body temperature decreases TSH, which lowers the metabolism to limit a further increase in body temperature.

Regulation of Body Fluid

ADH forms in the hypothalamus and is secreted by the posterior pituitary gland. ADH retains water in the body by increasing water reabsorption in the kidneys, thus decreasing urine volume. Exercise increases ADH secretion when baroreceptors, which are sensitive to pressure, detect a decrease in blood pressure from a decrease in blood volume (eg, loss of fluid volume through sweating) and the hypothalamus detects an increase in blood solutes.[9] Maintaining adequate hydration during activity inhibits this secretion of ADH because, when properly hydrated, there is no need to retain water.

Hormonal Response to Exercise

Exercise, or any other physical stress, causes a release of hypothalamic, pituitary, and adrenal hormones (Table 10-2).[9] As an adaptation, the exercise-related release of these hormones decreases as the level of conditioning and fitness improves.

Relatively intense exercise stimulates the release of GH, and this release actually increases with higher levels of fitness.[9] The intensity of exercise rather than its duration or frequency appears to be the most important factor stimulating GH release. By contrast, endurance exercise increases the level of cortisol, which decreases GH secretion.[9] Thus, a potential effect of overtraining is a net decrease in GH. Adverse effects, such as stunted height and physical development problems, can occur with combined overtraining and nutritional deficiencies among young athletes.

Secretion of the catecholamines, epinephrine and norepinephrine, occurs with onset of exercise and does not appear to adapt with conditioning. Frequent, intense exercise decreases FSH and LH and, subsequently, decreases secretion of estrogen and, to a lesser extent, testosterone. Decreased estrogen levels can produce amenorrhea among young female athletes, but usually only when excessive exercise is accompanied by a nutritional deficiency. Although circulating testosterone also decreases with high-volume endurance exercise, an associated delay of male puberty is very rare, possibly because extremely high exercise intensity is needed in males to depress testosterone release.

Neurotransmitters known as endorphins, or endogenous opioids, are released during exercise of moderate to high intensity. Endorphins may produce a mild analgesic effect to alleviate muscle pain during exercise and will counteract the increase in cortisol that occurs with exercise. Additionally, endorphins stimulate *lipolysis*, the breakdown of stored fat, to provide CHO to working muscles.

Table 10-2. Hormones Released During Exercise

HORMONE	RESPONSE TO EXERCISE
Growth hormone (GH)	Mobilizes free fatty acids; increases glycogenolysis (release glucose from the liver into the blood); inhibits uptake of glucose by the liver; stimulates release of insulin-like growth factor 1, which stimulates tissue growth
Adrenocorticotropic hormone (ACTH)	Stimulate cortisol release, which increases gluconeogenesis (increases blood glucose); increases protein synthesis; inhibits uptake of glucose by the liver
Follicle-stimulating hormone (FSH) and luteinizing hormone (LH)	Men: stimulate testosterone release, which increases protein synthesis Women: stimulate estrogen release, which inhibits uptake of glucose
Epinephrine	Increases glycogenolysis (release glucose from the liver into the blood); stimulates lipolysis (breaks down fat for conversion into glucose via gluconeogenesis)

SIGNS AND SYMPTOMS

The signs and symptoms listed next represent the general signs and symptoms associated with endocrine pathology. The clinical presentation of specific endocrine conditions or disorders may include various combinations of these signs and symptoms, depending on which gland or hormone is affected.

Skin Changes

Some endocrine disorders produce changes in the color, texture, or appearance of the skin. Hormones control the activity of melanin, a skin pigment, and can affect skin color. Changes in skin thickness, flexibility, texture, and integrity may appear in response to pathological conditions of the endocrine system.

Diaphoresis-Hyperhidrosis

Diaphoresis (sweating) or *hyperhidrosis* (excessive sweating) occurs as metabolism increases. Diaphoresis is a normal response to exercise or increased body temperature. Metabolic imbalance or endocrine disorders, however, can cause diaphoresis or hyperhidrosis at rest. Release of epinephrine and norepinephrine into the bloodstream can also cause profuse sweating.

Body or Breath Odor

High blood glucose levels, as occurs with insufficient circulating insulin (diabetes mellitus), produces a very sweet odor on the breath and from the body. Metabolic breakdown of ingested or absorbed toxins and organic substances (eg, alcohol, drugs) can be exhaled or secreted in breath, sweat, and urine, where they can often be detected by smell.

Polydipsia and Polyuria

Excessive thirst (*polydipsia*) or excessive urination (*polyuria*) can be caused by inadequate secretion of ADH from the posterior pituitary or thyroid disorders. These 2 symptoms may also be a sign of elevated sugars (diabetes mellitus).

Arthralgia and Myalgia

Pain in joints (*arthralgia*) and muscles (*myalgia*) is common with disturbance of endocrine function or metabolism. Multiple joints or muscles are usually involved, and the pattern is symmetric bilaterally.

Muscle Atrophy and Weakness

Changes in muscle function and structure are results of insufficient nutrition, from either starvation or chronic disease, or the long-term presence of hormones that increase metabolic demand (eg, cortisol, epinephrine). Many endocrine disorders also affect muscle energy metabolism, causing unusual weakness and atrophy.

Amenorrhea and Impotence

Function of the reproductive organs can be affected by disorders affecting the hypothalamus, pituitary gland, ovaries, or testes because these glands control the activity of those organs.

Confusion or Change in Mental Status

Cognitive function can be affected by many endocrine-metabolic disorders, including hypoglycemia, dehydration, abnormal body temperature, or insufficient nutrition.

Paresthesia

Long-term endocrine or metabolic disorders can damage nerve cells, axons, or myelin, causing progressive peripheral paresthesias.

Edema and Pitting Edema

Extracellular fluid can accumulate with certain endocrine or metabolic system disorders that cause water retention.

Polyphagia

Excessive intake of food without weight gain suggests an overactive thyroid, nutritional deficits, or metabolic imbalances that create a large caloric deficit.

Postural (Orthostatic) Hypotension

The endocrine system regulates fluid levels in the blood. If blood volume decreases significantly, as can occur with endocrine problems, leading to excessive urination or dehydration, blood pressure decreases rapidly with a change in posture from lying or sitting to standing.

Lethargy and Fatigue

Because the endocrine system regulates the metabolism, disorders in this system affect the availability and utilization of oxygen and energy. Fatigue and lethargy (abnormal sluggishness, drowsiness, or indifference) result either from an overactive metabolism requiring large energy expenditures or from an underactive metabolism that does not provide the body with enough energy. In addition, many endocrine conditions directly or indirectly affect sleep quality and duration (eg, through nocturia), leading to fatigue from sleep deprivation.

PAIN PATTERNS

The endocrine glands rarely produce pain directly. The signs and symptoms of hormonal imbalances, such as those previously listed, are usually more relevant than reports of pain. Large

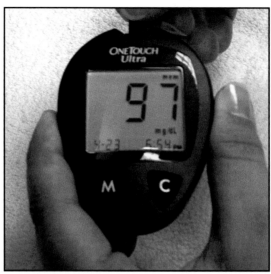

Figure 10-2. Glucometer.

tumors in the hypothalamus and pituitary glands may produce headaches or visual disturbances if they compress the brain. Pathology of the thyroid or parathyroid glands may cause tenderness in the anterior and inferior aspect of the throat and neck, especially during extension of the head and neck. Adrenal disorders can produce widespread myalgia and arthralgia. As discussed in Chapter 8, extensive pancreatic disease produces upper left quadrant or generalized epigastric pain.

MEDICAL HISTORY AND PHYSICAL EXAMINATION PROCEDURES

Family and Personal History

Certain metabolic disorders, such as diabetes mellitus, have a strong genetic component that may be evident in a family history. Metabolic disturbances can also be caused by environmental factors (eg, temperature, toxins, chronic physical stress), so these should be investigated during the medical history. Many endocrine disorders produce a characteristic pattern or progression of symptoms that may be detected through a careful medical history.

Physical Examination

Skin or hair changes, secondary sex characteristics, muscle atrophy, hyperhidrosis, odor of breath or perspiration, edema, postural hypotension, and paresthesia may all be related to endocrine system disorders. Depending on the condition, the observation, palpation, and assessment of vital signs may be the only physical examination procedures that indicate potential endocrine pathology. An enlarged thyroid can be seen and palpated lateral to the trachea, just above the clavicles.[10] An abnormally enlarged thyroid, called a *goiter*, is a sign of thyroid toxicity, iodine deficiency, or thyroid pathology. Most endocrine diseases require medical laboratory testing to confirm the diagnosis.

A *glucometer* can be used by an athletic trainer to monitor or quickly assess a patient's blood glucose level (Figure 10-2). These units are easy to use and can play a vital role in the management of patients with diabetes. When purchased, each glucometer kit includes disposable test strips and lancets, and replacement strips and lancets can be purchased as needed. The units run on batteries and many of them contain a memory chip that allows for the storage of multiple glucose values, which can be helpful in tracking an individual's measures over time. Although each glucometer may differ

Table 10-3. Measuring Blood Glucose Levels Using a Glucometer

STEP 1	Check that the glucometer's battery is good.
STEP 2	Check that the glucometer is coded correctly for the test strips to be used.
STEP 3	Wipe the fingertip with an alcohol prep pad.
STEP 4	Insert the lancet in the automatic lancet device.
STEP 5	Stick the fingertip with the lancet device.
STEP 6	Squeeze a small drop of blood onto the test strip.
STEP 7	Insert the test strip into the glucometer.
STEP 8	Read the digital display of the blood glucose level.
STEP 9	Remove the lancet from the device and dispose in an appropriate sharps container.

slightly, the steps for measuring blood glucose levels are very similar across the different brands. Table 10-3 provides a list of the general step-by-step instructions for measuring blood glucose levels using a glucometer. Normal blood glucose levels should be between 70 and 110 mg/dL. Normal fasting (nothing to eat or drink other than water for at least 8 hours) glucose levels should be between 60 and 80 mg/dL, and postprandial (2 hours after a meal) levels should be between 100 and 140 mg/dL. Newer devices can be attached to diabetic patients while allow for continuous glucose monitoring. Athletic trainers should be familiar with all these devices and its restrictions/limitations.

A routine *urinalysis* can be used by the athletic trainer to screen for glucose and ketones, which are products of fat metabolism (when cells are using fat instead of glucose as an energy source). When blood glucose levels become excessively high (> 250 mg/dL), glucose spills over into the urine (*glucosuria*). The presence of ketones in the urine is a sign of impending ketoacidosis, a potentially life-threatening condition. The procedures for performing a urinalysis were described in Chapter 9.

Rectal temperature is considered the criterion standard for assessing core body temperature in individuals exercising in the heat. Other sites for temperature assessments (oral, aural, axillary, temporal, and forehead) have been shown to be inaccurate in measuring core temperature in hyperthermic individuals exercising outdoors in the heat.[11] This is due to sweat dissipation along with blood flow changes during workouts. Rectal temperature can be easily assessed using a flexible rectal probe attached to an electronic thermometer. When measuring rectal temperature, the athlete should be rolled into a side-lying position with the superior hip and knee slightly flexed. The rectal probe should be inserted to a depth of 10 cm.[12] It may be necessary to slightly lift the superior gluteal cheek to insert the probe. Also, it is helpful to have this 10 cm point pre-marked on the probe with a piece of tape or permanent marker. The remaining portion of the probe can be "lassoed" and tucked into the athlete's shorts or pants. Rectal temperatures of 104°F to 105°F (40°C to 40.5°C) indicate exertional heat illness and warrant immediate cooling via full-body submersion. The rectal probe can be left in throughout the rapid cooling to identify when it is safe to transport the athlete (102°F [38.8°C]) to the nearest emergency facility.[13]

PATHOLOGY AND PATHOGENESIS

Diabetes Mellitus

There are 3 types of diabetes mellitus: *type 1*, formerly called insulin-dependent diabetes mellitus or juvenile diabetes; *type 2*, formerly known as noninsulin-dependent diabetes mellitus or adult onset diabetes; and *gestational*, which can occur during pregnancy. This chapter will address type 1 and type 2 diabetes.

Table 10-4. Diagnostic Criteria for Diabetes Mellitus

TEST	NORMAL	PREDIABETES	DIABETES
Random plasma glucose (RPG)	70 to 126 mg/dL	127 to 199 mg/dL	≥ 200 mg/dL with symptoms[a]
Fasting plasma glucose (FPG)	< 99 mg/dL	100 to 125 mg/dL	≥ 126 mg/dL with symptoms[a]
A1c	< 5.6%	5.7 to 6.4%	≥ 6.5%
Oral glucose tolerance test	< 140 mg/dL	140 to 199 mg/dL	≥ 200 mg/dL

mg/dL = milligrams of glucose in 1 deciliter (100 millimeters) of blood.

[a] Symptoms of diabetes include polydipsia, polyurea, polyphagia, and weight loss.

Type 1 Diabetes Mellitus

Type 1 diabetes mellitus is an autoimmune disease that destroys the insulin-producing cells of the endocrine pancreas (beta cells in the islets of Langerhans).[14] This condition affects approximately 1 in 500 children and adolescents.[5,6] and currently represents approximately 10% of all diabetes cases. Without insulin, the body cannot regulate blood glucose and, as a result, blood glucose levels become very high. Because there is no cure for this condition, people with type 1 diabetes mellitus must learn to maintain a balance between self-administration of insulin, diet, and exercise. An inability to maintain this balance can lead both to acute life-threatening complications (hypoglycemia and hyperglycemia)[15] and long-term health concerns (cardiovascular disease, impaired or delayed wound healing, peripheral neuropathies).

Type 1 diabetes mellitus is typically diagnosed in individuals prior to age 25 years. In most cases, individuals will present clinically with polydipsia, polyphagia, polyuria, and weight loss. It should be noted, however, that some individuals with type 1 diabetes mellitus, particularly young children, may experience no signs or symptoms prior to an initial diabetic crisis (ketoacidosis). Definitive diagnosis of diabetes mellitus requires a laboratory blood test. Table 10-4 outlines the types of blood glucose tests and criterion values for normal, prediabetes, and diabetes. The diagnosis is made based on the latest American Diabetes Association criteria. These criteria includes: A1c > 6.5% OR fasting plasma glucose > 126 mg/dL OR 2-hour plasma glucose > 200 mg/dL during an oral glucose tolerance test OR a patient with above symptoms with a random plasma glucose > 200 mg/dL.[16]

Type 1 diabetes mellitus is treated by administering insulin on a regular basis. There are several types of insulin available for use, ranging from fast acting to slow acting. Fast-acting insulin will generally produce effects within 5 to 30 minutes, with a peak effect occurring between 1 and 4 hours and a duration of 4 to 8 hours. Slow-acting insulin will produce longer-lasting effects within 2 to 4 hours, with a peak level obtained somewhere between 8 and 14 hours. The duration of effects produced by long-lasting insulin may be up to 24 hours. Patients will have specific instructions and precautions from their physician regarding administration of insulin that should be followed strictly. The patient and athletic trainer should also be aware of guidelines and restrictions on transporting glucose, which may require additional security screening. Packing insulin in checked luggage will likely expose it to extreme temperature fluctuations and affect its quality and function and is generally not recommended.[17] Adequate supplies for the duration of the trip, including insulin doses and supplies, should be taken.[17]

Individuals with type 1 diabetes mellitus require several injections of insulin each day. Many physicians will recommend alternating injections of short- and long-acting insulin or use a

Table 10-5. Components of an Individualized Diabetic Care Plan

COMPONENT	INFORMATION TO BE INCLUDED
Blood glucose monitoring	Frequency for monitoring
	Values that warrant exclusion from activity
Insulin therapy guidelines	Type of insulin used by athlete
	Delivery method (ie, manual injection, insulin pump)
	Normal dosages, as well as adjustment dosages for specific events and correction dosages for high glucose values
Other medications	Information related to any additional medications prescribed for management of athlete's diabetes
Hypoglycemia guidelines	Physician's recommendations for preventing hypoglycemia
	Athlete's specific signs and symptoms related to hypoglycemia
	Instructions for use of glucagon
Hyperglycemia guidelines	Physician's recommendations for preventing and treating hyperglycemia
	Athlete's specific signs and symptoms related to hyperglycemia

Adapted from Jimenez CC, Corcoran MH, Crawley JT, et al. National Athletic Trainers' Association position statement: management of the athlete with type 1 diabetes mellitus. *J Athl Train*. 2007;42:536-545.

short- and long-acting insulin mix. These injections are administered subcutaneously and are usually given before breakfast and again before the evening meal.[18] It is generally recommended that athletes inject their insulin into a non-exercising body part, such as the subcutaneous fat layer of the abdomen, because intramuscular injection and subsequent muscle contraction may increase the insulin absorption rate.[17] Athletic trainers should have an individualized diabetic care plan for each of their diabetic athletes.[17] Table 10-5 outlines the information that should be included in the diabetic care plan.

Some individuals may use an insulin pump to administer their insulin. The pump is a pocket-sized device that administers subcutaneous insulin continuously in varying doses depending on the individual's meal times and activity schedule. The pump provides more consistency for those individuals who have difficulty balancing their insulin doses with meals and exercise.[18] Although small, the pump can still be somewhat cumbersome for athletes during practice and competition. The pump may need to be removed prior to swimming or some contact sports.[18] Decisions regarding its use during athletic competition should be made by the individual's physician.

People who have difficulty regulating glucose levels through insulin and diet have a higher risk of severe complications.[19] Long-term health consequences of type 1 diabetes mellitus include peripheral and autonomic neuropathies, retinopathy leading to blindness, cardiovascular disease, hypertension, kidney disorders, chronic skin ulcers, and poor healing capability.[14] Diabetes mellitus (type 1 and type 2) also increases risk of tendon pathology, joint problems in the hands and feet, osteomyelitis, postoperative infection, osteoporosis, and fractures—which may be attributable to higher fall risk with development of compromised peripheral sensation.[20]

Regular aerobic exercise indirectly inhibits the development or advancement of some complications among people with type 1 diabetes mellitus, such as cardiovascular disease. People who have diabetes should wear appropriate shoes to protect their feet from injury, and their feet should be inspected daily to identify and treat any skin wounds. Impaired sensation and high risk of infection can result in severe infections and tissue loss from a seemingly minor foot injury (eg, a blister).[19]

Table 10-6. Signs of Hyperglycemia and Hypoglycemia in Individuals With Diabetes Mellitus

HYPERGLYCEMIA (DIABETIC KETOACIDOSIS, DIABETIC "COMA," OR DIABETIC HYPEROSMOLAR STATE)	HYPOGLYCEMIA (INSULIN SHOCK)
Blood glucose > 200 mg/dL	Blood glucose < 70 mg/dL
Gradual onset	Sudden onset
Abdominal pain	Headache
Thirst but not hunger	Hunger but not thirst
Fruity odor on breath (acetone)	Blurred vision
Dehydration	Dizziness
Lethargy	Decreased performance
Confusion	Autonomic signs (pallor, diaphoresis, tachycardia, tremors)
Loss of consciousness (coma)	Fatigue
	Slurred speech
	Confusion

Generally, significant health problems do not occur for at least 10 years after onset of the disease in patients who can maintain good glucose control. The risk for complications increases with age.

Athletic trainers should be aware of which of their patients have diabetes mellitus. The National Athletic Trainers' Association (NATA) has published a position statement on the "Management of the Athlete with Type 1 Diabetes Mellitus" to guide practice.[17] The preparticipation examination is the ideal time to identify diabetic athletes, to determine the level of control they have over their disease, and to develop an individualized management plan for glucose monitoring, insulin use, and specified treatment for hypoglycemic or hyperglycemic episodes.[15,17,21] Long-term control of blood glucose can be monitored by measuring glycosylated hemoglobin (HbA1c), which indicates the concentration of glucose over the prior 8 to 12 weeks. HbA1c levels in healthy individuals ranges between 4% and 6%; recommended levels for adults with diabetes mellitus on insulin therapy is less than 7% (7.5% in adolescents).[17] The reported frequency of hypoglycemia (low blood sugar) or hyperglycemia (high blood sugar) bouts can also provide a clear indication of the patient's level of control over their diabetes. As mentioned previously, both of these conditions can be potentially life threatening, so athletic trainers must be able to recognize and treat these emergencies.[15] Table 10-6 compares and contrasts the signs and symptoms of hypoglycemia and hyperglycemia.

Hypoglycemia is much more common than hyperglycemia among people with type 1 diabetes mellitus.[22] Hypoglycemia occurs during physical exertion when there is a high level of circulating insulin, which most commonly occurs when an individual injects insulin before exercise and then fails to eat.[23,24] Athletes must learn to estimate the correct insulin dosage based on the expected intensity and duration of the practice or competition. Injecting too low of an insulin dose prior to a high-intensity workout or failing to take in CHOs during an extremely long event can lead to hypoglycemia when energy demand exceeds the glucose supply in the blood. Athletes should use a glucometer to monitor their blood glucose levels 2 to 4 times per day. Most individuals will begin showing signs and symptoms of hypoglycemia when their blood glucose levels drop to 50 to 60 mg/dL. If an individual recognizes an impending hypoglycemic attack, they should stop activity immediately and consume 15 to 20 g of CHOs.[17] Table 10-7 provides examples of snacks that contain

Table 10-7. Examples of Fast-Acting Sources of Carbohydrates (~15 grams)

SNACK ITEM	QUANTITY
Glucagon gel	Follow instructions on label for quantity that provides 15 g
Glucagon tablets	Follow instructions on label for quantity that provides 15 g
Apple or orange juice	4 ounces (0.1 kg) (1/2 cup)
Raisins	2 tablespoons
Sugar or honey	1 tablespoon

approximately 15 g of CHOs. After 15 minutes, the individual should recheck their blood glucose level. If the levels are still below normal, the individual should consume another 15 g of fast-acting CHOs. If after another 15 minutes, the individual's blood glucose level is still below normal, the athletic trainer should activate the emergency action plan.[17] Once the blood glucose levels have returned to normal, the individual should eat a snack (eg, sandwich or bagel).[17]

Hypoglycemia can progress very quickly, therefore, athletic trainers, coaches, and parents should monitor their athletes closely for signs of a problem. Individuals experiencing hypoglycemia will often times exhibit changes in behavior such as mood swings, increased frustration, agitation, or increased aggression. Severe hypoglycemia that results in the athlete losing consciousness requires activation of the emergency action plan and the injection of glucagon.

Hyperglycemia is caused by excessively high levels of glucose, which is associated with low levels of insulin. There are a number of factors that can increase glucose levels, including emotional stress, illness or injury, a change in activity level, addition of a new medication that might stimulate glucose release, or a missed insulin dose. Hyperglycemia will usually develop slowly but can lead to a dangerous state of metabolic acidosis referred to as *diabetic ketoacidosis* (DKA). DKA occurs with extreme depletion of insulin and can result in coma and possible death.

When low levels of insulin prevent the body from moving glucose from the blood to the cells, the cells begin to use fats as an energy source. Ketones are then produced as a by-product of the breakdown of fats. These toxic acids build up in the blood and eventually spill over into the urine. Ketones are responsible for the fruity odor noticed on the breaths of persons experiencing extreme hyperglycemia and DKA.

Blood glucose testing and urine ketone testing are required to determine the patient's current glycemic status. A glucose reading over 250 mg/dL may prohibit exercise and requires a urinalysis to screen for ketones. If ketones are not present in the urine, the individual can still exercise.[17] The presence of ketones in the urine is a sign of impending diabetic ketoacidosis; therefore, exercise is contraindicated. Insulin should be administered immediately and the person should be transported for medical examination and monitoring.[6,14,24] Medically supervised treatment involves rehydration and restoration of electrolyte balance to correct the acidosis.

Type 2 Diabetes Mellitus

Type 2 diabetes mellitus is characterized by normal or high levels of insulin but decreased insulin receptor sensitivity. Glucose uptake by the liver and muscles is substantially impaired because the insulin receptors do not respond to circulating insulin.[5,6] As a result, blood glucose levels remain higher than normal. Until recently, type 2 diabetes was primarily a disease of adults, but the disorder has been gradually increasing among children. Type 2 diabetes mellitus is 9 or 10 times more common than type 1 diabetes, affecting at least 30 million people in the United States, many of whom are unaware they have the condition.[25]

The chronically elevated blood glucose level eventually produces hyperlipidemia (increased fat in blood), arteriosclerosis (hardening of arteries), peripheral neuropathy, chronic infections, and bone changes (eg, osteoporosis).[10] A positive family history of type 2 diabetes mellitus and the presence of obesity are strong predictors of this condition.[6] Polydipsia and polyuria are the most common symptoms of type 2 diabetes mellitus.[10] Increased fluid intake (polydipsia) occurs to dilute blood glucose concentration, but the increased fluid intake causes an increase in fluid excretion by the kidneys (polyuria).

The most severe metabolic consequence in type 2 diabetes mellitus is hyperosmolar hyperglycemic nonketotic coma. This potentially fatal complication occurs most often in older patients who have a concurrent illness, such as influenza or gastroenteritis, that predisposes them to dehydration.[22] This condition is a result of an extreme hyperglycemic state (>600 mg/dL) that results in the blood being hyperosmolar—meaning that it has too much particulate relative to the amount of fluid. The hyperosmolarity causes a flow of fluids from the tissues into the blood in an effort to dilute the particulate level. The result is a severe state of dehydration that is self-perpetuating; clinical signs include seizure, coma, delirium, lethargy, and vision changes.[22] Treatment involves hydration, restoring electrolyte balance, insulin to reduce hyperglycemia, and addressing any underlying illness.

Exercise and a controlled diet are mainstays in the prevention and treatment of type 2 diabetes mellitus.[6,19] Exercise directly affects blood glucose level by increasing metabolic demand of muscle, which burns more glucose as fuel, and increasing the effectiveness of insulin receptors. Low- to moderate-intensity exercise thus facilitates muscle glucose uptake among people with type 2 diabetes mellitus.[19,26] In contrast to type 1 diabetes mellitus, hyperglycemia is more common than hypoglycemia in type 2 diabetes mellitus.[22] In type 2 diabetes mellitus, the person's resting state is hyperglycemic. Exercise may lead to hypoglycemia if the person is using hypoglycemic agents to control their high glucose levels.[22]

Diabetes and Exercise

Aerobic exercise such as walking has certain advantages for persons with diabetes: no increase in blood pressure (which would increase the risk of retinopathy or nephropathy); a low potential for skin wounds; increased insulin receptor sensitivity; cardiovascular benefits (eg, lowering blood lipids); and weight control (particularly for type 2 diabetes mellitus).[5,19] Children and adolescents who maintain a good regimen and controlled diet can participate in most sports with few or no precautions.[6,19] Adults with poorly controlled type 1 diabetes mellitus are at substantial risk for cardiovascular pathology and should exercise only under medical advice and guidelines.[23]

Because exercise affects glucose levels, athletes with type 1 diabetes mellitus should discuss the adjustment of insulin type, dose, and/or regimen with their physician.[19,21,23] Preparticipation meals and insulin should be adjusted both for expected exercise intensity and blood glucose level at the time of the meal.[23] Immediately before exercise, a blood glucose level below 100 mg/dL requires a CHO snack to raise blood glucose.[27] Approximately 15 to 30 g of CHO per 30 minutes of athletic exercise may be needed to prevent hypoglycemia.[6,14,27] A source of quick glucose, such as fruit juice, glucose tablets or gel, sectioned oranges, or hard candy, should be available during practice and competition to counteract acute hypoglycemia during exercise.[6,14,19,21,24] A plan for glucagon and insulin availability and administration in the event of hypoglycemia or hyperglycemia, respectively, should be established between the patient, patient's parents (if the patient is a minor), athletic trainer, physician, and coaches.[14,21] Table 10-8 outlines the management of patients with diabetes mellitus. The International Society for Pediatric and Adolescent Diabetes has developed guidelines for individualized treatment and management planning (http://www.ispad.org).

Any athlete or patient who has diabetes should be allowed to stop activity at the first sign of a hypoglycemic attack. Should the individual lose consciousness (and IV access cannot be obtained) or begin to have a seizure, the athletic trainer must quickly administer glucagon (which is only effective for suspected insulin-mediated hypoglycemia). All athletic trainers should be familiar with

Table 10-8. Managing the Athlete With Diabetes Mellitus

Obtain frequency of hypoglycemia episodes in preparticipation examination.

Communicate with doctor relative to adjusting insulin dose and schedule specific to type of exercise.

Take blood glucose before practice or competition and take appropriate action:

< 100 mg/dL	> 200 mg/dL = no practice
Eat a carbohydrate snack before practice (30 to 40 g CHO)	Urinalysis for ketones (ketones = emergency)
	Insulin injection

Communicate with athlete and coach to be excused from practice immediately at the first sign of hypoglycemia.

Have a ready source of simple CHO (hard candy, fruit juice) available at all times.

Establish an emergency plan for severe hypoglycemia with athlete and athlete's physician or team physician, including injection of glucagon or intravenous glucose if available.

CHOs = carbohydrates; g = gram; mg/dL = milligrams of glucose in 1 deciliter (100 millimeters) of blood.

their patient's glucometers and emergency glucagon kits should they need to use them in an emergency situation. Most emergency glucagon kits will include a glucagon powder and dissolving liquid to produce a single dose of 1 mg of glucagon. Once dissolved completely, the glucagon is injected intramuscularly or subcutaneously. Unconscious individuals experiencing hypoglycemia will usually regain consciousness within 5 to 20 minutes after a glucagon injection.[18] Once conscious, the athlete should eat a small snack made up of CHO and proteins.

In addition, people with type 1 diabetes mellitus may have a significant hypoglycemic response 6 to 24 hours after strenuous exercise.[5,6,23,24] After exercise, the body's muscle and liver glycogen stores must be restored. This process, which uses circulating blood glucose to synthesize glycogen, leads to a further depletion of blood glucose levels. The post-exercise insulin dose may need to be decreased and the post-exercise meal should ensure adequate caloric intake.[6] Conversely, failure to inject insulin after exercise causes hyperglycemia because glucose released during exercise is not countered by an insulin secretion response in individuals with type 1 diabetes mellitus. Additional potential risks for patients with diabetes are orthostatic hypotension and dehydration, both consequences of polyuria and the associated decrease in blood volume.[6,24]

Competitive athletes must adhere to specific regimens to maintain blood glucose control, including injection schedules, frequent blood glucose monitoring, and strict dietary constraints.[6,14,19,23] With awareness and simple precautions, most patients with diabetes can participate in sports without restriction or complications.[6,23] Again, the athlete's physician should guide any medical or dietary adjustments.

Disorders of the Pituitary Gland

Diabetes Insipidus

Inadequate secretion of ADH from the pituitary gland causes diabetes insipidus (DI). Decreased ADH level prevents water from being reabsorbed in the kidneys, and the result is large amounts of dilute urine. *Central DI* refers to decreased release of ADH, whereas *nephrogenic DI* results from resistance of the action of ADH leading to a decrease in urine concentrating ability. Polyuria and polydipsia in the presence of a normal blood glucose level characterize this disorder. Most cases are *idiopathic* (no discernable cause) but can be caused by tumors, infections, or vascular problems that affect the hypothalamus or pituitary gland. Medical examination to find an explanation is warranted. Return to play and sports is based on the cause and treatment plan.

Acromegaly

Overproduction of GH causes a condition called acromegaly.[10] Excess GH causes continual growth of bones and soft tissues. Persons with acromegaly are usually tall, have a thick prominent mandible, protruding frontal bone, large thick hands and feet, a "barrel" chest, and thoracic kyphosis.[10] Some organ systems, including cardiovascular, renal, and digestive, are affected both by the excess GH and the metabolic stress of maintaining a large, continually growing body. The life span is shortened and the most common causes of death are cardiovascular disease (from cardiomyopathy, hypertension, and hyperlipidemia) and cancer (from overstimulation and overproduction of organ cells). Abuse of human GH as an ergogenic aid can produce similar physical characteristics and clinical syndromes.

Disorders of the Thyroid and Parathyroid

Hyperthyroidism

An excess of thyroid hormone impairs glucose metabolism by interfering with insulin function and changing glucose absorption rate. The result is that muscles may have difficulty maintaining exercise.[28] In addition, core body temperature increases to above normal both at rest and with exercise as a result of thyroid hormone increasing overall metabolism. Monitoring for signs of hyperthermia during exercise is warranted.[28] Heart rate response to exercise may also be greater than normal. Other symptoms include nervousness, anxiety, diaphoresis, and insomnia.[29] Hyperthyroidism is treated with medication, radiation, or surgery to inhibit or remove the thyroid gland, depending on the severity and stage of disease.

Graves' disease is the most common form of hyperthyroidism and is 8 times more common in women than men. Graves' disease causes tremors, weakness, difficulty swallowing or speaking, fatigue, and facial or eye motor disorders (called tics).[10] Other signs and symptoms include an enlarged thyroid gland (goiter), heat intolerance, nervousness, sweating, weight loss, and protrusion of the eyes. Diagnosis is made based on symptoms, laboratory blood tests, and a thyroid scan. Treatment is similar to that for hyperthyroidism.

Hypothyroidism

After diabetes mellitus, hypothyroidism is the second most common endocrine disorder and affects the functioning of multiple organ systems. Hypothyroidism is caused by a deficiency of the thyroid hormones T3 and T4, with T4 being the primary hormone involved. Inadequate thyroid hormone decreases cardiac output by limiting heart rate (bradycardia) and left ventricle contractility, and thus limiting physical activity.[28] Furthermore, the normal peripheral vasodilation during exercise may not occur. The net effect is decreased oxygen and glucose available to exercising muscle, thus limiting endurance.[28] Signs and symptoms of hypothyroidism include dry skin, weakness, myalgia, bilateral paresthesias, impaired deep tendon reflexes, peripheral nonpitting edema, bradycardia, cold intolerance, memory problems, and slowed cognition.[29]

Hypothyroidism is diagnosed based on symptoms and the results of laboratory blood tests measuring the hormone blood levels of TSH and T4. Elevated TSH levels with lowered T4 values indicate *primary hypothyroidism*. High TSH levels demonstrate that the pituitary is functioning normally by continuing to secrete TSH but the thyroid is unable to produce normal levels T4. Low TSH levels with normal T4 levels indicate that the pituitary gland may not be functioning properly, causing *central hypothyroidism*. Further work-up is needed to differentiate between *secondary hypothyroidism* (pituitary) and *tertiary hypothyroidism* (hypothalamus).

Hypothyroidism is treated with levothyroxine (Levothyroid; Synthroid), a synthetic thyroid hormone (T4). In addition, there are other forms of thyroid replacement including desiccated thyroid abstract (ie, Armour Thyroid) and liothyronine (Cytomel), another synthetic thyroid hormone (T3). Because there is no cure for hypothyroidism, individuals with this disorder must take thyroid hormone for the rest of their lives. It may take 6 months to 1 year to effectively regulate the thyroid hormone levels and treatment regimen.

Parathyroid Hormone

Hyperparathyroidism and hypoparathyroidism, or an excess or inadequate secretion of PTH, respectively, are rarely encountered in athletes because they both limit muscle function. PTH regulates calcium metabolism. Hyperparathyroidism causes excess calcium release, primarily from bone, into the bloodstream. The most obvious consequences are muscle weakness, arthralgia in the hands and feet, and hyperactive reflexes. If untreated, kidney stones, peptic ulcers, and cognitive changes occur.[10] Hypoparathyroidism, by contrast, creates a deficiency of blood calcium, leading to muscle spasms during activity, cardiac arrhythmia, thin hair, and brittle nails. Hyper- and hypoparathyroidism also cause symptoms in the GI, neurological, and urogenital systems. Surgical removal of the glands is the treatment of hyperparathyroidism, whereas calcium and vitamin D supplementation are used for hypoparathyroidism.[10]

Disorders of the Adrenals

Addison's Disease

Addison's disease results from inadequate production of the hormones aldosterone and cortisol by the adrenal glands. Hyperpigmentation ("bronzing") of the skin, fatigue, hypotension, weakness, GI symptoms, and joint pain are common signs and symptoms. Fluid and electrolyte imbalances from decreased aldosterone secretion causes dehydration and impaired cardiac output. Tolerance for physical or emotional stress decreases, coordination is impaired, and hypoglycemia may occur between meals.

If untreated, Addison's disease is fatal. Lifetime prescription corticosteroids are usually prescribed as treatment. Fluid and electrolyte levels should be maintained, particularly during exercise. The treatment side effects of long-term corticosteroid therapy (see Cushing's syndrome next) become more prominent with age. Individuals with Addison's disease should have ready access to hydrocortisone to counteract acute adrenal crisis, which exhibits signs of shock and hypoglycemia. Recognition of adrenal crisis and subsequently immediate transfer to a hospital is important for the athletic trainer.

Cushing's Syndrome

Cushing's syndrome, in contrast to Addison's disease, occurs as a result of overproduction of cortisol by the adrenal glands. This syndrome can also occur in individuals who must take glucocorticoids for extended periods of time, such as prescriptions of prednisone for the treatment of asthma, lupus, rheumatoid arthritis, or other chronic inflammatory conditions. Classic signs and symptoms include "moon face," upper body obesity, a pendulous abdomen with stretch marks (sometimes called "central obesity" with "purple striae"), muscle atrophy, easy and frequent bruising, fatigue, and impaired wound healing. Cortisol acts as a very potent anti-inflammatory agent and in large amounts may mask signs of infection or tissue damage. In addition, emotional disturbances, decreased libido, and type 2 diabetes mellitus (from inhibition of insulin receptors) eventually occur.[10]

Diagnosis is usually made based on the patient's history, physical examination, and the results of laboratory tests. Surgery, radiation, and medication to cause adrenal suppression are the treatments.[10] If extended use of glucocorticoids is the cause of the Cushing's syndrome, the patient's dose may be reduced by the treating physician to obtain more controlled levels of cortisol. The patient's glucocorticoid dose will then be gradually increased, again but with doses taken every other day rather than every day.

Thermoregulation and Environmental Conditions

Thermoregulatory mechanisms are less effective in very young and very old people. Nutrition, drugs, alcohol use,[30] and fitness level also affect the ability of the body to disperse or retain heat.[7,31] Individuals with seizure disorders or sickle cell anemia may be predisposed to conditions caused by thermoregulatory disorders.[31]

During exercise in hot (>95°F [>35°C]) and humid environments, large amounts of sweat are produced in an effort to cool the body by evaporation. Simultaneously, peripheral vasodilation supplies muscles with additional oxygen and glucose. Vasodilation also provides an increased surface area to dissipate heat through the skin by convection. These mechanisms, sweating and vasodilation, create a relative hypovolemia in the vascular system, which decreases the heart's stroke volume. As a result, heart rate increases to maintain cardiac output. At lower environmental temperatures (<95°F [<35°C]) excess body heat is dissipated primarily through radiation to transfer heat from the skin to the environment.[32]

If hypovolemia continues to increase as a result of dehydration, reflex peripheral vasoconstriction occurs, which then impairs the heat dissipation mechanisms. Central ("core") body temperature increases as a consequence. If hydration is not restored to allow appropriate vasodilation, further vasoconstriction and a further increase in body temperature results. Heart rate continues to increase as cardiac output continues to decrease and blood pressure decreases, eventually producing shock and, in extreme cases, death.[30] Several stages of this pathological process theoretically exist (heat cramps, heat exhaustion, and heat stroke), and these are collectively referred to as heat illness. Other heat-related conditions exist, including heat syncope and exertional hyponatremia.

Heat Cramps

Heat cramps occur in the leg and trunk muscles during exercise in hot weather after mild dehydration. Associated signs and symptoms include fatigue, thirst, and profuse sweating.[33] Athletes who are accustomed to exercising in heat ("acclimatized") produce very dilute sweat, which preserves salts. Unacclimated athletes, however, secrete a relatively high concentration of salt with the fluids in their sweat. Attempts by unacclimated athletes to replace fluid loss with plain water may further dilute the blood and worsen muscle spasms as a result of the relative lowering electrolyte (sodium and potassium) levels.[7]

Gradual acclimatization is usually preventive. During an attack of heat cramps, cooling, rehydration, and a dilute (0.1% to 1.0%) saline solution can be used.[33,34] Adding one-quarter teaspoon of table salt to a sports drink can be very effective. Ice, stretching, and massage can help alleviate the pain associated with heat cramps. Return-to-play decisions should be based on the individual's ability to perform at the necessary level and their hydration status.[35] Increased dietary salt intake is not necessary, and may actually contribute to heat cramps by stimulating sweat glands to secrete more salt, thus compounding the problem.[7]

Heat Syncope

This condition, also in the spectrum of exercise associated collapse, typically occurs within the first few days of returning to exercising in hot, humid conditions. The combined effects of peripheral vasodilation, hypovolemia, and dehydration causes pooling of the blood in the lower limbs, leading to decrease cardiac output, depriving the brain of blood.[32,33,36,37] When the blood flow to the brain is inadequate, syncope results. Contributing factors include standing for several hours (as often occurs during practices in sports), stopping strenuous exercise suddenly, and rapidly standing up from sitting. The person usually recovers consciousness within minutes and may report feeling dizzy or having tunnel vision just before fainting. Skin may be pale or sweaty, heart rate is generally slowed, and body temperature is elevated as a result of exercising but is not excessive. Treatment is moving the person into the shade, elevating the legs (Trendelenberg position), and rehydrating.[32,37] Vital signs should be monitored to ensure that the condition does not progress.

Heat Exhaustion

Advanced dehydration, usually from a failure to adequately replace fluid or sodium, produces heat exhaustion.[31,36] The signs and symptoms, although variable, include profuse sweating, increased body temperature (100°F to 103°F [37.8°C to 39.4°C]), tachycardia, hyperpnea, hypotension, headache, fatigue, and nausea.[7,31,34] The person may report muscle cramping, weakness, or dizziness.[33] Changes in mental status are usually not present, although physical collapse may occur.[7] Remember, at this point, thirst is not a reliable source of hydration status.

Rapid cooling using cool towels or a cool shower, removing excess clothing, resting in shade or air conditioning, and rehydration with a dilute electrolyte drink (0.1% saline content) usually precipitate recovery.[7,34] Rehydration with large amounts of plain water may dilute the blood, thus accentuating the existing electrolyte depletion.[31] Symptoms usually resolve within 2 to 3 hours, and transport to a physician for intravenous rehydration is recommended if recovery does not progress rapidly.[33,37] Avoiding extreme heat, ensuring a reasonable acclimatization period at the beginning of the season, and proper rehydration during exercise can prevent heat exhaustion. Following heat exhaustion, individuals should be fully hydrated and free of symptoms before returning to activity, usually at least 24 to 48 hours later.[34,35]

Exertional Heat Stroke

Heat stroke is a medical emergency with a very high rate of mortality. Heat stroke occurs with body temperatures higher than 104°F (40°C) (*hyperthermia*).[15,33,35,36] It is the third leading cause of sport-related death, after head and neck trauma and cardiac failure.[31] When severe dehydration and hypovolemia inhibits the sweating mechanism, the peripheral vascular system collapses in an attempt to preserve blood pressure and supply to the central vital organs.[7,38] Once this transition occurs, the body has no mechanism to dissipate heat, and central body temperature increases very quickly. Lactic acid and potassium levels build in the blood and muscle tissue breaks down (rhabdomyolysis), flooding the bloodstream with proteins that eventually block the kidneys and cause acute renal failure. Cardiac output eventually falls so low it cannot maintain blood flow to the brain and kidneys, which produces a reflex systemic vasodilation in a vascular system that is already lacking in fluid volume. Vasodilation greatly increases cardiac demand on the insufficient cardiovascular system, which results in acute heart failure. Loss of consciousness, convulsions, coma, and death can result.[7,38]

An individual exercising in a hot environment who has tachycardia, very high core body temperature (> 104°F [> 40°C]), lack of coordination, physical collapse, and altered cognitive ability (ie, disorientation, confusion, seizure, hallucination) has all of the signs of heat stroke. The central nervous system (CNS) symptoms in addition to the high core temperature distinguish exertional heat stroke from heat exhaustion. The NATA recommends that athletic trainers assess rectal temperatures to obtain the most accurate measure of core temperature.[15,39] When exertional heat stroke is suspected, drastic emergency measures should be undertaken immediately.

Rapid cooling by immersion in cold water (35°F to 58°F [1.7°C to 14.4°C]) is the preferred method for reducing core temperature, and cooling should occur prior to emergency transportation to a hospital.[15,34,39] Once core temperature has reduced to 101°F to 102°F (38.3°C to 38.9°C), the individual should be transported immediately to the closest emergency room.[37] If onsite cooling by immersion is not available, then the individual should be transported immediately with cooling performed in route to the hospital using cold towels or ice bags.[7,33] Intravenous fluids need to be administered under medical direction to prevent forced overhydration, which can cause pulmonary or cerebral edema. Following heat stroke, return-to-play decisions should be made by the treating physician with a minimal 7-day withdrawal from all activities.[34] Once clearance is obtained, the individual should begin a very gradual return to activity and environmental heat, allowing time for re-acclimatization. Full recovery, in which responses to activity in the heat normalize, may require up to 1 year.

Exertional Hyponatremia

This type of heat-related illness has signs and symptoms that are similar to exertional heat stroke. Exertional hyponatremia is a dangerous condition in which the sodium level in the blood falls below 130 mmol/L.[33,40] Exercise lasting 4 hours or longer during which a person drinks a large amount of water, much more than they have lost through sweat (so-called water intoxication, in which the person may actually drink so much water that they gain weight during exercise), or fails to replace sodium lost through sweat, or both, lead to this condition.[15,36] The result of low blood sodium is a movement of water out of the vascular system and into the tissues. The cells in the tissues swell to the point of bursting, causing a severe impairment of cell function. Fluid shifts into the lungs and brain can cause death quickly.

Exertional hyponatremia produces headache, nausea, impaired cognition, loss of consciousness, seizures, and swollen extremities.[15] The CNS signs and symptoms of hyponatremia are similar to those of exertional heat stroke, except that the core body temperature is typically not elevated above 104°F (40°C). The person with exertional hyponatremia should never be given fluids until a physician has properly diagnosed the condition and an appropriate hypertonic saline solution is determined. Suspicion of hyponatremia warrants immediate referral to the hospital.[15] Restoration of normal sodium levels is required, such as intravenous administration of a hypertonic (3% to 5%) solution,[15] as well as close monitoring by a physician. Return-to-play decisions following exertional hyponatremia should be made by the treating physician and should include an appropriate hydration plan to prevent another episode.

Prevention of Heat Illness

Deaths during exercise or activity that are attributable to environmental heat are preventable. Preparticipation examinations can be used to identify people at risk for heat illness, such as a history of previous exertional heat illness.[15] Coaches, participants, and others involved in organized outdoor activities should be educated regarding the prevention and recognition of heat illness, and a protocol for adverse environmental conditions should be established before the season begins.[13,15,41] The NATA position statements on exertional heat illness, preseason heat acclimatization, fluid replacement for athletes, and safe weight loss and maintenance, as well as other consensus statements for preventing sudden death in athletes, list several other preventive measures.[13,15,33,39,42-44] The International Olympic Committee has developed a similar set of recommendations.[8]

First, a period of acclimatization should be allowed, during which the cardiovascular system and sweating mechanism can adapt.[7,8,13,15,32,33,39,44] Usually physiological acclimatization adaptations begin within several days but take 2 weeks or longer to become effective.[31,33,44] Second, vigorous exercise during the hottest part of the day should be avoided, and drills and practice should be moved indoors whenever feasible.[33] The largest determining factor related to the body's ability to cool itself is the ambient temperature and humidity.[34] Wet bulb globe temperature (WBGT) combines temperature, humidity, wind velocity, and sunlight radiation into a single measure that indicates the environmental heat risk.[34] Current recommendations for modifying activity are based on the WBGT, with suggestions to reschedule outdoor activities or proceeding with extreme caution and continuous monitoring of participants when the WBGT exceeds 82°F (28°C).[33] When exercise in hot weather cannot be avoided, reasonable precautions are usually possible, such as providing accessible and appropriate hydration; modifying type, intensity or duration of activities; scheduling frequent breaks in the shade; and having shorter practices.[8,29,33,38] Third, wearing appropriate clothing that allows evaporation and cooling, avoiding the consumption of diuretics such as alcohol and caffeine, and the continuous monitoring of athletes during practice can prevent many heat illnesses.[7,8]

Proper hydration maintains thermoregulatory and cardiovascular function.[42] Individuals should be fully hydrated when they begin exercise. Pre-hydration guidelines recommend the consumption of 17 to 20 ounces (0.5 to 0.6 L) of water or sports drink 2 to 3 hours before exercise and an additional 7 to 10 ounces (0.2 to 0.3 L) of fluids 10 to 20 minutes before exercise.[42] Fluid intake during exercise is also essential for preventing dehydration.[7,30] During shorter, less-intense events (up to 1 hour), plain water can be used to rehydrate. Replacement of electrolytes, and to some extent CHOs, in addition to water becomes more important as intensity and duration of exercise increases.[7,30] Cooler beverages may help to prevent an excessive core temperature increase and to maintain performance.[45] During endurance events and in between practices, however, plain water increases urine output even when mildly dehydrated. Thus, a CHO-electrolyte drink (solute content between 3% and 6%) may be preferred.[30,42] An athlete who has lost 3% or more of their body weight during an exercise session or across several sessions in heat should be held from subsequent practices until body weight is restored. Remember that thirst is not an adequate source to determine hydration status and typically, athlete should replenish 16 ounces (500 mL) for every pound loss during exercise.

Exposure to Cold

Prolonged exposure to cold environmental temperatures can also cause medical problems, some of which are life threatening, particularly if moisture and wind are also present. Water has 25 times the heat conductance of air, so wet clothes, rain or sleet, or immersion in cold water quickly removes body heat.[7] Wind chill removes heat from the skin by convection and can substantially reduce body temperature, which is compounded if running or moving into the wind.[7,46] In addition, at least half of the body's expelled heat radiates through the head and neck during exercise in cooler environments. Appropriate clothing or protective gear should protect against rain, snow, and wind and cover the head and neck to prevent excessive heat loss during prolonged exposure.

Hypothermia

Prolonged exposure to cold environmental temperatures can produce a potentially fatal condition called *hypothermia*, which is a central body temperature of 95°F (35°C) or less.[36,46,47] As central body temperature decreases, metabolism decreases, blood viscosity (resistance to flow) increases, and heart rate and cardiac output decrease.[7,47] Uncontrollable shivering may occur and changes in cognitive function occur, such as confusion, psychosis (loss of reasoning), lethargy, or coma.[7,31] Physical signs include facial erythema and edema, ataxia (uncoordinated gait), bradycardia, and hypotension.[31]

Treatment of hypothermia takes precedence over frostbite.[47] Passive rewarming, or removing wet clothing and placing the victim in a warm environment (indoors with blankets), is preferred to applying heating pads or immersion in warm baths.[34,37] Rapid reheating of a person with hypothermia can cause a paradoxical reaction known as "after drop," wherein peripheral vasodilation and subsequent rush of cold fluids from the extremities actually causes core temperature to decrease even further.[31,47] The risk of after drop can be reduced by heating the trunk, armpits, and groin rather than the extremities or the entire body.[46] For severe cases of hypothermia, emergency department techniques are required to prevent cardiac fibrillation.[31] At very low body temperatures (< 90°F [< 32°C]), vital signs may not be detectable but resuscitation may still be possible, even after a prolonged period of time. Thus, cardiopulmonary resuscitation and emergency transportation to a hospital should occur so that physicians can determine the status of the patient.

Prevention of hypothermia and other problems related to cold environments primarily involves avoidance of cold, wet, windy environments and wearing appropriate clothing. Similar to prevention of heat injuries, protocols for cold weather should be established before conditioning and the season begins.[46] The guidelines should be based on the windchill temperature, which accounts for the added effect of wind on ambient temperature, and provide for monitoring changing conditions during an event. Windchill temperatures below 25°F (−4°C) require additional clothing and breaks for rewarming. When windchill temperatures fall below 0°F (−18°C), rescheduling the event or moving activity indoors should be strongly considered.[46] Clothes should be layered, with a light, wicking material near the skin, a water-resistant layer on the outside, and insulating materials in the layers in between.[7,46]

Altitude Sickness

Exercise in altitude can cause several pathological conditions due to decreased barometric pressure, low partial pressure of oxygen, decreased ambient temperature, higher intensity sunlight, and dehydration, and a failure of the body's systems to respond and adapt appropriately.[36,48] Within 6 to 24 hours of ascent to over 12,000 feet (3.7 km), headache along with at least one other symptom such as loss of appetite, nausea, irritability, dizziness, fatigue, sleep disturbance, and mild confusion characterizes acute altitude sickness.[8,32,37,49] Although bothersome, this condition is seldom serious at altitudes below 15,000 feet. Most cases resolve in a few days with rest and maintaining adequate hydration. Slow or gradual ascent to high altitudes may prevent or substantially decrease symptoms.

Some people experience pulmonary or cerebral edema in high altitude, particularly with rapid ascent to at least 8000 feet (2.4 km).[49] Pulmonary edema is recognized by dyspnea, cough, cyanosis, tachycardia, hyperpnea, and rales on auscultation.[36] Cerebral edema impairs cognitive and other CNS functions, causing confusion, ataxia, hallucination, and loss of consciousness.[32] Early recognition of these serious conditions allows descent from altitude in a timely manner. Oxygen supplementation and corticosteroids may be needed in more severe cases.[32,37,49]

At very high altitude (over 15,000 feet [4.6 km]), retinal hemorrhage and retinopathy may occur. Exercise may exacerbate this situation, which is recognized by blurring vision and aching in the orbits. The condition is usually self-limiting with no permanent complications if descent occurs quickly.[49]

High altitude also increases the risk for sickle cell crisis in individuals with sickle cell trait. The increased oxygen demand at altitude leads to an increased rate of red blood cell production, which in turn leads to an increased viscosity of the blood. This thickened blood increases the risk for clumping or clotting of the abnormally shaped red blood cells associated with sickle cell trait. Anyone relocating to a high-altitude environment should allow time for gradual acclimatization.

Metabolic Disorders

Obesity

Obesity, the presence of excess adipose (fat) tissue, has become a major health concern in the United States and the world. Obesity has been increasing across the entire United States over the last 25 years. Current estimates indicate that approximately 39.8% of adults (and 18.5% of children are obese.[50-52] Obesity rates are about equal between men and women, and older Americans have higher obesity rates than young and middle-aged adults. Black and Hispanic patients have substantially higher obesity rates compared to non-Hispanic White patients. Obesity is more frequent in populations with lower socioeconomic status and less education and is most prevalent in the southeastern part of the United States. The excess medical cost attributable to obesity-related health problems is estimated to be hundreds of billions of dollars per year.[53]

For an individual, obesity occurs after a sustained positive energy imbalance in which energy intake exceeds energy expenditure.[54,55] Excess body fat is associated with risk of many chronic diseases, including heart disease, hypertension, stroke, type 2 diabetes mellitus, and certain cancers. These risks increase proportionately as excess body fat increases, such that individuals who have some excess body fat may be at no or only slightly increased risk, whereas those with morbid obesity are at high risk for serious health problems.[56]

Obesity contributes to development of disease in a number of ways. Large amounts of excess fat tissue create a physical, physiological, and metabolic strain on virtually all organ systems. Fat tissue secretes signaling proteins (adipokines) that stimulate widespread chronic inflammatory and immune responses. When a large fat mass is present, these adipokines appear in large enough concentration to interfere with endocrine responses and functions in other tissues, such as endothelium, blood, and muscle, and systems, including the GI, hepatobiliary, and immune. For example, several of these adipokines impair insulin binding in various tissues, thus blunting transport of glucose from the blood into tissues. This impairment of insulin function and the resulting hyperglycemia is called insulin resistance. Chronic insulin resistance is one of the defining signs of type 2 diabetes mellitus, thus demonstrating a physiological mechanism linking obesity to risk of that condition.

Identifying obesity requires measuring body fat or body weight accurately. In terms of body fat as a percentage of total body mass in young and middle-aged adults, obesity is generally considered as a body fat percentage > 25% in men and > 33% in women.[57] When evaluating individuals clinically, body fat can be estimated using a variety of methods, including dual-energy X-ray absorptiometry, skinfold thicknesses from different body regions, air displacement plethysmography, bioelectrical impedance analysis, near-infrared interactance, underwater weighing, ultrasound, and circumferential measures. Each method has different advantages, disadvantages, and costs, but when used properly all are reasonably accurate estimates of body fat.

For estimating the prevalence of obesity in a population rather than an individual, measuring body fat for thousands of people is impractical. Instead, population-level obesity rates are estimated using body mass index (BMI), which is the ratio of body weight (kg) to height (m) squared (kg/m^2). Measures of height and weight are readily available for many populations, which facilitates the computation and use of BMI. The World Health Organization defines BMI categories for adults as follows: underweight, < 18.5; normal weight, 18.5 to 24.9; overweight, 25.0 to 29.9, class I obesity, 30.0 to 34.9; class II obesity, 35.0 to 39.9; and class III obesity, ≥ 40.0.[56] Risk of chronic disease increases with higher classes of obesity.

For children, BMI is computed the same way but must be interpreted relative to sex and age. because height and weight develop at different rates, BMI changes as children grow, and boys and girls grow at different rates. To account for these sex- and age-related changes, a child's BMI is compared to the Centers for Disease Control and Prevention's growth charts from the year 2000.[59] These charts plot the range of BMI seen in the United States population of children using the 2000 growth charts as a reference point to convert a child's BMI into a percentile. Overweight is defined as a sex- and age-referenced percentile value of 85.0 to 94.9, and obesity is defined as a percentile value of 95 or greater.[59] For example, a 5-year-old boy who is 109 cm (43 inches) tall and weighs 21 kg (46 pounds) would have a BMI of 17.7, which corresponds to a percentile of 93.5. A percentile value of 93.5 lies between 85 and 94.9, so this child would be classified as overweight.

For adults and children, caution is warranted when interpreting BMI for individuals. Individuals who have proportionately more fat-free tissue, which has a higher density than fat, will have higher BMIs despite having a lower percentage of body fat compared to another person with proportionately more fat mass. Also, the relation of BMI to relative fat mass varies between men and women, by age, by ethnicity, and perhaps by a number of other as yet unidentified factors. Consequently, interpreting BMI in terms of an absolute health risk for any given individual is difficult. A person with a high BMI may require further assessment to determine percentage of body fat and other health risk factors in order to provide appropriate guidance for weight control and health.

The determinants of energy imbalance leading to obesity are complex, with potential influences from many genetic, biological, behavioral, socioeconomic, cultural, and environmental factors.[60,61] As a result, prevention and treatment of obesity are also complex. At the individual level, the key is balancing adequate intake and nutrition to maintain health with adequate physical activity to maintain healthy fat-free mass (muscle and bone) and a healthy fat mass. While even a small sustained positive energy balance (eg, 25 kcal/day intake > expenditure) is associated with the development of obesity,[61] maintaining either extreme positive or negative energy imbalances can increase health risk. A healthy energy balance may be difficult to achieve when influences beyond individual behavior are considered, such as comorbid health conditions, poverty, low availability of nutrient-dense foods, limited opportunities for physical activity (eg, poorly maintained or dangerous neighborhoods), and cultural norms (eg, food traditions, variable perceptions of what foods and behaviors are "healthy"). To address this wide array of contributing factors, current obesity prevention and treatment programs are targeting families, environments, communities, and systems (eg, health care, public schools, legislative) rather than only behaviors of the individual.[62-68]

Gout

Gout is caused by a defect in the breakdown of an amino acid called purine that causes accumulation of uric acid in the blood. As uric acid concentration increases, it cannot be efficiently excreted by the kidneys and forms crystals in the joints and other tissues. The typical first manifestation of gout is sudden, severe pain and swelling in one or more joints. More than 90% of patients with gout have symptoms in the great toe (eg, podagra). The foot, knee, elbows, and wrist are also commonly involved. Surgery, fatigue, rich diet, stress, infection, or certain medications can precipitate gout attacks. Chalky crystal deposits may erupt through the skin of a gouty joint. Unless treated, the attacks recur with increasing frequency and severity, although remissions lasting years may also be experienced. Treatment is prescription medication and dietary lifestyle changes.

Metabolic Bone Diseases

Osteoporosis

A pathological decrease in bone density is called osteoporosis.[69] Many factors contribute to the development of osteoporosis, including hormonal disturbances (decreased estrogen), nutritional deficiencies (primarily of calcium), and age.[69] With continued loss of density, the bones eventually become very fragile and fracture easily. Frequently, compression fractures of the vertebrae cause permanent deformities such as severe thoracic spine kyphosis ("Dowager's hump"), loss of height, and back pain.[69] Accidents or falls may fracture the femur, tibia, humerus, or radius. For people at risk for osteoporosis (female, postmenopausal, older than age 75 years), precautions should be taken when applying manual mobilization techniques, exercising the spine, or performing load-bearing exercises. As mentioned in Chapter 9, osteoporosis can also occur in females who have an eating disorder and amenorrhea (female athlete triad syndrome).[70] Screening guidelines are now in place for various populations.

Paget Disease

Paget disease (osteitis deformans) is an abnormality of bone remodeling, with alternating excess deposition or resorption of bone during various stages of the disease. The etiology is unclear, but the pathophysiology involves a deposition-resorption cycle that happens many times faster than normal. The disease begins in a destructive phase, in which bone resorption dominates. The second phase displays an acceleration of bone formation to counter the high rate of resorption. The final phase involves osteosclerotic changes in which the bone becomes thickened and dense. The disease may affect one bone or many. Although many patients are asymptomatic or have minor aching pains, in others the thickening of bone leads to neural compression, particularly of the cranial nerves. The abnormal bone is also prone to deformity, particularly in the spine (kyphosis) and long bones of the legs (bowing), and fracture.

The condition occurs most frequently in the flat and long bones of older adult men.[69] Over time, Paget disease produces bony deformities, functional disability, head or face pain, and pathological fractures.[69] Treatment involves control of symptoms with anti-inflammatory medications and administration of hormones that control bone metabolism. Treatment precautions, such as avoiding heavy loads or extreme motions, are necessary to lower the risk of fracture.

Pediatric Concerns

Osteogenesis Imperfecta

Osteogenesis imperfecta (OI) is an inherited, autosomal dominant (most frequently, but autosomal recessive and spontaneous mutation forms also occur) condition that interferes with bone formation by affecting the quantity, quality, or both of synthesis of type I collagen.[71] OI makes the bones very brittle and susceptible to fracture, even during normal activities. People with OI are nearly always diagnosed in early childhood and rarely participate in athletics because of the high risk of injury. Several variants of OI, from mild to severe, exist and there is no cure.[71] Signs of OI are due to the collagen defect and include heart valve disorders, stunted growth, blue eye sclera, dental problems, joint laxity, and scoliosis. Fractures may be surgically stabilized or treated nonoperatively with casting or splinting. Many patients become progressively disabled and acquire bony deformities from multiple fractures, and lifespan may be shortened. Treatment consists primarily of prevention and management of fractures and bony deformities.

SUMMARY

The endocrine system regulates the functions of many organ systems including normal metabolism and homeostasis. Pathology of the endocrine glands can produce signs and symptoms in many organ systems, including the GI, cardiovascular, neurological, urogenital, and musculoskeletal. The personal medical history, which can reveal distinct patterns of endocrine dysfunction, is the most important aspect of assessment for endocrine or metabolic disorders. Diabetes, thyroid hormone imbalance (hypo- and hyper-), and Cushing's syndrome (either primary or a result of long-term corticosteroid use) are the most common endocrine disorders in the general population. Treatment of endocrine disorders is complicated and may involve many side effects that impair physical activity. Pathological metabolic conditions that are most frequently encountered include adverse environmental exposure (heat, cold, and altitude) and bone diseases. Pathology resulting from environmental conditions is treated by prevention (avoiding extreme environments) or removal from the hazardous environment.

CASE STUDY: PART 1

Scott, one of your high school junior varsity football athletes, has recently been diagnosed with type 1 diabetes mellitus. He is having trouble regulating his blood glucose levels, particularly now during 2-a-day practice sessions. You notice during the second workout of the day that Scott is starting to look a little sluggish. You ask him how he feels, and he insists that he is fine. Still suspecting a problem, you continue to watch him closely. Just before the next water break, you see Scott stumble and then collapse on the field. As you reach him, you find that he is pale, clammy, confused, and slurring his words.

Critical Thinking Questions

1. Based on Scott's medical history and the current signs and symptoms, what condition(s) do you suspect?
2. How would you treat the condition(s), both on the field and after removing Scott from the field?
3. What could you have done differently to prevent the condition(s) from occurring?

CASE STUDY: PART 2

Scott's physician has decided to have him use an insulin pump to better regulate his blood glucose levels. For the next 3 weeks, he wants Scott wearing his pump during all practices and games.

Critical Thinking Question

1. How would you modify Scott's football equipment to accommodate and protect the insulin pump?

REFERENCES

1. National Athletic Trainers' Association. *Athletic Training Education Competencies*. 5th ed. The Commission on Accreditation of Athletic Training Education; 2011.
2. Ganong WF. *Review of Medical Physiology*. 22nd ed. McGraw-Hill Medical; 2005.
3. Gould BE. Endocrine disorders. *Pathophysiology for the Health-Related Professions*. W.B. Saunders Company; 1997:377-395.
4. Martini FH, Timmons MJ, McKinley MP. The endocrine system. *Human Anatomy*. 3rd ed. Prentice-Hall; 2000:499-521.
5. Hough DO. Diabetes mellitus in sports. *Med Clin North Am*. 1994;78(2):423-437.
6. Landry GL, Allen DB. Diabetes mellitus and exercise. *Clin Sports Med*. 1992;11:403-418.
7. Thein LA. Environmental conditions affecting the athlete. *J Orthop Sports Phys Ther*. 1995;21(3):158-171.
8. Bergeron MF, Bahr R, Bartsch P, et al. International Olympic Committee consensus statement on thermoregulatory and altitude challenges for high-level athletes. *Br J Sports Med*. 2012;46:770-779.
9. Allen DB. Effects of fitness training on endocrine systems in children and adolescents. *Adv Pediatr*. 1999;46:41-66.
10. Boissonnault JS, Madlon-Kay D. Screening for endocrine system disease. In: Boissonnault WG, ed. *Examination in Physical Therapy Practice: Screening for Medical Disease*. Churchill Livingstone; 1995:155-173.
11. Casa DJ, Becker SM, Ganio MS, et al. Validity of devices that assess body temperature during outdoor exercise in the heat. *J Athl Train*. 2007;42:333-342.
12. Mazerolle SM, Casa TM, Casa DJ. Heat and hydration curriculum issues: part 1 of 4—hydration and exercise. *Athl Ther Today*. 2009;14:39-44.
13. Casa DJ, Anderson SA, Baker L, et al. The inter-association task force for preventing sudden death in collegiate conditioning sessions: best practices recommendations. *J Athl Train*. 2012;47:477-480.
14. Jimenez CC. Diabetes and exercise: the role of the athletic trainer. *J Athl Train*. 1997;32:339-343.
15. Casa DJ, Guskiewicz KM, Anderson SA, et al. National Athletic Trainers' Association position statement: preventing sudden death in sports. *J Athl Train*. 2012;47:96-118.
16. American Diabetes Association. Standards of Medical Care in Diabetes 2011. *Diabetes Care 2011*; 34:S11.
17. Jimenez CC, Corcoran MH, Crawley JT, et al. National Athletic Trainers' Association position statement: management of the athlete with type 1 diabetes mellitus. *J Athl Train*. 2007;42:536-545.
18. Landry GL, Burnhardt DT. Diabetes mellitus. *Essentials of Primary Care Sports Medicine*. Human Kinetics; 2003:37-53.
19. Bell DS. Exercise for patients with diabetes: benefits, risks, precautions. *Postgrad Med*. 1992;92:183-184,187-190,195-198.
20. Wilder RP, Cicchetti M. Common injuries in athletes with obesity and diabetes. *Clin Sports Med*. 2009;28:441-453.
21. Draznin MB. Managing the adolescent athlete with type 1 diabetes mellitus. *Pediatr Clin North Am*. 2010;57:829-837.
22. Jimenez CC. Recognizing and managing diabetes-related emergencies. *Athl Ther Today*. 2004;9(2):6-10.
23. Fahey PJ, Stallkamp ET, Kwatra S. The athlete with type I diabetes: managing insulin, diet and exercise. *Am Fam Physician*. 1996;53(5):1611-1617.
24. Martin DE. Glucose emergencies: recognition and treatment. *J Athl Train*. 1994;29:141-143.
25. Dabelea D, Mayer-Davis EJ, Saydah S, et al. Prevalence of type 1 and type 2 diabetes among children and adolescents from 2001-2009. *JAMA*. 2014 May;311(17);1778-86.
26. Petrella RJ. Exercise for older patients with chronic disease. *Phys Sportsmed*. 1999;27(11):79-104.
27. Fincher AL. Managing diabetic emergencies. *Athl Ther Today*. 1999;4:45-46.
28. McAllister RM, Delp MD, Laughlin MH. Thyroid status and exercise tolerance: cardiovascular and metabolic considerations. *Sports Med*. 1995;20:189-198.
29. Duhig TJ, McKeag D. Thyroid disorders in athletes. *Curr Sports Med Rep*. 2009;8:16-19.
30. Murray R. Dehydration, hyperthermia, and athletes: science and practice. *J Athl Train*. 1996;31:248-252.
31. Bracker MD. Environmental and thermal injury. *Clin Sports Med*. 1992;11:419-436.
32. Dhillon S. Environmental hazards, hot, cold, altitude, and sun. *Infect Dis Clin North Am*. 2012;26:707-723.

33. Binkley HM, Beckett J, Casa DJ, Kleiner DM, Plummer PE. National Athletic Trainers' Association position statement: exertional heat illnesses. *J Athl Train.* 2002;37(3):329-343.

34. Noonan B, Bancroft RW, Dines JS, Bedi A. Heat- and cold-induced injuries in athletes: evaluation and management. *J Am Acad Orthop Surg.* 2012;20:744-754.

35. Interassociation Task Force on Exertional Heat Illness. Consensus statement. Available at: nata.org.

36. Seto CK, Way D, O'Connor N. Environmental illness in athletes. *Clin Sports Med.* 2005;25:695-718.

37. DeFranco MJ, Baker CL 3rd, DaSilva JJ, Piasecki DP, Bach BR Jr. Environmental issues for team physicians. *Am J Sports Med.* 2008;36:2226-2237.

38. Epstein Y, Roberts WO. The pathopysiology of heat stroke: an integrative view of the final common pathway. *Scand J Med Sci Sports.* 2011;21:742-748.

39. Casa DJ, Almquist J, Anderson SA, et al. The Inter-Association Task Force for Preventing Sudden Death in Secondary School Athletics Programs: best practices recommendations. *J Athl Train.* 2013; 48(4):546-553.

40. Hew-Butler T, Almond C, Ayus JC, et al. Consensus Statement of the 1st International Exercise-Associated Hyponatremia Consensus Development Conference, Cape Town, South Africa 2005. *Clin J Sport Med.* 2005;15:208-213.

41. Almquist J, Valovich McLeod TC, Cavanna A, et al. Summary statement: appropriate medical care for the secondary school-aged athlete. *J Athl Train.* 2008;43:416-427.

42. Casa DJ, Armstrong LE, Hillman SK, et al. National Athletic Trainers' Association position statement: fluid replacement for athletes. *J Athl Train.* 2000;35:212-224.

43. Turocy PS, DePalma BF, Horswill CA, et al. National Athletic Trainers' Association position statement: safe weight loss and maintenance practices in sport and exercise. *J Athl Train.* 2011;46:322-336.

44. Casa DJ, Csillan D, Inter-Association Task Force for Preseason Secondary School Athletics Participants, et al. Preseason heat-acclimatization guidelines for secondary school athletics. *J Athl Train.* 2009;44(3):332-333.

45. Burdon CA, O'Connor HT, Gifford JA, Shirreffs SM. Influence of beverage temperature on exercise performance in the heat: a systematic review. *Int J Sport Nutr Exerc Metab.* 2010;20:166-174.

46. Cappaert TA, Stone JA, Castellani JW, et al. National Athletic Trainers' Association position statement: environmental cold injuries. *J Athl Train.* 2008;43:640-658.

47. Grace TG. Cold exposure injuries and the winter athlete. *Clin Orthop Relat Res.* 1987;(216):55-62.

48. Woods DR, Stacey M, Hill N, de Alwis N. Endocrine aspects of high altitude acclimatization and acute mountain sickness. *J R Army Med Corps.* 2011;157:33-37.

49. Mountain RD. High-altitude medical problems. *Clin Orthop Relat Res.* 1987;(216):50-54.

50. Flegal KM, Carroll MD, Kit BK, Ogden CL. Prevalence of obesity and trends in the distribution of body mass index among US adults, 1999-2010. *JAMA.* 2012;307:491-497.

51. Ogden CL, Carroll MD, Kit BK, Flegal KM. Prevalence of obesity in the United States, 2015-2016. *NCHS Data Brief.* 2017;288:1-8.

52. Ogden CL, Carroll MD, Kit BK, Flegal KM. Prevalence of obesity and trends in body mass index among US children and adolescents, 1999-2010. *JAMA.* 2012;307:483-490.

53. Finkelstein EA, Brown DS, Wrage LA, Allaire BT, Hoerger TJ. Individual and aggregate years-of-life-lost associated with overweight and obesity. *Obesity (Silver Spring).* 2010;18:333-339.

54. Hill JO, Wyatt HR, Peters JC. Energy balance and obesity. *Circulation.* 2012;126:126-132.

55. Goran MI. Energy metabolism and obesity. *Med Clin North Am.* 2000;84:347-362.

56. Flegal KM, Kit BK, Orpana H, Graubard BI. Association of all-cause mortality with overweight and obesity using standard body mass index categories: a systematic review and meta-analysis. *JAMA.* 2013;309:71-82.

57. Okorodudu DO, Jumean MF, Montori VM, et al. Diagnostic performance of body mass index to identify obesity as defined by body adiposity: a systematic review and meta-analysis. *Int J Obes (Lond).* 2010;34:791-799.

58. World Health Organization. BMI classification. Available at: http://apps.who.int/bmi/index.jsp?introPage=intro_3.html. Accessed June 23, 2013.

59. Centers for Disease Control and Prevention. CDC growth charts: United States. Available at: http://www.cdc.gov/growthcharts/background.htm. Accessed June 23, 2013.

60. Bleich SN, Ku R, Wang YC. Relative contribution of energy intake and energy expenditure to childhood obesity: a review of the literature and directions for future research. *Int J Obes (Lond).* 2011;35:1-15.

61. Goran MI, Weinsier RL. Role of environmental vs. metabolic factors in the etiology of obesity: time to focus on the environment. *Obes Res.* 2000;8:407-409.

62. Foltz JL, May AL, Belay B, Nihiser AJ, Dooyema CA, Blanck HM. Population-level intervention strategies and examples for obesity prevention in children. *Annu Rev Nutr.* 2012;32:391-415.

63. Bahr DB, Browning RC, Wyatt HR, Hill JO. Exploiting social networks to mitigate the obesity epidemic. *Obesity (Silver Spring).* 2009;17:723-728.

64. Crombie IK, Irvine L, Elliott L, Wallace H. Targets to tackle the obesity epidemic: a review of twelve developed countries. *Public Health Nutr.* 2009;12:406-413.

65. Fuemmeler BF, Baffi C, Masse LC, Atienza AA, Evans WD. Employer and healthcare policy interventions aimed at adult obesity. *Am J Prev Med.* 2007;32:44-51.

66. Hammond RA. Complex systems modeling for obesity research. *Prev Chronic Dis.* 2009;6:A97.

67. Khambalia AZ, Dickinson S, Hardy LL, Gill T, Baur LA. A synthesis of existing systematic reviews and meta-analyses of school-based behavioural interventions for controlling and preventing obesity. *Obes Rev.* 2012;13:214-233.

68. Mitchell NS, Catenacci VA, Wyatt HR, Hill JO. Obesity: overview of an epidemic. *Psychiatr Clin North Am.* 2011;34:717-732.

69. Boissonnault WG, Bass C. Pathological origins of trunk and neck pain: Part III-diseases of the musculoskeletal system. *J Orthop Sports Phys Ther.* 1990;12(5):216-221.

70. Thein-Nissenbaum JM, Carr KE. Female athlete triad syndrome in the high school athlete. *Phys Ther Sport.* 2011;12:108-116.

71. Myers GJ. Congenital anomalies: musculoskeletal abnormalities. In: Beers MH, Berkow R, eds. *The Merck Manual of Diagnosis and Therapy.* 17th ed. Merck Research Laboratories; 1999:2218-2222.

ONLINE RESOURCES

◊ **American Diabetes Association**

    ¤ www.diabetes.org

◊ **Best Practices Recommendations**

    ¤ http://www.nata.org/sites/default/files/preventingsuddendeath-consensusstatement.pdf

◊ **Centers for Disease Control and Prevention-Division of Diabetes Translation**

    ¤ www.cdc.gov/diabetes

◊ **Inter-Association Task Force on Exertional Heat Illnesses Consensus Statement**

    ¤ http://www.nata.org/sites/default/files/inter-association-task-force-exertional-heat-illness.pdf

◊ **Inter-Association Task Force for Preseason Heat-Acclimatization Guidelines for Secondary School Athletics**

    ¤ https://www.nata.org/sites/default/files/HeatFactSheet.pdf

◊ **Inter-Association Task Force for Preventing Sudden Death in Collegiate Conditioning Sessions: Best Practice Recommendations**

    ¤ http://www.nata.org/sites/default/files/preventingsuddendeath-consensusstatement.pdf

◊ **Juvenile Diabetes Research Foundation International**

    ¤ www.jdrf.org

◊ **National Diabetes Education Program**

    ¤ www.ndep.nih.gov

◊ **National Heart, Lung, and Blood Institute**

    ¤ www.nhlbi.nih.gov

◊ **National Institute of Diabetes and Digestive and Kidney Diseases**

    ¤ www.niddk.nih.gov

◊ **NATA Age-Specific Task Force Issue on Youth Football and Heat-Related Illness**

    ¤ http://www.nata.org/sites/default/files/HeatRelatedIllness.pdf

◊ **NATA Position Statement on Exertional Heat Illnesses**

    ¤ http://www.nata.org/sites/default/files/ExternalHeatIllnesses.pdf

◊ **NATA Position Statement on Management of the Athlete with Type 1 Diabetes Mellitus**

    ¤ http://www.nata.org/sites/default/files/MgmtOfAthleteWithType1DiabetesMellitus.pdf

◊ **NATA Position Statement on Preventing Sudden Death in Sports**

  ¤ http://www.nata.org/sites/default/files/Preventing-Sudden-Death-Position-Statement_2.pdf

◊ **NATA Position Statement on Environmental Cold Injuries**

  ¤ http://www.nata.org/sites/default/files/EnvironmentalColdInjuries.pdf

Please visit www.routledge.com/9781630917234
to access additional material.

CHAPTER 11

Eye, Ear, Nose, Throat, and Mouth Disorders

CHAPTER OUTLINE AND OBJECTIVES

Introduction

Review of Anatomy, Physiology, and Pathogenesis

◊ Describe the basic functional anatomy eye, ear, nose, throat, and mouth.

Signs and Symptoms

◊ Identify the general signs and symptoms of injuries and illnesses involving the eye, ear, nose, throat, and mouth.

Pain Patterns

◊ Identify the referred pain patterns associated with injuries and illness of the eye, ear, nose, throat, and mouth.

Medical History and Physical Examination Procedures

◊ Discuss the medical history findings relevant to injuries and illnesses involving the eye, ear, nose, throat, and mouth.

◊ Describe the physical examination procedures associated with common illnesses and injuries involving the eye, ear, nose, throat, and mouth.

  ¤ Medical History
  ¤ Palpation
  ¤ Inspection
  ¤ Special Tests
    • Visual Acuity
    • Pupillary Shape and Reaction
    • Eye Movements
    • Peripheral Vision

Bhojani RA, O'Connor DP, Fincher AL. *Clinical Pathology for Athletic Trainers: Recognizing Systemic Disease, Fourth Edition* (pp 295-323).
© 2022 Taylor & Francis Group.

- Fluorescein Strips and Cobalt Blue Light
- Ophthalmoscope
- Otoscope

Pathology and Pathogenesis

◊ Discuss the signs, symptoms, interventions, medical referral guidelines, and, when appropriate, return-to-participation criteria for eye pathology.
  ¤ Eye Injuries
   - Subconjunctival Hemorrhage
   - Corneal Abrasions
   - Hyphema
   - Ruptured Globe
   - Orbital Fracture
   - Detached Retina
  ¤ Eye Infections and Disorders
   - Conjunctivitis
   - Stye
   - Glaucoma
◊ Discuss the signs, symptoms, interventions, medical referral guidelines, and, when appropriate, return-to-participation criteria for ear pathology.
  ¤ Ear Injuries
   - Auricular Hematoma
   - Ruptured Tympanic Membrane
  ¤ Ear Infections and Disorders
   - Otitis Externa
   - Otitis Media
   - Impacted Cerumen
◊ Discuss the signs, symptoms, interventions, medical referral guidelines, and, when appropriate, return-to-participation criteria for nose pathology.
  ¤ Nose Injuries
   - Epistaxis (Nose Bleed)
   - Nasal Fracture
  ¤ Nasal Allergies and Infections
   - Allergic Rhinitis
   - Sinusitis and Sinus Infections
◊ Discuss the signs, symptoms, interventions, medical referral guidelines, and, when appropriate, return-to-participation criteria for throat infections.
  ¤ Laryngitis, Pharyngitis, and Tonsillitis
◊ Discuss the signs, symptoms, interventions, medical referral guidelines, and, when appropriate, return-to-participation criteria for mouth pathology.
  ¤ Gingivitis
  ¤ Periodontitis
  ¤ Dental Caries
  ¤ Oral Candidiasis
  ¤ Oral Cancer

Summary

Case Study

◊ Develop critical-thinking and clinical decision-making skills.

Online Resources

This chapter addresses the following knowledge and skills from the *Athletic Training Education Competencies, Fifth Edition*[1]:

Content Area	Knowledge and Skills
Prevention and Health Promotion (PHP)	24
Clinical Examination and Diagnosis (CE)	1; 7; 13–15; 17–19; 20 a–c, j; 21 m, n; 22
Therapeutic Interventions (TI)	30

INTRODUCTION

Regardless of their setting, athletic trainers may encounter injuries or illnesses involving the eye, ear, nose, throat, and mouth. Although most of these conditions are relatively benign in nature, others have the potential for serious complications (loss of sight or hearing) if not managed properly. This chapter will review the pertinent anatomy, signs and symptoms, evaluation procedures, referral guidelines, and, when appropriate, return-to-participation criteria for the common injuries and illnesses involving the eye, ear, nose, throat, and mouth.

REVIEW OF ANATOMY, PHYSIOLOGY, AND PATHOGENESIS

Eye

The eye globe, or eyeball (Figure 11-1), is composed of many individual structures, some of which can be easily viewed by the naked eye and others that require an ophthalmoscope to view. The *sclera*, also referred to as "the white of the eye," forms the outer protective layer of the eye. It covers the posterior five-sixths of the globe with openings in the front and back for the cornea and optic nerve, respectively. The clear *cornea* is located in the center of the most anterior portion of the eye. The *conjunctiva* is a thin mucous membrane that covers the anterior eye and lines the eyelids. The *iris* contains pigment cells, which give the eye its color, and includes muscles that work to constrict or dilate the pupil. Located in the center of the iris, the *pupil* is often compared to the aperture lens of a camera, controlling the amount of light allowed into the eye. The *anterior chamber* is formed by the space between the cornea and the iris and is filled with aqueous humor. The *lens* is a clear, biconvex structure located just posterior to the pupil and the iris. It is surrounded by the *ciliary body*, a ring of muscular tissue, which through contraction and relaxation controls the shape of the lens and the degree of focus on near and far objects. The ciliary body also produces the aqueous humor that fills the anterior chamber of the eye. The *retina* is a multilayer tissue that lines the inner, posterior portion of the eye (Figure 11-2). The space within the globe is composed of a gelatinous substance called vitreous humor. The *macula* is located in the center of the retina and

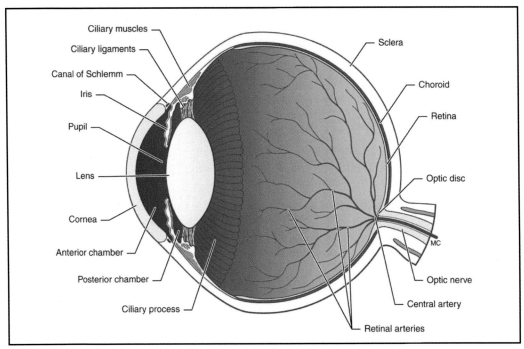

Figure 11-1. Anatomy of the eye.

Figure 11-2. Retina.

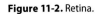

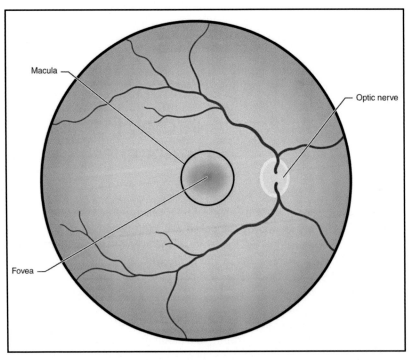

provides detailed central vision. Located within the center of the macula, the *fovea* is responsible for the sharpest detail in central vision. The *optic nerve* is located at the back of the eye and transmits nerve impulses from the eye to the brain. A portion of the optic nerve, the optic disc, is visible when viewed with an ophthalmoscope.

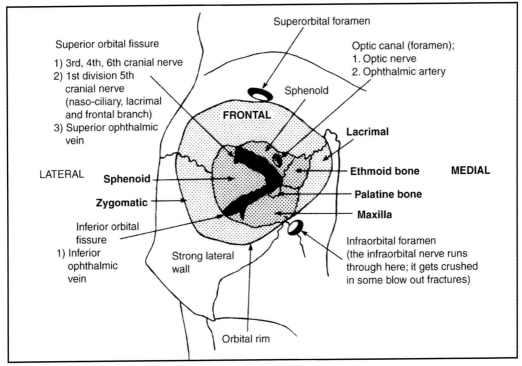

Figure 11-3. Bony orbit.

The paired orbits, or eye sockets, that surround and protect the eyes are formed by 7 bones: frontal, zygomatic, maxillary, ethmoidal, sphenoid, lacrimal, and palatine (Figure 11-3). The orbital floor and medial walls are the weakest portion of the bony socket and are therefore often fractured with external periorbital forces (blow-out fractures). Movement of the eyes are controlled by the 6 extraocular muscles. These muscles include 4 rectus muscles, which function to adduct, abduct, elevate, and depress the eye globe, and 2 oblique muscles that control circular movements (Figure 11-4). The lacrimal apparatus, which functions to produce, distribute, and collect tears, can also be damaged with lacerations involving the medial portion of the eyelids.

Ear

The ear is divided into 3 main sections: the external ear, middle ear, and inner ear (Figure 11-5). The *external ear* includes the auricle (Figure 11-6), which is visible to the naked eye, and the external auditory canal. The outermost portion of the external canal is funnel-shaped, which helps to move sound waves toward the tympanic membrane (ear drum). The *tympanic membrane* forms the outermost border of the middle ear, (Figure 11-7) separating the external canal from the 3 tiny ossicle bones: the *malleus*, *incus*, and *stapes*. The tympanic membrane vibrates when sound waves strike it, initiating the process of converting sound waves to electrical nerve impulses. Damage to the membrane can result in some degree of hearing loss. The *inner ear* contains the cochlea and semicircular canals, which function to continue the conversion of sound waves to nerve impulses for the brain to interpret and to maintain balance, respectively. The *eustachian tube* connects the middle ear to the nasal passages and regulates the amount of pressure within the middle ear.

Nose

The nasal complex is composed of the bones and cartilage that form the nasal cavity and the paranasal sinuses (frontal, sphenoid, ethmoidal, maxillary; Figure 11-8). The upper one third of the

Figure 11-4. Extraocular muscles.

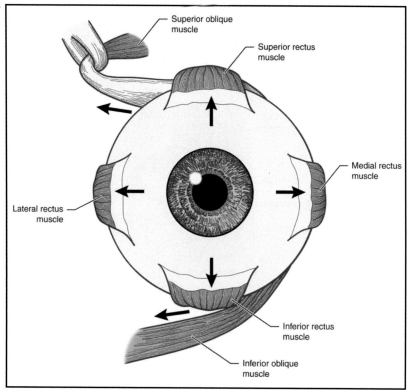

Figure 11-5. Ear anatomy.

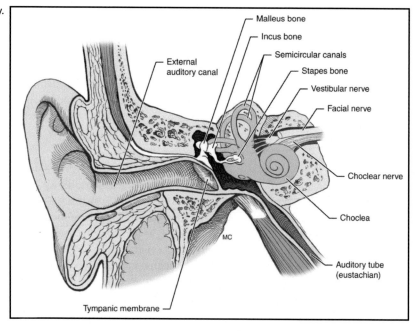

nose is formed by the nasal bones, while the lower two thirds is supported by cartilage. The nasal cavity includes 3 curved bony structures called *turbinates*, which are covered in a highly vascularized mucous membrane. Air enters the nose through the paired nares (nostrils), vestibule, and nasal cavity where it is filtered, warmed, and humidified before passing on to the nasopharynx, trachea, and lung.

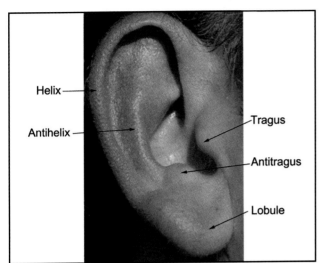

Figure 11-6. Auricle.

Helix

Antihelix

Tragus

Antitragus

Lobule

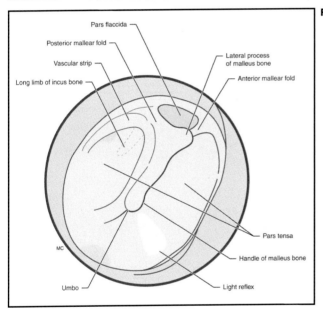

Figure 11-7. Tympanic membrane.

Pars flaccida

Posterior mallear fold

Vascular strip

Long limb of incus bone

Lateral process of malleus bone

Anterior mallear fold

Pars tensa

MC

Handle of malleus bone

Umbo

Light reflex

Throat

The throat, or pharynx, includes the tonsils, adenoids, uvula, epiglottis, and esophagus. The *tonsils* are located on both sides of the back of the mouth and the *adenoids* are on the back of the nasal cavity. Both structures are composed of lymphoid tissue and function to help fight infection. The *uvula* hangs at the back of the throat between the 2 tonsils. Functionally, the pharynx provides the pathway for food and fluids to pass from the mouth to the esophagus and for air to pass to the lungs. The pharynx is divided into 3 sections: the nasopharynx, oropharynx, and laryngopharynx (Figure 11-9). Like the nose and mouth, the pharynx is also lined with mucous membranes and cilia to warm, filter, and humidify inspired air. Below the laryngopharynx, the pharynx becomes the esophagus. The *epiglottis* lies between the oropharynx and laryngopharynx and functions to prevent food from entering the larynx. The larynx has 3 main functions: (1) prevent food and fluids from entering the trachea, (2) produce sound vibrations, and (3) to assist in the cough mechanism.

Figure 11-8. Nasal anatomy. (A) Frontal cross-section. (B) Sagittal cross-section.

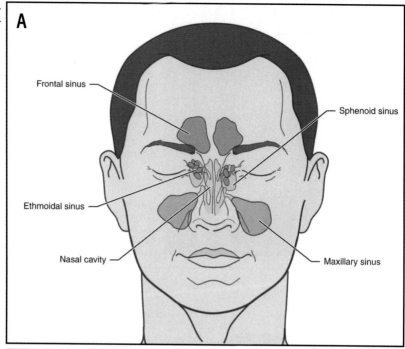

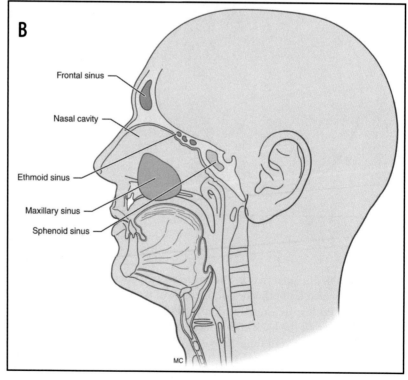

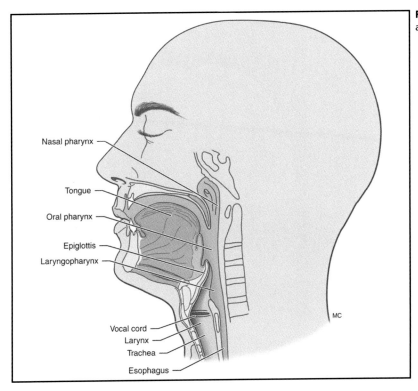

Figure 11-9. Throat anatomy.

Mouth

The oral cavity (Figure 11-10) is lined with mucous membranes and in the adult contains 32 teeth: 16 in the upper jaw and 16 in the lower jaw (Figure 11-11). The visible portion of each tooth is referred to as the crown and is made of enamel (Figure 11-12). The *dentin* forms a layer just below the enamel and is harder than bone. The tooth fits into an individual socket in the jawbone and is surrounded at its base by the gums. The *root* of the tooth, which sits below the gum line in the bony socket, contains the blood vessels and nerves that provide circulation and sensation to the tooth.

SIGNS AND SYMPTOMS

Eye

Pain

Eye pain can occur periocular, ocular, or retrobulbar (behind the globe). The location of the pain, along with its intensity, onset, and duration, can provide clues regarding the possible pathology. Severe eye pain accompanied by systemic symptoms (eg, nausea) or significant changes in vision (eg, severe photophobia, blurring, flashing, "floaters," partial loss of visual field) suggest serious pathology, such as acute glaucoma (increased pressure in the eye). In such situations, a risk of permanent loss of vision exists and, therefore, immediate medical care is indicated.

Discharge

With eye allergies and infections, the eye will often present with a discharge or drainage. This discharge can range from a clear, watery substance to a white or yellowish pus. Clear drainage is associated with allergies and viral infections, whereas white or yellow colored discharge suggests a

Figure 11-10. Mouth anatomy.

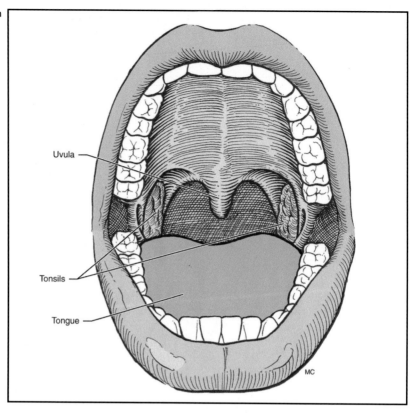

Figure 11-11. Dental anatomy.

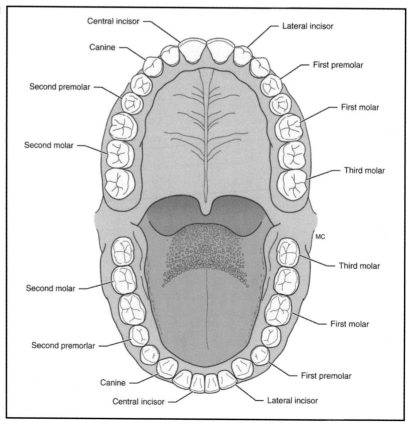

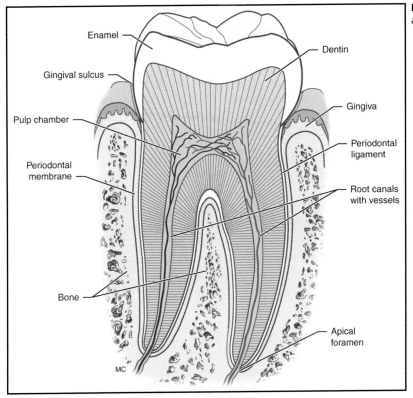

Figure 11-12. Tooth anatomy.

Enamel

Dentin

Gingival sulcus

Pulp chamber

Gingiva

Periodontal ligament

Periodontal membrane

Root canals with vessels

Bone

Apical foramen

MC

bacterial infection. Typically, allergies and viral infections affect both eyes, whereas bacterial infections start with one eye and may migrate to the other eye.

Double Vision

Patients with double vision (*diplopia*) will see 2 images of the same object, one from each eye. Normally the images seen by both eyes are fused into a single image. Double vision can result from a variety of disorders including a head injury. Systemic conditions associated with double vision include multiple sclerosis, diabetes, and myasthenia gravis. Patients complaining of diplopia should be referred to an ophthalmologist.

Itching

Itching of the eyes is commonly associated with allergy; however, some eye infections may also cause itching.

Photophobia

Photophobia, or sensitivity to light, is a common symptom reported with corneal abrasions; of note, photophobia may also be indicative of neurological conditions (see Chapter 13).

Ptosis

Drooping of the eyelid, or *ptosis*, can occur with some eye pathologies as well as endocrine and neurological pathologies.

Tearing

Increased tearing can occur due to an irritation of the anterior eye surface. Injury or illness involving the lacrimal apparatus can cause either increased or decreased tearing.

Halos

Halos around lights at night are often reported by patients with glaucoma, corneal edema, corneal scarring, or a dislocated intraocular lens and therefore require referral to an ophthalmologist.

Light Flashes and Floaters

Brief light flashes (*photopsia*) or a sudden increase in "floaters" are common symptoms reported by patients with a retinal tear or detachment and warrant immediate referral.

Anisocoria

Unequal pupils are referred to as *anisocoria*. Differences in pupil size less than 0.5 mm are found normally in approximately 20% of the general population. Differences greater than 0.5 mm, particularly when accompanied by abnormal papillary reactions and a history of head or eye trauma, are considered abnormal and warrant immediate referral.

Nystagmus

Nystagmus can occur with a head injury or other neurological pathology and presents as a rhythmic oscillation of the eyes. Persons with nystagmus should be examined by a physician to identify the cause.

Protruding Eyes

Retraction of the eyelids can cause the appearance of protruding eyes (*exophthalmos*) and is a common sign associated with Grave's disease (see Chapter 10).

Curtain Over Vision

Patients may report having a curtain suddenly drop down over their eye blocking either their direct vision or their peripheral vision. This curtain is associated with a detached retina or detached vitreous and warrants emergency medical evaluation and treatment.

Ear

Tinnitus

A sensation of ringing in the ears is referred to as *tinnitus*. Patients may report tinnitus when they experience a ruptured tympanic membrane. Of note, low-pitched tinnitus is usually pathological and warrants immediate referral to the physician.

Pain

Pain is a common symptom with most ear pathologies. The typical earache can occur with ear infections and is difficult for the patient to localize (ie, middle ear or external ear). Both palpation of the tragus and traction of the ear lobe will often cause ear pain in patients with otitis externa. A blocked Eustachian tube or middle ear infection (otitis media) can result in increased pressure behind the tympanic membrane which can cause a sensation of pressure or pain.

Loss of Hearing

Damage to middle and inner ear structures can result in partial to complete hearing loss. The degree of hearing loss is usually related to the severity of injury.

Nasal Cavity

Runny Nose

Inflammation of the mucous membranes within the nasal cavity can lead to the production of a clear, watery drainage (*coryza*).

Congestion and Pressure

Accumulation of mucus and drainage within the nasal cavity and sinuses can lead to congestion and a feeling of pain and pressure within the sinuses.

Throat

Pain

Throat infections are associated with throat pain.

Difficulty Swallowing

Throat pain can make it difficult for patients to swallow.

White or Red Spots

Throat infections can produce white or red spots on the tonsils and soft palate.

Mouth

Pain

Pain is one of the most common symptoms of mouth disorders. Mouth pain can be local and specific to the disorder (eg, cavity, tooth fracture, infection) or be referred from another area (sinuses) or to another area (ear).

Swollen, Red, or Bleeding Gums

Inflammation and infection from gingivitis can produce swollen and red gums that may bleed when brushed.

Sensitivity to Hot and Cold Food or Beverages

Demineralization of the teeth secondary to plaque or cavities can lead to sensitivity to hot or cold food and beverages.

Bad Breath (Halitosis)

Poor dental hygiene and periodontal disease lead to bad breath.

White or Yellow Plaques

Plaques may develop on the tongue, buccal mucosa (inside the cheek), and palate with fungal infections of the mouth such as oral candidiasis.

PAIN PATTERNS

The pain associated with most eye, ear, nose, throat, and mouth pathology is very localized. Sinus infections can involve referred pain to the teeth and some tooth disorders can refer pain to the ipsilateral ear.

MEDICAL HISTORY AND
PHYSICAL EXAMINATION PROCEDURES

Medical History

With the exception of glaucoma, most disorders involving the eye, ear, nose, throat, and mouth do not have a genetic factor associated with them. Findings from a personal history however can be very important in the assessment of these disorders, especially eye and ear conditions.

Palpation

Palpation of the bony orbit and surrounding facial bones is an essential part of a thorough eye or nose exam. Also, when evaluating the ear, pain with palpation of the tragus or traction of the earlobe is associated with otitis externa.

Inspection

Unlike many of the other systemic disorders within this text, injuries and illnesses involving the eye, ear, nose, throat, and mouth require close visual inspection. Inspection of the facial anatomy is critical for detecting deformity or abnormalities.

Physical Examination

Eye

Visual Acuity

Examination of the eye typically begins with an assessment of visual acuity. This assessment should include testing the patient's ability to see an object at 20 feet (6 m) and the ability to focus and read text at 14 to 16 inches (35.5 to 40.6 cm). In the clinical setting, visual acuity is most often tested using a *Snellen eye chart* (Figure 11-13) to test distant vision and the *Rosenbaum pocket card* to test near vision. The eye chart is hung on a wall at eye level, and a mark is then made on the floor 20 feet (6 m) from the wall. Each eye should be tested separately by covering the opposite eye. If the patient wears glasses or contacts, then they should be tested with these on. The patient should start at the smallest line on the eye chart and move upward until they are able to correctly read more than half of the letters. If the patient is unable to read the top line at 20 feet, then place them closer to the chart (15, 10, or 5 feet [4.6, 3, or 1.5 m]) and the test is repeated. Distant visual acuity is recorded as a fraction, with the numerator containing the patient's distance from the chart and the denominator representing the distance that a "normal" person would read that line. For example, if a patient reads a line at 15 feet (4.6 m) that a normal person could read at 40 feet (12.2 m), this visual acuity would be recorded at 15/40.

The Rosenbaum pocket card is used in a similar fashion to test near vision. The card should be held approximately 14 to 16 inches (35.5 to 40.6 cm) from the face. If a Snellen eye chart or Rosenbaum packet card is not available, other objects can be used to screen visual acuity, although an acuity value will not be obtained. For example, when on the sideline, the athletic trainer can ask the athlete to read the score board or other object in a distance. Also, a game program or magazine can be used to assess near vision. Any loss of visual acuity secondary to an eye injury warrants immediate referral. Athletic trainers should consider having an ocular first aid kit on the sideline of all events and in the athletic training facility. Table 11-1 provides a list of items that should be included in this kit.

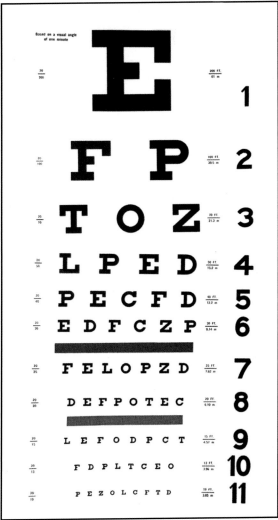

Figure 11-13. Snellen eye chart.

Pupillary Shape and Reaction

Following a head injury or isolated ocular injury, the pupils should be inspected for size, shape, and reaction to light. As mentioned above, anisocoria can occur normally in some individuals; however, unequal pupil size following a head or ocular injury suggests neurological involvement and warrants immediate referral. A tear-drop shape or an irregularly peaked pupil suggests possible globe rupture and is considered a medical emergency.

The pupils' response to light should be checked both for direct and consensual response. To check direct response to light, the penlight should be directed from an angle lateral to the eye to shine directly into the eye. Normally, the pupil should constrict in response to the light. The opposite eye is then tested in the same fashion. Failure of the pupil to constrict is considered abnormal and warrants referral. To test consensual response, again shine the penlight directly into one eye; however, observe the reaction of the opposite eye. When the penlight is directed into one pupil, the other pupil should also constrict. Failure of the opposite pupil to constrict is considered abnormal. Lastly, the penlight is rapidly swung from one eye to the other without allowing time between eyes (swinging flashlight test). Each pupil should constrict as the light hits it. If one of the pupils dilate

Table 11-1. Ocular First Aid Kit

Penlight with cobalt blue filter

Fluorescein strips

Rosenbaum pocket eye card or similar near vision chart

Sterile irrigation fluid (squeeze bottle of saline works well)

Sterile tipped applications

Sterile eye patch (soft) or shield (hard)

Contact case with contact solution

Visual occluder (to cover opposite eye when testing visual acuity)

Topical anesthetic

Topical antibiotic drops or ointment

Gloves

Sterile gauze pads

Tape

Phone numbers for local hospital, team physician, and team ophthalmologist

instead of constricting, this is considered a positive test and indicates a problem with the nerve between the eye and the brain (*afferent pupil defect*).

Eye Movements

Assessment of the extraocular muscles should be performed following any traumatic eye injury. Using a penlight or a finger, the athletic trainer should instruct the patient to follow the object without moving the head. The patient's ability to look laterally, medially, upward, downward, diagonally up and out, and diagonally down and out should be tested. Orbital blowout fractures can entrap the inferior vastus muscle, preventing the patient from being able to look up. Normal eye movement can also be affected with head injuries or other neurological conditions. It is important to remember which muscles control the directional movements as well as the nerves associated with these 6 muscles.

Peripheral Vision

The patient's peripheral field of vision can be tested by asking them to cover one eye with the hand. The examiner also covers their eye (same as the patient's—right or left) to compare the patient's peripheral vision with their own. On the same side as the eye being tested, the examiner will place their hand out laterally to the patient with one or more fingers held up. The examiner slowly brings their hand inward toward the patient's direct vision and asks the patient to say when they can see the hand and to state how many fingers they see. This test would then be repeated on the opposite side. Of note, you can test peripheral vision in multiple planes.

Fluorescein Strips and Cobalt Blue Light

Staining the eye with fluorescein dye can enable the athletic trainer to visualize corneal abrasions or clear foreign objects in the eye such as glass or contact lens fragments. The dye stains the eye orange and highlights areas of abrasion within the cornea or conjunctiva. When viewed with a cobalt blue light, the dye appears yellowish green, further enhancing the visual identification of abrasions or foreign objects. The proper steps for performing the fluorescein dye test are outlined in Table 11-2. The fluorescein dye is water soluble and can be easily flushed from the eye using saline irrigating solution.

Table 11-2. Fluorescein Dye Test for Corneal Abrasions

1. Remove a single fluorescein strip from the package
2. Wet the tip of the strip with sterile saline.
3. Pull the lower lid out slightly, forming a pouch.
4. Touch the wet tip of the strip within the lower lid pouch. (The strip should not touch the cornea directly.)
5. Instruct the patient to blink several times to spread the orange-colored dye across the eye.
6. Dim the lights in the room if possible.
7. Attach the cobalt blue filter to the end of the penlight.
8. Shine the cobalt blue light in the involved eye.
9. Under the blue light, the fluorescein dye will appear yellowish green.
10. Carefully inspect the eye for abrasions or foreign objects.
11. A corneal abrasion will pick up the dye, causing it to appear green with the cobalt blue light.

Ophthalmoscope

A hand-held direct ophthalmoscope (Figure 11-14) uses a battery-powered light source and a series of magnifying lens to look inside the eye to view the cornea, lens, and central portion of the retina. This evaluation instrument can provide the athletic trainer with valuable information when assessing the eye (Figure 11-15). The steps for using an ophthalmoscope to evaluate the eye are outlined in Table 11-3. Both eyes should be examined and typically examining the unaffected eye will allow for a better exam for the affected eye.

Otoscope

Injuries or illnesses involving the external auditory canal or the tympanic membrane can be evaluated using an otoscope (Figure 11-16). These hand-held units include a handle, light source, and several specula of varying sizes. Units with halogen bulbs and magnifying lenses provide the most optimal viewing of the tympanic membrane. Table 11-4 outlines the proper steps for using an otoscope. To prevent cross-contamination, the unaffected ear should always be evaluated first. This practice also provides a basis for comparison when viewing the affected ear. The otoscope can also be used to inspect the nose for injury.

PATHOLOGY AND PATHOGENESIS

Eye Injuries

Subconjunctival Hemorrhage

Bleeding under the clear conjunctiva can be caused by trauma, forceful coughing, high blood pressure or some bleeding disorders. In some cases, the etiology is never known. Although this condition may look serious, in the absence of trauma, it is generally benign. Most cases of subconjunctival hemorrhaging will resolve on their own within 1 to 3 weeks. Referral should be made for recurrent subconjunctival hemorrhages or other visual symptoms observed by the patient.

Corneal Abrasions

Corneal abrasions are one of the most common sports-related eye injuries. These injuries are usually the result of a direct blow to the eye by an external object (eg, ball, elbow, hockey stick,

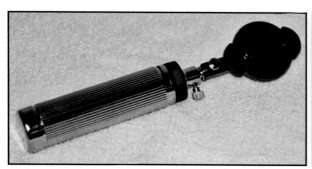

Figure 11-14. Ophthalmoscope.

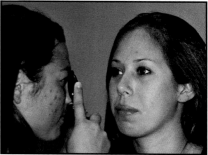

Figure 11-15. Examining the eye with an ophthalmoscope.

finger). Corneal abrasions can also be caused by foreign objects becoming trapped between the upper lid and the cornea, particularly when the eye is rubbed in an attempt to remove the object. Patients with a corneal abrasion will complain of photophobia, eye pain, and a sensation of "grittiness" or of a foreign body being in the eye. Inspection of the eye may find increased tearing, redness, and possible swelling, depending on the severity of the abrasion. As described earlier in the chapter, a corneal abrasion can be diagnosed using a fluorescein strip and cobalt blue penlight (see Table 11-2).

Patients with corneal abrasions should be referred to a physician or ophthalmologist immediately. Deep or large abrasions or lacerations can be very serious and can lead to vision loss. Eye patches are not recommended for the treatment of corneal abrasions as they may decrease oxygen delivery to the abrasion, increase moisture, and increase the infection rate.[2] Physicians will typically prescribe topical antibiotic ointment or drops to prevent infection. Topical nonsteroidal anti-inflammatory drugs (NSAIDs) have been shown to be slightly more effective in reducing eye pain associated with corneal abrasions as compared to the use of oral NSAIDs.[3] Patients with a corneal abrasion should be re-evaluated by their physician or ophthalmologist at 24 hours. Patients who wear contact lenses should refrain from wearing them during the healing period. These patients should also be re-evaluated 3 to 4 days later. Most corneal abrasions heal within 24 to 72 hours; however, deeper lesions may take 4 to 5 days to heal.

Hyphema

A *hyphema* injury results from a direct blow to the globe and results in bleeding within the anterior chamber. The bleeding associated with a hyphema injury will be contained within the anterior chamber and should not be confused with subconjunctival bleeding. Patients will usually complain of eye pain, photophobia, and blurred vision.[4] Forces great enough to cause a hyphema can also rupture the globe; therefore, a thorough eye exam should be performed to rule out a ruptured globe. Patients with sickle cell trait are at risk for complications with a hyphema injury, such as increased ocular pressure and the potential for a secondary bleeding incident.[5] Patients with a hyphema should be immediately referred to an ophthalmologist or the local emergency room. Hyphema injuries are usually treated with a topical corticosteroid, a rigid eye shield, analgesics for eye pain (NSAIDs should be avoided), and elevation of the head of the head approximately 30 degrees.[6] Bed rest may also be recommended, depending on the severity of the injury. Patients should be reassessed daily by their ophthalmologist to check for rebleeding or other complications. As previously mentioned, patients should be instructed to avoid the use of NSAIDs during this treatment period. Return to play decisions will be made by the ophthalmologist depending on the sport and severity.

Ruptured Globe

Any eye injury caused by blunt or penetrating trauma to the orbit or globe can result in a *ruptured globe*. The rupture may not be apparent on inspection because most ruptures occur at sites that

Table 11-3. Steps for Using an Ophthalmoscope to Evaluate the Eye

STEP 1	Darken the examination room
STEP 2	Turn on the ophthalmoscope with the lens disc set on large round beam.
	Shine the beam of light on your hand to check the level of brightness and the charge of the ophthalmoscope.
STEP 3	Turn the lens disc to the 0 diopter setting, keeping your index finger on the lens disc to adjust the setting later.
STEP 4	Hold the ophthalmoscope in the right hand when examining the right eye and the left hand when examining the left eye.
STEP 5	Rest the head of the ophthalmoscope on the medial aspect your orbit, with the handle tilted laterally approximately 20 degrees (Figure 11-15).
STEP 6	Instruct the patient to focus on a point on the wall up and over your shoulder.
STEP 7	Start at a position approximately 15 inches (38 cm) away from the patient and in a plane approximately 15 degrees lateral to the patient's line of vision.
	Shine the light beam into the patient's eye and look for the red reflex, which will appear as an orange glow in the pupil.
STEP 8	While keeping the light beam focused on the red reflex, move slowly toward the patient in the 15-degree plane until you are almost touching the patient's eyelashes.
STEP 9	Keep both eyes open as you begin to look into the eye.
	If the brightness of the light beam is uncomfortable for the patient, adjust it slightly.
STEP 10	As you look through the eye, locate the optic disc, which will appear as a round, yellowish-orange structure.
	If you are unable to find the optic disc initially, locate a blood vessel and follow it centrally to the disc.
STEP 11	Once you locate the optic disc, adjust the sharpness of the image by turning the lens disc.
STEP 12	Inspect the optic disc for clarity and color. (It is not abnormal to find the edge on the nasal side of the disc to be slightly blurry.)
	The normal disc is yellowish-orange to creamy pink; however, the outer ring may be white.
STEP 13	Inspect the retina looking for lesions.
	Move the ophthalmoscope and your head as one unit as you attempt to view all areas of the retina.
STEP 14	To view the macula and fovea, instruct the patient to look directly into the light beam. (A light reflection off of the fovea helps identify these structures.)
	The macula surrounds the fovea.

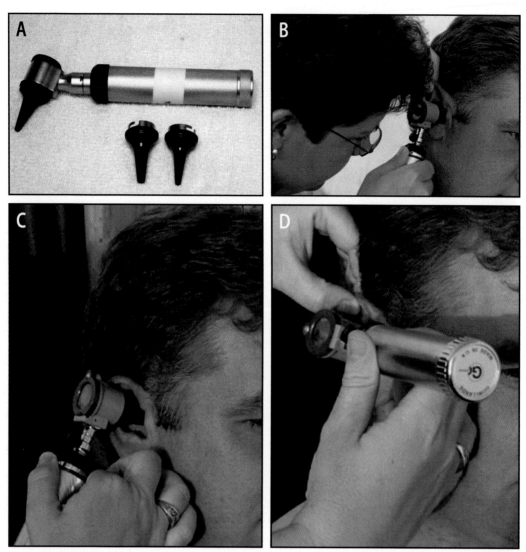

Figure 11-16. (A) Otoscope with additional specula. (B) Examining the ear with an otoscope. (C) Hammer grip. (D) Pencil grip.

are not visible. Patients will usually complain of eye pain, decreased vision, and possible diplopia. Key signs to watch for include excessive subconjunctival bleeding, swelling, irregular pupil shape, asymmetry in the depth of the anterior chamber, and *enophthalmos* (recession of the globe within the orbit) or *exophthalmos* (protrusion of the globe beyond the orbit). The eye should be protected from any type of pressure or contact; therefore, a hard eye shield should be applied rather than a pressure eye patch. Any penetrating foreign body should be left in place during transport to the emergency room. Ruptured globes are medical emergencies that require surgical repair as soon as possible.

Orbital Fracture

Blunt trauma to the bony orbit can result in an orbital fracture. Because the orbital floor and medial wall are the thinnest and weakest part of the orbit, fracture to this area, referred to as *blowout fractures*, occurs most often. Forces great enough to produce an orbital fracture can also cause soft tissue damage to the eye and surrounding areas, as well as potentially rupture the globe.

Table 11-4. Steps for Using an Ophthalmoscope to Evaluate the Ear

STEP 1	Place your patient in a seated position with their head turned slightly downward and away from the ear to be examined.
STEP 2	Select the largest possible speculum that can be comfortably inserted into the ear.
	When inserted, the speculum should fit snugly in the outer one third of the canal and rest against the tragus and anterior wall of the canal.
	Choosing a speculum that is too small will cause movement within the canal.
	Excessive movement can cause discomfort for your patient.
STEP 3	Hold the otoscope with the same hand as the ear you are examining. • Right hand for right ear • Left hand for left ear
STEP 4	Stabilize the otoscope by placing the ring and little finger resting on the patient's cheek or temple using 1 of 2 grips: • Hammer grip (see Figure 11-16C) • Pencil grip (see Figure 11-16D)
STEP 5	Pull the pinna upward and backward to straighten the canal.
STEP 6	While maintaining traction on the pinna, place the speculum of the otoscope at, but not in, the ear canal.
STEP 7	"Watch your way into the ear." Never insert the otoscope blindly.
	If the patient experiences pain, reposition the canal by adjusting the angle and degree of traction on the pinna.
	If the patient's discomfort persists even after readjustment of the canal, halt the examination and refer the patient to a physician.
STEP 8	Once the tympanic membrane comes into view, rotate the speculum to view as much of the membrane as possible. This is like trying to view the corners of a room through a key hole.
STEP 9	Inspect the membrane for color, clarity, and position.

STEP 10	Identify key landmarks (see Figure 11-7).
	• Malleus:
	   ◦ Manubrium (angles toward 2-o'clock in right ear, angles toward 10-o'clock in left ear)
	   ◦ Short process
	   ◦ Umbo
	• Light reflex
	• Pars flaccida
	• Pars tensa
	• Annulus
	• Stapes
	• Incus

STEP 11	Look for abnormalities. • Fluid • Perforations

Patients will typically complain of pain and diplopia. Clinical presentation will include periorbital swelling, ecchymosis, and enophthalmos. Palpation may detect a bony step-off and point tenderness along the orbital rim, as well as subcutaneous emphysema (air under the skin) and numbness in the upper cheek area. Assessment of the extraocular muscles should be performed. Eye movement may be limited and painful. Entrapment of the inferior rectus muscle will often prevent the patient from looking upward.

All suspected orbital fractures should be referred immediately. Soft tissue entrapment or extensive damage to the bony orbit will require surgical repair. Athletes with orbital fractures will typically be out of participation for several months, and possibly permanently, depending on the severity of the injury.[4]

Detached Retina

As described previously, the retina forms the inner lining of the back wall of the eye and is responsible for sending visual images to the brain. A sudden jarring of the head can cause the retina to pull away from the back wall causing a *detached retina*. In some cases, a sneeze has been the reported cause of a torn or detached retina, while with other cases, there has been no apparent cause. Patients with detached retinas will most commonly report floaters, blind spots or shadows, bright flashes of light, or describe a curtain falling over their field of vision.[4] A suspicion of retinal injury warrants immediate referral to an ophthalmologist. The longer the retina is detached from its blood supply, the greater the potential is for permanent damage.[4] In most cases, the torn retina will need to be repaired surgically. Athletes with torn retinas will typically be held out of contact sports for an extended period of time. Any additional trauma to the eye can result in reoccurrence of retinal injury and increased chance for permanent damage.

Eye Infections and Disorders

Conjunctivitis

Inflammation of the conjunctiva can result from allergens or infection (bacterial or viral). Itching (allergy) or burning (infection) with mucoid (allergy) or purulent (infection) drainage from the eye occurs. The "white" of the eyeball appears swollen and reddened, thus the layman's term *pink eye*. Allergic reactions usually affect both eyes, whereas an infection begins unilaterally. Infectious conjunctivitis, however, spreads quickly to the opposite eye, usually after rubbing first the infected eye and then the other. This eye infection is highly contagious; therefore, infected individuals should not share towels with anyone else or rub their eyes during sports participation. Athletes who participate in high-contact sports (eg, wrestling, rugby) or swimming and diving should be held out of practice and competition until the infection is resolved.

Allergic conjunctivitis is usually treated with antihistamines or anti-inflammatories. Treatment of infectious conjunctivitis includes antibiotic eyedrops or ointment. The person must be instructed not to touch the eyedrop or ointment applicator to the eye, to avoid rubbing the face, and to practice meticulous hand-washing to avoid spreading the disease.

Athletes who wear contacts should have a pair of glasses as a backup should they develop an eye infection. Wearing disposable lenses beyond their recommended time frame can lead to eye infections. Also wearing infected lenses can lead to repeated infections and possible scarring of the cornea.

Eye infections associated with significant pain or photophobia suggest a more serious condition such as corneal injury or a herpes viral infection. Medical referral for definitive diagnosis and treatment is indicated.

Stye

Infection of an eyelid duct or follicle is called a *stye* or *hordeolum*. Caused most often by *Staphylococcal* bacteria, the stye produces localized pain on the margin of the eyelid. Lacrimation (tears) and a sensation of "something in the eye" also occur. Visual inspection usually reveals a round, red lump on the lid margin. A stye can be treated with warm, moist compresses for 10 minutes a few times per day and should completely resolve in a few days. Athletes who wear makeup should also be told to discontinue makeup use when a stye is present. Lesions observed in other parts of the eyelid or eye or no resolution of symptoms within 1 to 2 weeks requires prompt referral to an ophthalmologist.

Glaucoma

Glaucoma is an eye disease that is caused by optic nerve damage secondary to increased intraocular pressure. As discussed in the anatomical section, the anterior chamber is filled with aqueous fluid. The level of fluid in this area is constantly being produced and then drained away to maintain a healthy level of pressure within this chamber. If the draining mechanism becomes damaged, then the intraocular pressure in the eye will increase. This increased pressure is then transmitted to the back of the eye, causing damage to the optic nerve. The optic nerve damage first leads to a loss of peripheral sight. Because this loss of sight may occur gradually, glaucoma is sometimes referred to as the "sneaky thief of sight" Risk factors for glaucoma include (1) positive family history, (2) age (40 or over), (3) nearsightedness, (4) diabetes, (5) hypertension, and (6) Black race.[7] Although there is no cure, glaucoma can be treated through the use of drops or other medications to reduce the intraocular pressure and surgery to improve or replace the drainage system for the aqueous fluid. People in the high-risk group should have their eyes checked yearly. Not at-risk individuals should have their eyes examined every 2 years starting at age 40 years. Early detection is the key to preventing the loss of sight from glaucoma.

Ear Injuries

Auricular Hematoma

Repeated trauma or friction to the external ear can lead to an *auricular hematoma* between the thin layer of skin that covers the ear and the cartilage that composes the ear. As the hematoma develops, the skin will separate from the cartilage, forming a palpable collection of fluid. Ice and compression can be used to limit the size of the hematoma. Prompt referral to a physician for drainage of the hematoma is recommended to prevent scarring. The development of scar tissue within the hematoma can produce a cauliflower-like appearance on the external ear known as *cauliflower ear*. To prevent rebleeding within the space, the physician will typically apply some form of compression to the area such as a button sutured to the front and back of the ear, a silicone splint or cast applied to the ear, or dental rolls applied with gauze. The compression is left in place for 7 to 14 days to ensure proper healing without scarring. Athletes who participate in noncontact sports can usually return to play right away. Those individuals who participate in contact sports can return to play if protective head gear is worn. If the compression bandage is held in place with sutures, return to play may be delayed until the sutures are removed. Auricular hematomas are most prevalent in wrestlers; however, they can be prevented by wearing protective headgear.

Ruptured Tympanic Membrane

Sudden changes in pressure within the ear or insertion of foreign objects, such as cotton-tipped applicators, into the ear can cause the tympanic membrane to rupture. Signs and symptoms of a ruptured or perforated tympanic membrane include sudden ear pain, sudden relief of ear pain followed by drainage from the ear, tinnitus, and a decrease in hearing. The degree of hearing loss is typically related to the size of the perforation. Common causes of membrane rupture include a direct blow to the ear, increased pressure in the middle ear as a result of infection, changes in cabin pressure when flying in an airplane (such as with ascent and descent), or a sudden loud noise (as might occur with an explosion or gunshot). When a tympanic membrane rupture is suspected, a thorough ear evaluation should be performed including the use of an otoscope. Inability to visualize the membrane because of wax or drainage or visual confirmation of a hole or tear in the membrane warrants referral to a physician. Membrane ruptures will usually heal on their own within 2 to 3 weeks; however, occasionally, surgery is required to repair the opening. During the healing period, patients should wear earplugs during showers or baths to prevent water from getting into the ear. Tylenol or over-the-counter NSAIDs can be taken if the patient experiences ear pain. The ability of swimmers to return to play should be determined by the treating physician.

Ear Infections and Disorders

Otitis Externa

Frequent exposure to water (eg, competitive swimmers) flushes the protective cerumen (wax) from the ear and can cause infections of the external ear canal; this infection is called *otitis externa*. The constant moisture also softens the ear canal's tissue, providing further opportunity for infection by bacteria or fungi. Using cotton swabs to scour the ear can further irritate the canal and increase the risk of infection. Lakes, rivers, or improperly chlorinated pools commonly contain bacteria responsible for these infections.

Otitis externa produces ear drainage, canal swelling, and erythema that can be visualized with the otoscope. These effects decrease hearing, cause itching, and produce pain when the auricle is gently pulled or the tragus is palpated (see Figure 11-6). Treatment involves irrigation with sterile saline or hydrogen peroxide, inserting antibiotic or antifungal eardrops, and discontinuing swimming. Prior to any treatment mentioned, please ensure that the tympanic membrane is not ruptured. Usually within 3 days the pain and erythema decrease and swimming can be resumed. Using earplugs while swimming, carefully drying the ears, using drying agents (eg, boric acid solution), and avoiding the use of swabs are some simple protective measures.

Otitis Media

Otitis media (interna) is an infection of the middle ear and often follows or accompanies upper respiratory infections (URIs). Signs and symptoms include ear pain without tenderness to touch, fever, a feeling of pressure in the ear, slight loss of hearing, and occasionally dizziness. Otoscopic examination will usually reveal a red tympanic membrane that may be bulging or retracted. If the membrane bulges, the light reflex may become diminished or absent; when retracted, the bony prominences of the inner ear may become more apparent. In some cases of otitis media, the membrane will appear yellowish in color with possible fluid or bubbles visible behind the membrane. Otitis media requires referral and is treated with antibiotics and analgesics. Patients with otitis media can return to participation as long as they are free of fever. Also, patients with otitis media may be restricted from flying because of the risk for pressure changes during ascent and descent from altitude.[8] Patients with otitis media that cause increased pressure may result in rupture of the tympanic membrane.

Impacted Cerumen

Impacted cerumen can cause symptoms similar to otitis externa, including itching, pain, and impaired hearing. A physician may remove the cerumen by scraping with a blunt tool under direct visualization or suctioning the ear canal. Irrigation with saline or other solutions is not recommended if a history of ear infection or drainage exists. Self-application of cotton swabs or solvents to remove the cerumen may irritate the skin, creating opportunity for infection to develop, and should be avoided.

Nose Injuries

Epistaxis (Nosebleed)

Nosebleeds can result from a variety of conditions, including trauma (nasal or facial fracture), infection, dry nasal passages, allergies, or hypertension. In most cases, nosebleeds can be easily controlled by instructing the patient to lean forward slightly and pinch the nostrils between the tip and the bridge of the nose. Leaning the head forward will allow the blood to drain from the nose rather than running down the back of the throat. Swallowing the blood from a nosebleed can cause nausea and vomiting in some individuals. Applying an ice bag to the nose can also help control a nosebleed. In cases that do not respond to this treatment or in cases involving a nasal fracture, the nose can be packed with rolled gauze or tampons cut into small sections to control the bleeding. Patients who experience frequent unexplained nosebleeds should be referred to a physician for follow-up. Nosebleeds accompanied by occipital headaches are classic signs and symptoms for hypertension.

Nasal Fracture

Nasal fractures are common in sports and typically involve epistaxis. Once the bleeding is controlled, the nose and surrounding facial bones should be visually inspected and palpated for deformity. Fractures involving a deviated septum can impair breathing within one nostril. Ice can be applied to the nose to reduce the pain and swelling, and the patient should be referred to a physician for follow-up. Repeat exam may be needed within 24 to 48 hours to ensure there is no evidence of *septal hematoma* formation. This will look like a shiny blue ball in the nare and warrants immediate referral to a physician.

Nasal Allergies and Infections

Allergic Rhinitis

There are 2 types of allergic rhinitis: seasonal and perennial. *Seasonal allergic rhinitis* occurs most often during particular seasons, such as during the peak pollen season in the spring. As the name suggests, *perennial allergic rhinitis* occurs throughout the year and is often caused by animal dander, dust, cockroach droppings, or mold. Both types of rhinitis are caused by specific triggers or allergens that produce a histamine response that leads to sneezing, congestion, and itchy, watery eyes. Treatment should focus on avoiding known triggers and medication to relieve the symptoms. As discussed in Chapter 3, antihistamines are commonly used to treat the symptoms caused by rhinitis. Athletes who suffer from nasal allergies should take a second-generation antihistamine (eg, loratadine [Claritin], fexofenadine [Allegra]) that does not produce drowsiness as a side effect. In addition, intra-nasal corticosteroids such as Flonase, Nasonex, and Rhinocort have been shown to be superior to the other treatments for control of nasal symptoms.

Sinusitis and Sinus Infections

When the mucous membranes that line the sinus cavities become irritated and inflamed, sinusitis can occur. Sinusitis and sinus infections often occur secondary to an URI. Patients with sinusitis may complain of congestion or drainage from the sinuses, headache, and sinus pressure. When the sinus drainage thickens and accumulates within the sinuses, a bacterial or viral infection can develop, leading to a sinus infection. In addition to the symptoms associated with sinusitis, patients may experience pain in the teeth and over the sinuses. Decongestants, analgesics, and antibiotics are typically used to treat a sinus infection. As long as an athlete does not have a fever and feels like playing, they can still participate in the sport.

Throat Infections

Pharyngitis and Tonsillitis

Throat infection or inflammation can accompany other immune system pathology (eg, URI, allergies); however, they can also occur as isolated conditions. *Pharyngitis* and *tonsillitis* both produce throat pain, painful or difficult swallowing (and subsequent avoidance of food), and pain in the ears when swallowing. Inspection reveals a red (*erythematous*) throat with purulent or mucoid spots or exudate on the pharynx (pharyngitis) or tonsils (tonsillitis). In cases of tonsillitis, the tonsils will be notably swollen, sometimes to the point that they press on the uvula. Palpation may reveal swollen and/or tender anterior cervical lymph nodes.

The origins of pharyngitis and tonsillitis can be viral or bacterial. Bacterial infections will typically present with higher fever and more systemic signs of infection (fatigue, malaise, arthralgia). Patients who present with fever, white spots or exudate on the throat or tonsils, systemic symptoms of infection, or signs and symptoms that have not resolved within 5 to 7 days should be referred to a physician. The physician will typically order a throat culture and complete blood count laboratory test to determine if the throat infection is bacterial or viral. Streptococcal pharyngitis (*"strep throat"*) is contagious and requires antibiotics and temporary isolation (24 to 36 hours) to prevent communicating the infectious organism to others. Individuals with strep throat will typically present with multiple symptoms and use of the Centor Criteria may help guide the diagnosis. The 4 criteria (fevers, tender cervical lymph nodes, tonsillar exudate/pus, and absence of cough) along with age modifiers has a score system that guides culture and/or antibiotic therapy. Bacterial tonsillitis will also require antibiotics for resolution. Of note, infectious mononucleosis may also mimic pharyngitis/tonsillitis and is discussed separately in this book.

Return-to-participation decisions for athletes recovering from pharyngitis or tonsillitis should be based on the "neck rule." As long the signs and symptoms are all above the neck (runny nose, congestion, sore throat) and the athlete does not have a fever, they can perform a 10-minute test period of light-intensity exercise. If the activity increases the symptoms, the athlete is not ready to return to participation. If the exercise does not increase symptoms, the athlete may continue working out at a subnormal intensity, gradually increasing the duration and intensity over several days.[8]

Laryngitis

Laryngitis is caused by an inflammation of the larynx and therefore presents with changes in the quality of the voice, such as hoarseness or complete inability to speak. Itching may require frequent throat clearing. Fever, difficulty or pain with swallowing, or even dyspnea may occur with severe laryngitis. A physician may observe purulent exudate on the larynx with a laryngoscope.

Treatment for laryngitis includes resting the voice, analgesics for throat pain, fluids, and a vaporizer to maintain moisture within the larynx. Antihistamines should be avoided as they may produce a drying effect. Throat lozenges and throat sprays may also improve symptoms. Athletes with laryngitis can return to participation as long as they do not have a fever, feel well enough to exercise, and have no difficulty breathing at rest or with exertion.

Mouth Disorders

Gingivitis

Gingivitis is a bacterial infection of the gums and typically presents with swollen, red, and bleeding gums along with bad breath. People with gingivitis should be treated by a dentist to prevent the progression of the infection. Maintaining good oral hygiene (ie, brushing and flossing teeth, regular dental check-ups) is essential for oral health. There are no restrictions for participation in athletics or group exercise for individuals with gingivitis.

Periodontitis

Periodontitis occurs when the inflammation and infection from gingivitis spreads to the ligaments and bones that support the teeth. Signs and symptoms include those of gingivitis along with infections or abscesses along the gums and partially loose teeth. Individuals with periodontitis should be referred to a dentist for evaluation and treatment. There are no restrictions for participation in athletics or group exercise for individuals with periodontitis.

Dental Caries

Dental caries refers to general tooth decay associated with demineralization of the tooth enamel. Plaque (formed from food, saliva, bacteria, and mucus) begins to develop within 20 minutes of eating and then begins to adhere to the teeth. The plaque's acidity causes demineralization that can progress to holes in the teeth (cavities). Patients will complain of sensitivity to hot and cold beverages and may also have bad breath (halitosis). A chalky white spot on a tooth is the first sign of dental caries. Treatment options vary depending on the extent of the disease, but will generally include fillings, crowns, root canals, or tooth extraction. Dental caries is not associated with any activity restrictions.

Oral Candidiasis

Oral candidiasis is a fungal infection involving the mucous membranes in the mouth and is most commonly caused by the fungus *Candida albicans*. Extensive antibiotic use and immunosuppression are the most common causes of this fungal infection. Patients will typically present with creamy white to yellow plaques on the tongue, buccal mucosa (inside of check), and palate, which later develop into raw, tender lesions. Topical or systemic antifungal medications are the standard treatment for this disorder. Individuals with oral candidiasis are not restricted from athletics or other exercise.

Oral Cancer

Each year, more than 42,000 people are diagnosed with oral cancer and 8,000 individuals die from this disease.[9] There is a direct link between tobacco use and oral cancer, and the combined use of tobacco products and alcohol increases the risk for developing oral cancer by 15 times. The human papilloma virus version 16 (HPV-16 virus) has also been linked to be a cause of oral cancer. Table 11-5 provides a list of risk factors for developing oral cancer, which includes lip and pharyngeal cancer.

Signs and symptoms include hoarseness that lasts for an extended period of time, pain or difficulty swallowing or chewing, and masses in the mouth or neck. The lip, tongue, and floor of the mouth are the most common sites for oral cancer. Treatment will vary depending on the location and stage of the cancer, but may include surgery, chemotherapy, and radiation. Oral cancer will not prohibit an individual from participating in athletics or recreation; however, the treatments and their associated side effects may temporarily limit or prevent physical activity.

SUMMARY

Although injuries or illnesses involving the eye, ear, nose, throat, and mouth are not the most common conditions encountered by the athletic trainer, they have the potential for serious complications such as loss of sight or hearing. Athletic trainers should be skilled in evaluating the eye, ear, nose, throat, and mouth including the use of an otoscope and ophthalmoscope. Early recognition and prompt referral are important aspects of the management of these conditions.

Table 11-5. Risk Factors for Oral and Pharyngeal Cancer

Tobacco use

Alcohol use

Heavy use of tobacco and alcohol combined

Exposure to human papilloma virus (HPV) virus (pharyngeal cancer)

Age (greater risk after 44 years of age)

Sex (men have twice the risk as women)

Ultraviolet light exposure (lip cancer)

Diet low in vegetables and fruits

Adapted from American Cancer Society. Oral Cavity and Oropharyngeal Cancer [Web site]. Available at: http://www.cancer.org/cancer/oralcavityandoropharyngealcancer/index. Accessed August 26, 2014.

CASE STUDY

One of your basketball athletes reports to you after having a teammate accidentally poke her in the eye during a one-on-one drill. She says that it feels like something is in her eye and the bright lights in the hallway hurt her eye.

Critical Thinking Questions

1. What steps would you take in evaluating this athlete?

2. Given the information provided at this time, what eye conditions would you include in your differential diagnosis?

3. What factors would determine whether you allow this athlete to return to play or refer her to an ophthalmologist?

REFERENCES

1. National Athletic Trainers' Association. *Athletic Training Education Competencies.* 5th ed. The Commission on Accreditation of Athletic Training Education; 2011.

2. Wilson SA, Last A. Management of corneal abrasions. *Am Family Phys.* 2004;70:123-128.

3. Weaver CS, Terrell KM. Evidence-based emergency medicine. Update: do ophthalmic nonsteroidal anti-inflammatory drugs reduce the pain associated with simple corneal abrasion without delaying healing? *Ann Emerg Med.* 2003;41:134-140.

4. Weber TS. Training room management of eye conditions. *Clin Sports Med.* 2005;24:681-693.

5. Tsaras G, Owusu-Ansah A, Boateng FO, Amoateng-Adjepong Y. Complications associated with sickle cell trait: a brief narrative review. *Am J Med.* 2009;122:507-512.

6. Walton W, Von Hagen S, Grigorian R, Zarbin M. Management of traumatic hyphema. *Surv Ophthalmol.* 2002;47:297-334.

7. Ledford J, Pineda R. *The Little Eye Book: A Pupil's Guide to Understanding Ophthalmology.* Slack Incorporated; 2002.

8. Hosey RG, Rodenberg RE. Training room management of medical conditions: infectious diseases. *Clin Sports Med.* 2005;24:477-506.

9. American Cancer Society. Oral Cavity and Oropharyngeal Cancer [Web site]. Available at: http://www.cancer.org/cancer/oralcavityandoropharyngealcancer/index. Accessed August 26, 2014.

ONLINE RESOURCES

◊ **American Academy of Family Physicians: Family Doctor Online**
  ¤ http://familydoctor.org/
◊ **American Academy of Ophthalmology**
  ¤ http://www.aao.org
◊ **American Dental Association**
  ¤ http://www.ada.org
◊ **Eye Care America**
  ¤ http://www.eyecareamerica.org/
◊ **The Merck Manual for Health Care Professionals: Eye Disorders**
  ¤ http://www.merckmanuals.com/professional/eye_disorders.html
◊ **The Merck Manual for Health Care Professionals: Ear, Nose and Throat Disorders**
  ¤ http://www.merckmanuals.com/professional/ear_nose_and_throat_disorders.html
◊ **National Eye Institute**
  ¤ http://www.nei.nih.gov/
◊ **National Institute of Dental and Craniofacial Research**
  ¤ http://www.nidcr.nih.gov/
◊ **Prevent Blindness America**
  ¤ http://www.preventblindness.org/

Please visit www.routledge.com/9781630917234
to access additional material.

CHAPTER 12

Dermatological Conditions

CHAPTER OUTLINE AND OBJECTIVES

Introduction

◊ Describe the common types of lesions associated with most common skin injuries and illnesses.

Review of Anatomy and Physiology

◊ Describe the basic anatomy of the integumentary system.

Mechanical Trauma

◊ Describe the clinical presentation, differential diagnosis, treatment, prevention, and return-to-participation guidelines for common skin injuries and illnesses caused by mechanical trauma.

   ¤ Blisters

   ¤ Calluses

   ¤ Acne Mechanica

   ¤ Talon Noir

Skin Infections

◊ Describe the clinical presentation, differential diagnosis, treatment, prevention, and return-to-participation guidelines for common bacterial skin infections.

   ¤ Community-Acquired Methicillin-Resistant *Staphylococcus Aureus*

   ¤ Impetigo

   ¤ Cellulitis and Erysipelas

   ¤ Furuncles and Carbuncles

   ¤ Folliculitis

◊ Describe the clinical presentation, differential diagnosis, treatment, prevention, and return-to-participation guidelines for common viral skin infections.

Bhojani RA, O'Connor DP, Fincher AL. *Clinical Pathology for Athletic Trainers: Recognizing Systemic Disease, Fourth Edition* (pp 325-350).
© 2022 Taylor & Francis Group.

- ¤ Herpes Simplex Virus
- ¤ Herpes Labialis
- ¤ Herpes Gladiatorum
- ¤ Warts
- ¤ Plantar Warts

◊ Describe the clinical presentation, differential diagnosis, treatment, prevention, and return-to-participation guidelines for common fungal skin infections.

- ¤ Tinea Pedis
- ¤ Tinea Cruris
- ¤ Tinea Unguium
- ¤ Tinea Corporis
- ¤ Tinea Versicolor

◊ Describe the clinical presentation, differential diagnosis, treatment, prevention, and return-to-participation guidelines for common parasitic skin infections.

- ¤ Scabies
- ¤ Pediculosis

◊ Describe the clinical presentation, differential diagnosis, treatment, prevention, and return-to-participation guidelines for common inflammatory skin conditions.

- ¤ Acne Vulgaris
- ¤ Contact Dermatitis
- ¤ Chronic Eczema
- ¤ Psoriasis

◊ Describe the clinical presentation, differential diagnosis, treatment, prevention, and return-to-participation guidelines for common skin conditions caused by environmental conditions.

- ¤ Cold Urticaria
- ¤ Frostnip
- ¤ Frostbite
- ¤ Sunburn
- ¤ Skin Cancer

Summary

Case Study

◊ Develop critical-thinking and clinical decision-making skills.

This chapter addresses the following knowledge and skills from the *Athletic Training Education Competencies, Fifth Edition*[1]:

Content Area	Knowledge and Skills
Prevention and Health Promotion (PHP)	24
Clinical Examination and Diagnosis (CE)	19, 21o
Therapeutic Interventions (TI)	30

INTRODUCTION

Skin injuries or illnesses tend to occur more frequently in athletes and other active individuals than in sedentary individuals. Regardless of their patient population, athletic trainers should be familiar with the more common dermatological conditions and how to manage them. Also to prevent the spread of contagious skin infections, athletic trainers should be familiar with the return-to-participation guidelines associated with these conditions.

Most skin conditions will present with a specific lesion (macules, papules, plaques, nodules, pustules, bullae, vesicles, wheals, or scales) (Figure 12-1). Also, some conditions are known to present with one type of lesion and then transition to a second type of lesion. Recognition of the type of lesion involved and the history of the skin condition will help the athletic trainer develop a differential diagnosis as well as communicate to physicians the description of the lesion. The common types of lesions, their descriptions, and examples of actual pathology are provided in Table 12-1.

A discussion of all dermatological conditions is well beyond the scope of this textbook. This chapter will address the conditions that athletic trainers are most likely to encounter in their clinical practice. These conditions are grouped into 5 categories: (1) those caused by mechanical trauma, (2) those associated with an infection (bacterial, viral, fungal, or parasitic), (3) those associated with localized inflammatory reactions (acne vulgaris, contact dermatitis, chronic eczema, and psoriasis), (4) those caused by environmental exposure (frostnip, frostbite, sunburn, and skin cancer), and (5) those caused by an allergic reaction (urticaria, insect bites). The discussion of each skin condition will include the clinical presentation, differential diagnosis, treatment, prevention, and return-to-participation guidelines, when applicable.

REVIEW OF ANATOMY AND PHYSIOLOGY

The skin is the largest organ of the body and, along with its derivatives (sweat and oil glands, hair, and nails), forms the integumentary system. The skin performs many functions, including protecting the body against germs, helping in the regulation of body temperature, and assisting with the elimination of wastes through sweat. It is divided into 2 layers, the epidermis and dermis (Figure 12-2). The *epidermis* is composed of keratinized, stratified, squamous epithelial tissue that consists of 4 distinct layers: stratum corneum, stratum granulosum, stratum spinosum, and stratum basale. The *dermis* is composed of strong, flexible connective tissue.

The sweat glands are located throughout the skin and help to regulate body temperature and excrete wastes. Each coiled, tubular gland has a secretory portion that lies within the dermis and a duct that travels to the surface of the skin where it forms a funnel-shaped pore.

The sebaceous, or oil glands, are located in all areas of the skin except over the palms of the hands and feet. These glands secrete an oily substance called sebum. Blockage of a sebaceous gland duct leads to an accumulation of sebum, which causes a "whitehead" to form. Acne is caused by an inflammation of the sebaceous glands and appears as pustules (pimples) and cysts on the skin.

Hair follicles extend from the dermis up to the epidermal surface. Infection of the hair follicle can lead to folliculitis. The nails provide a protective covering for the dorsal aspect of the fingers and toes. Each fingernail and toenail consist of a free edge, body, and root. The skin surrounding the nail forms the eponychium (cuticle), and proximal and lateral nail folds.

MECHANICAL TRAUMA

Mechanical trauma accounts for a large number of skin conditions among athletes and other active individuals. These conditions are usually caused by either acute trauma, such as lacerations and abrasions, or repetitive trauma, such as blisters, calluses, acne mechanica, and talon noir. The proper treatments for lacerations and abrasions are covered in most introductory athletic training

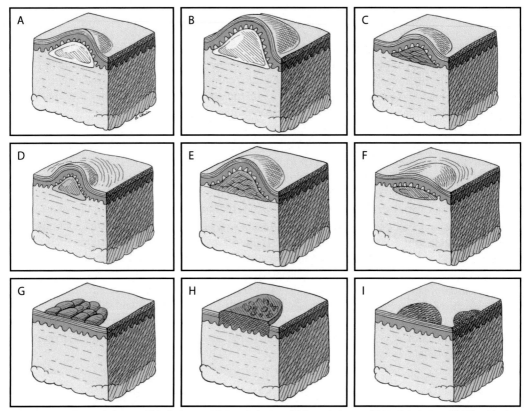

Figure 12-1. (A) Vesicle lesion. (B) Bulla lesion. (C) Papule lesion. (D) Pustule lesion. (E) Nodule lesion. (F) Wheal lesion. (G) Scale lesion. (H) Plaque lesion. (I) Macule lesion.

textbooks, therefore, this chapter will address only those conditions caused by repetitive trauma. It should be noted, however, that all open skin wounds, including acute lacerations and abrasions, are susceptible to bacterial infection. For this reason, athletic trainers should educate their patients that all skin conditions should be thoroughly evaluated.

Blisters

Blisters occur most frequently on the soles of the feet and the palms of the hands. Appearing as tender vesicles filled with either clear or serous fluid, blisters are typically caused by a combination of moisture and repetitive friction. Just prior to the development of a blister, individuals may complain of a "hot spot."

To prevent blisters on the feet, individuals should wear absorbent socks, or 2 pairs of socks made up of 2 different materials, and properly fitted shoes. Gradually increasing the intensity of a workout or slowly breaking in new shoes can help to develop calluses rather than blisters. Lubricating the skin or applying moleskin to a friction site can also help prevent blisters.

When treating small blisters, the roof of the blister should be left intact to help protect against infection and prevent friction to the tender skin below. When treating large blisters that are prone to tearing or rupture with further friction, the fluid should be drained by puncturing the blister with a sterile needle or scalpel. The puncture should be made at the base of the blister. When punctured with a scalpel, the fluid can be milked out of the blister using a sterile gauze pad. When using a sterile needle, the fluid can be suctioned or drained into the attached syringe. Once drained, the blister should be covered with antibiotic ointment and a sterile dressing. When covering a blister prior to physical activity, possible dressings might include a doughnut pad with lubricating gel or antibiotic

Table 12-1. Common Skin Lesions Associated With Infections and Allergic Reactions

LESION	DESCRIPTION	EXAMPLE
Vesicles	Small, fluid-filled blister; < 10 mm	Impetigo; herpes labialis; herpes gladiatorum
Bullae	Thin-walled sacs of fluid; > 10 mm (large blisters)	Blister
Papules	Solid, round bumps; < 5 mm	Warts; molluscum contagiosum
Nodules	Solid, raised bumps; > 10 mm	Late stages of acne mechanica; furuncles
Pustules	Small, inflamed, pus-filled blister-like lesions	Acne mechanica; acne; furuncles
Wheals	Circumscribed lesions of inflamed skin	Urticaria
Scales	Excess epidermis forming small flakes	Eczema; tinea pedis
Plaques	Broad, raised (palpable) area on the skin	Psoriasis
Macules	Small, flat (not palpable) spots or blemishes	Tinea versicolor

ointment, a piece of "second-skin," or moleskin. A drained blister or a blister whose roof becomes torn should be treated as an open wound. As with all open wounds, caution should be taken to prevent a bacterial infection. Wound location and care given will guide activity level by sport.

Calluses

Like blisters, calluses occur most often on the plantar surface of the foot and the palms of the hands. These thickened areas of skin occur in response to repetitive friction. Ensuring that shoes fit properly, and hand grips are soft can prevent many calluses. Most calluses remain asymptomatic unless they become overly large. If calluses begin to impair an athlete's performance, or should a blister develop under the callus, the callus can be pared down using a scalpel. An alternative treatment would include soaking the area and applying salicylic acid preparations followed by abrasion of the callus using a file or pumice stone. Calluses do not prevent an athlete from participating in practice or competition.

Acne Mechanica

Acne mechanica typically presents as either papules or pustules in mild to moderate cases and may transition to cysts or nodules in more severe cases.[2] This condition is not to be confused with acne vulgaris, which is discussed later in this chapter. Acne mechanica is typically caused by the combination of pressure, friction, heat, and occlusion, which often occurs under protective equipment. Acne mechanica is sometimes referred to as sports-induced acne because of its prevalence in athletes, and "football acne" because of its specific prevalence in football athletes. This condition may occur anywhere, but occurs most often on the forehead, chin, shoulders, and upper back. Acne mechanica is generally treated with topical or systemic antibiotics such as topical retinoids or benzoyl peroxide, depending on the severity.[2,3] To prevent this condition on their shoulders and

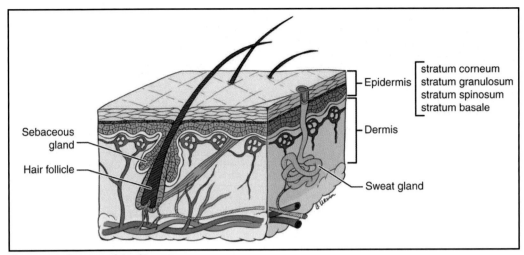

Figure 12-2. Anatomy of the skin.

upper backs, athletes should be encouraged to wear an absorbent, cotton T-shirt under their protective equipment, as well as remove their perspiration-soaked clothing and shower immediately after activity. Differential diagnosis might include contact dermatitis and certain forms of folliculitis.[3] Acne mechanica does not exclude an athlete from participation and will usually resolve on its own once the sports season ends.

Talon Noir

Talon noir, or black heel, is associated with sports involving sudden stops and starts, such as tennis and basketball. The lateral shearing forces cause intra-epidermal bleeding that presents as horizontally arranged rows of small dots along the posterior or posterolateral heel. The bluish-black dots that make up talon noir will often resemble the seeds of a plantar wart. Talon noir can also be seen on the palms of the hands in racket sports or weightlifting. Paring down the superficial skin layers using a scalpel will usually remove the pigmented black heel. It should be noted that when paring down the superficial skin layers does not remove the black dots, possible melanoma should be suspected. Talon noir does not prevent participation in any sports or recreational activity.

Skin Infections

Common skin infections affecting athletes and other active individuals can be classified as bacterial, viral, fungal, or parasitic. Also, skin infections can be categorized as primary or secondary. *Primary skin infections* involve an infectious agent entering and affecting normal skin, whereas a *secondary infection* results from an infectious agent entering an existing break in the skin (eg, cut, laceration, or other wound).[4] There are several risks factors that are common to each of these types of infections, including a warm, moist environment produced by perspiration and increased body temperature, occlusive clothing and equipment, close skin-to-skin contact, and acute and chronic trauma to skin. Many of these infectious skin conditions require restrictions on participating in sports, particularly in sports that involve direct skin-to-skin contact such as wresting.

Bacterial Infections

Most bacterial infections can be classified into 1 of 3 categories: (1) those that are contagious, like impetigo, (2) those to which continued competition can cause further tissue damage, like cellulitis, furuncles, and carbuncles, and (3) those that are neither contagious nor pose further risk to the

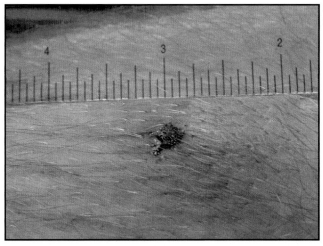

Figure 12-3. Community-acquired methicillin-resistant *Staphylococcus aureus* infection.

patient, like folliculitis.[5] The common bacterial infections that an athletic trainer might encounter in their practice are summarized next.

Community-Acquired Methicillin-Resistant Staphylococcus aureus

Methicillin-resistant Staphylococcus aureus (MRSA) skin and soft tissue infections were once associated only with hospitals; however, they are now becoming more prevalent in the community, with the first reported case in the athletic setting occurring in 1998. Community-acquired MRSA (CA-MRSA) infections are resistant to commonly prescribed β-lactam antibiotics, which include the penicillin group and the cephalosporin group, making them a challenge to treat.

The typical presentation of a CA-MRSA infection is similar to that of a common *Staphylococcus* ("staph") skin infection, making it difficult to distinguish without a bacterial culture. Both types of infections can present with small pimple-like lesions, pustules, or boils. In their early stage, these lesions are often mistaken for an insect bite, which leads to a delay in proper treatment. Both staph and CA-MRSA infections can quickly progress to a much larger inflamed, painful, indurated lesion (Figure 12-3).[6] CA-MRSA infections can also attack existing cuts and abrasions.

The Centers for Disease Control and Prevention describes the common risk factors for CA-MRSA infections as the 5 Cs, which are listed in Table 12-2. Without proper precautions, these infections can easily spread to an entire sports team. The National Athletic Trainers' Association (NATA) published an official statement on the prevention of CA-MRSA infections.[7] The NATA's recommendations are summarized in Table 12-3. It is important that all open wounds be covered at all times, and any individual suspected of having a CA-MRSA infection be referred to a physician for possible culture and treatment recommendations. Accurate diagnosis of CA-MRSA can help to determine the appropriate antibiotic to be used in treatment. Often the individual will need to be hospitalized for intravenous antibiotics depending on risk factors for systemic infection, failure of outpatient antibiotics, or rapid spread of the infection.

Repeated occurrences of staph or CA-MRSA infections within the same individual or among a single team warrants the performance of nasal swab testing to identify if someone is a carrier. Individuals who carry the bacteria in their noses, but are not ill, are said to be colonized. Approximately 30% of the general population is colonized with *S. aureus* and 1% are colonized with CA-MRSA.[6] These individuals may be treated for colonization including chlorhexidine daily washes or dilute bleach baths along with nasal mupirocin ointment.[8]

There are currently no published return-to-participation guidelines for the management of CA-MRSA infections in athletes. Many physicians are using the guidelines established for other bacterial infections and the National Collegiate Athletic Association's (NCAA's) rules for wrestlers to guide their decisions in returning athletes to practice and competition.

Table 12-2. CDC Risk Factors for CA-MRSA Infections—5 Cs

1. Close skin-to-skin contact
2. Contaminated items such as towels, razors, or soap
3. Crowding
4. Cleanliness (poor hygiene)
5. Compromised skin integrity

CA-MRSA = community-acquired methicillin-resistant *Staphylococcus aureus;* CDC = Centers for Disease Control and Prevention.

Table 12-3. Steps for Preventing CA-MRSA Infections

Wash hands thoroughly with soap and water or an alcohol-based hand cleaner before and after treating a wound.

Individuals should shower immediately after activity.

Do not treat individuals with open wounds in a common whirlpool or tub.

Individuals should not share towels, razors, athletic clothing, or equipment.

Athletic clothing and towels should be properly washed after each use.

Facilities and equipment should be kept clean.

Refer all individuals with active skin lesions that do not respond to initial therapy.

Proper first aid procedures should be followed when treating all wounds.

Individuals with suspicious lesions should be referred for a bacterial culture to establish a diagnosis.

All skin lesions should be covered before participation in sports activity.

CA-MRSA = community-acquired methicillin-resistant *Staphylococcus aureus.*

Adapted with permission from NATA Position Statement on MRSA Infections (www.nata.org).

Impetigo

Impetigo is most commonly caused by the S. aureus bacteria; however, some cases may involve the Group A *Streptococcus* bacteria. It typically presents with honey-colored, crusted, well-defined, erythematous vesicles and occurs most frequently on the face and other exposed areas (Figure 12-4). It is particularly common in wrestlers, swimmers, and gymnasts.[2] Football and rugby athletes are also considered at risk for developing impetigo because of their close skin-to-skin contact.[9] In its earliest stages, impetigo may be confused with tinea corporis, herpes simplex, or acneiform papules. Treatment of impetigo typically includes debridement with hydrogen peroxide and 7 to 10 days of antibiotics. Topical antibiotics such as mupirocin (Bactroban) are used for localized lesions, whereas oral antibiotics are recommended for the treatment of extensive or bullous impetigo.[2] It is prudent to rule out MRSA in athletes with impetigo.[9] Athletes with moist, crusted lesions should be withheld from practice or competition. Athletes may return to play when the lesion crusts have dried, they have completed 5 days of antibiotic treatment, and they have had no new lesions appear within the last 48 hours.[2] Following these guidelines, active lesions should not be covered to allow participation. Inactive lesions can be covered by a nonpermeable dressing during activity.

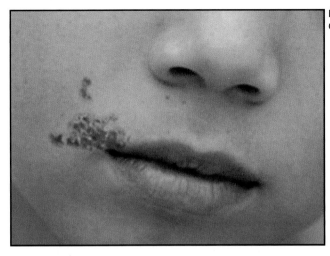

Figure 12-4. Impetigo. (Image from CNX OpenStax/used under CC BY 4.0.)

Cellulitis and Erysipelas

Cellulitis and erysipelas are acute bacterial infections involving the skin and subcutaneous tissues. These infections typically occur at the site of a previous wound (eg cut, laceration, insect bite) and are caused by either S.aureus or Group A Streptococcus. Both conditions will present with redness, swelling and warmth at the site of the infection, and may include systemic symptoms such as fever and malaise.[10]

Erysipelas is a more superficial infection typically involving the epidermis and upper portion of the dermis. The clinical presentation includes a raised, well-defined, expanding, red plaque.[4] Cellulitis also presents with a raised red plaque; however, it will typically take several days to fully develop.[4] Again, both conditions may also present with fever, chills, and malaise.

Both cellulitis and erysipelas are treated with antibiotics and may in some cases require an incision to drain the abscess for full resolution. Return-to-participation guidelines for these infections are similar to those for impetigo.[4]

Furuncles and Carbuncles

Furuncles, or boils, typically present as tender, red nodules that contain a core of necrotic tissue and pus. They may initially appear as a small nodule that turns into a 5- to 30-mm pustule. Open wounds pose an increased risk for the development of furuncles. All open wounds should also be covered. Single furuncles are treated with moist, hot compresses to promote drainage. At times, furuncles may require lancing to allow the wound to drain. Furuncles are not contagious (unless they become infected with S. aureus or MRSA); however, returning to play too soon may cause further tissue damage. Carbuncles are formed by clusters of furuncles and are treated similarly to furuncles. Generally, it is recommended that athletes complete at least 5 days of treatment and have no draining or moist lesions, as well as have no new lesions within the last 48 hours before returning to activity.

Folliculitis

Folliculitis is a gram-positive infection (S. aureus) of the hair follicles most often caused by friction from clothing or equipment.[2] Mild cases typically involve the superficial portion of the hair follicle, resolve on their own, and usually do not require treatment. More extensive cases involve the deeper portion of the hair follicle and are associated with redness and tenderness. Topical antibiotic therapy typically is sufficient for most cases of folliculitis.[11] Hot tub folliculitis is caused by *Pseudomonas aeruginosa* (gram-negative infection) and presents with papules and pustules on skin areas that were covered by a bathing suit.[2] These lesions usually appear 2 to 3 days after exposure to the hot tub or swimming pool and typically last for 7 to 10 days. The presence of skin abrasions

Figure 12-5. Herpes Labialis. ("Herpes labialis Ulcus" by Speifensender/used under CC BY-SA 3.0.)

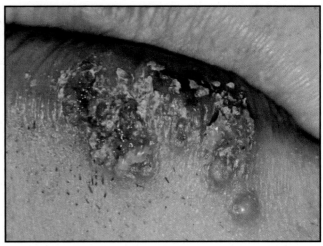

increases the risk for developing hot tub folliculitis as does poor maintenance of chlorine levels in pools and hot tubs.[9] Systemic signs and symptoms can be associated with hot tub folliculitis and may include fever, nausea, vomiting, headache, pharyngitis, and otitis externa. Systemic involvement warrants referral to a physician and the use of oral antibiotics.[3] Hot tub folliculitis can be prevented by maintaining chlorine and pH levels and regularly cleaning whirlpools and hot tubs. Folliculitis should not prohibit an athlete from sports participation.

Viral Infections

Most viral skin infections encountered by athletic trainers are caused by one of the following viruses: herpes simplex (HSV), *Molluscum contagiosum* (MCV), or human papilloma (HPV). Sweating, in combination with occlusive clothing and equipment, provides a perfect environment for viral skin infections. Spread of these infections requires direct skin contact with infected lesions or their secretions. Prevention of viral infections focuses on covering all abrasions and other open wounds, early detection through regular skin screenings, early treatment, and exclusion of athletes from participation when recommended by rules and guidelines.

Herpes Simplex Virus

There are 2 types of HSV: type 1 (HSV-1) and type 2 (HSV-2). HSV-1 is associated with herpes labialis and herpes gladiatorum, whereas HSV-2 is associated with the sexually transmitted genital herpes. Both HSV-1 and HSV-2 can produce primary and secondary infections. The primary episode is typically more severe and may produce systemic symptoms. HSV can become dormant in the neural ganglia, leading to periodic recurrences. These recurrent infections usually have a shorter duration and less severe symptoms.

Herpes Labialis

Herpes labialis (cold sore or fever blister) is caused by HSV-1 and can present as a single vesicle or a cluster of vesicles on the lips (Figure 12-5). Exposure to the sun and physical or emotional stress seem to be triggers for the development of cold sores or fever blisters. Individuals will usually report prodromal symptoms of tingling or burning prior to the appearance of the lesions. Treatments are intended to reduce pain or discomfort and to promote early healing. There are a variety of over-the-counter (OTC) ointments for treating the discomfort of herpes labialis; however, prescription oral antiviral medications are more effective in reducing the duration of the infection and may also be used in certain settings to prevent recurrent infections. Acyclovir, famciclovir, and valacyclovir are commonly prescribed oral antiviral medications use to treat herpes labialis.[12,13]

Athletes should be withheld from participation if they have moist lesions and their sport involves direct skin-to-skin contact with the involved area. The NCAA requires that wrestlers with a primary herpes labialis infection be withheld until they meet the following criteria: (1) the athlete is asymptomatic, (2) no new lesions have developed for 3 consecutive days, (3) all of the lesions are crusted, and (4) the athlete has been taking an appropriate dose of a systemic antiviral medication for at least 5 days.[14,15]

Herpes Gladiatorum

Herpes gladiatorum, also caused by HSV-1, commonly affects wrestlers, hence the name.[13,16] Open wounds such as abrasions or other cuts in the skin are necessary for HSV transmission to occur. Herpes gladiatorum typically presents with clustered vesicular lesions on an erythematous base. These lesions will usually progress to a crusty stage before resolving in 1 to 3 weeks. Many individuals will report itching or burning in the area of the lesions prior to the actual appearance of the vesicles.[16] Systemic symptoms of fever, chills, headache, sore throat, malaise, myalgia, and regional lymphadenopathy have also been reported with herpes gladiatorum.[13,16]

A differential diagnosis might include *Staphylococcal furunculosis*, herpes zoster, or contact dermatitis. The patient's history and location of the lesions may be helpful in identifying herpes gladiatorum. The head, face, and extremities are the most common sites affected by herpes gladiatorum; however, the trunk and eyes may also be involved.[16] Ocular HSV can be a serious complication leading to blindness; therefore, individuals with herpetic lesions close to the eyes should be referred to a physician as soon as possible. In isolated cases, it may be necessary to perform a cell culture to distinguish HSV from a bacterial infection. Although viral cultures are considered the gold standard in HSV diagnosis, it can take up to 4 to 5 days to get the results. A Tzanck test or direct fluorescent antibody test can provide a more rapid diagnosis.

As with herpes labialis, treatment with oral antiviral medications will often shorten the course of herpes gladiatorum.[13] All lesions should be kept clean and dry throughout treatment to prevent secondary bacterial infections. Prophylactic use of antiviral medications can be helpful in preventing recurrent HSV infections.[13]

The criteria for returning wrestlers with herpes gladiatorum to competition are the same as that for herpes labialis. It should be noted that the NCAA prohibits covering of an active HSV infection (moist lesions without proper treatment) to permit participation.[17]

Molluscum Contagiosum

MCV is caused by the poxvirus MCV and is spread in the sports environment through direct skin-to-skin contact. Wrestlers, rugby athletes, swimmers, and gymnasts are most commonly affected by this virus.[9,12] This virus is also transmitted through sexual contact and is therefore considered to be a common sexually transmitted disease.[18] Of note, this virus is commonly seen in children, but can also occur in adults.

MCV typically presents with a rash that includes white, pinkish, or skin-colored, dome-shaped papules with a center dimple (Figure 12-6).[18,19] The rash will usually be made up of individual or grouped lesions that range in size from as small as 3 to 5 mm to as large as 10 mm.[18,19]

Definitive diagnosis is made based on clinical appearance of skin lesions but also can be through histology.[20] Treatment of this lesion usually focuses on the destruction of the papules. Topical agents such as salicylic acid, trichloroacetic acid, phenol, podophyllin, and tretinoin can be used.[20] A quicker removal can be accomplished by physicians through curettage, laser therapy, or cryotherapy.[19]

The NCAA requires that these lesions be curetted or removed in order for a wrestler to compete in a meet or tournament. After the lesions have been removed, the area should be covered with a gas-permeable dressing held in place with pre-wrap and elastic tape.[17]

Figure 12-6. Molluscum contagiosum. (Published in *Color Atlas of Dermatology*, 3rd ed, White G, 52-53, Copyright Elsevier [2004].)

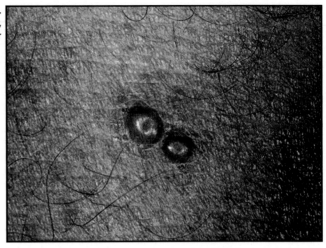

Warts

Warts are caused by HPV. There are several different types of warts that are categorized by their general appearance and location (Table 12-4). Warts are contagious and are spread by either skin-to-skin contact or contact with a contaminated surface. Warts that are located on an exposed area of skin will typically have a hard surface; those located in moist, occluded areas will typically be soft. The treatment for warts generally focuses on destroying the lesions by freezing, burning, electrocautery, or applying topical acids.[19]

Because warts are contagious, athletes should have their warts covered prior to practice or competition. Wrestlers with warts on their faces should be withheld from participation since these lesions cannot be effectively covered.[17]

Plantar Warts

Plantar warts are found on the soles of the feet and are probably the most common wart seen by the athletic trainer. They may commonly occur within calluses, where they hide the usual swirls or "fingerprints" of the callus (Figure 12-7). Because of the weight-bearing forces on the feet, plantar warts grow into the foot rather than growing above the skin surface. As a result, individuals with plantar warts will commonly report a sensation of walking on a pebble. When plantar warts become painful or hinder performance, they can be pared down with a scalpel. This removal of the superficial layers of the wart will reveal tiny blood vessels that appear as a pattern of pin-sized black dots. Paring down the plantar wart will also help differentiate this lesion from corns or calluses.[19] Applying a doughnut pad over the plantar wart will often alleviate the individual's discomfort and allow them to participate. OTC salicylic acid preparations can also be used to treat plantar warts. The effectiveness of these OTC treatments can be improved by soaking the plantar warts first and then paring down the dead skin with a pumice stone before applying the salicylic acid. More extensive treatments require referral to a physician and include cryotherapy, electrocautery, excision, and the application of chemicals. These treatments can limit the mobility of an athlete and therefore may result in time lost from workout or competition.

Keeping the feet dry and wearing shoes in locker rooms and showers can help prevent the spread of plantar warts.[9] Wrestlers with plantar warts are allowed to participate since their warts are covered by their shoes.[17]

Fungal Infections

Superficial fungal infections are the most common type of dermatological infections in athletes. These fungal infections are caused by dermatophytes and are named for the sites they attack: *tinea capitis* (scalp), *tinea barbae* (beard area), *tinea pedis* (feet), *tinea manum* (hands), *tinea cruris*

Table 12-4. Types of Warts

LESION	DESCRIPTION	COMMON LOCATION
Common	Irregularly surfaced, domed lesions	Hands and fingers
Flat	Smooth, flat-topped lesion	Face and extremities
Periungual	Abraded or peeling appearance	Nail margins of the toes and fingers
Filiform	Finger-like projections	Face
Plantar	Broad, raised (palpable) area on the skin	Soles of the feet

(groin area), *tinea unguium* (fingernails and toenails), and *tinea corporis* for infection of all other skin areas.[21] A warm, moist environment serves as the primary predisposing factor for all of these infections. This chapter will discuss tinea pedis, tinea cruris, unguium, tinea corporis, and tinea versicolor since they are the conditions that are most commonly encountered by athletic trainers.

Tinea Pedis

Tinea pedis is most commonly caused by the dermatophyte *Trichophyton rubrum*. There are 3 forms of tinea pedis, with each one having a distinct clinical presentation. The first and most common form, interdigital tinea pedis, occurs in the web spaces of the toes and presents with a scaly, peeling area that may also be erythematous, with maceration and fissuring (Figure 12-8).[22] It is not uncommon for these lesions to spread to either the dorsal or plantar surfaces of the foot. The second form of tinea pedis presents with vesicles or bullae on the midfoot, while the third involves hyperkeratotic scale on the plantar surface of the foot. Individuals with tinea pedis, regardless of the type, will complain of itching, especially after the removal of their socks.[22]

Mild, localized fungal infections usually respond well to a topical antifungal powder such as tolnaftate (Tinactin). Moderate cases usually respond better to a topical cream such as clotrimazole (Mycelex, Lotrimin), miconazole (Monistat), econazole (Spectazole), sulconazole (Exelderm), or terbinafine (Lamisil) twice daily for 2 to 4 weeks.[13] The athlete should be instructed to apply these topical medications at least 2 cm beyond the infected lesions onto the healthy skin around the area.[21] Extensive cases of tinea pedis may require oral antifungal medications such as terbinafine (Lamisil), fluconazole (Diflucan) or itraconazole (Sporanox) in addition to a topical cream.[22] If a bacterial infection occurs secondary to the fungal infection, oral antibiotics should be used in addition to the antifungal medications.

Tinea pedis can be prevented if individuals make a habit of wearing shower shoes or other types of shoes in gym locker rooms and shower areas. Athletes should also keep their feet dry by wearing breathable, synthetic socks and using tolnaftate powder (Tinactin). Tinea pedis should not restrict an individual from participation in athletics or other activities.

Tinea Cruris

Tinea cruris (jock itch) is most commonly caused by *T. rubrum* or *T. interdigitale* and typically involves the proximal medial thighs, inguinal folds of the groin, and buttocks.[18] This fungal infection will usually present with large, round, scaly plaques that have pustules and papules at the edges (Figure 12-9).[20] Tight clothing, obesity, male gender, diabetes, and chronic corticosteroid use are risk factors associated with developing tinea cruris.

Clinical diagnosis can be made by the appearance and location of the lesions. Topical OTC antifungal medications are usually very effective in treating tinea cruris. Individuals who do not

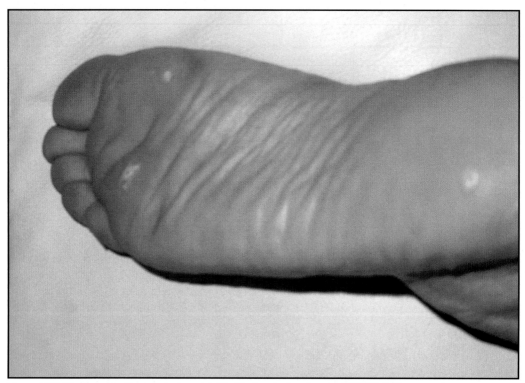

Figure 12-7. Plantar warts. ("Large plantar warts" by Marionette/used under CC BY-SA 3.0.)

Figure 12-8. Tinea pedis. (Image from Dr Hari K Kasi/ used under CC BY 4.0.)

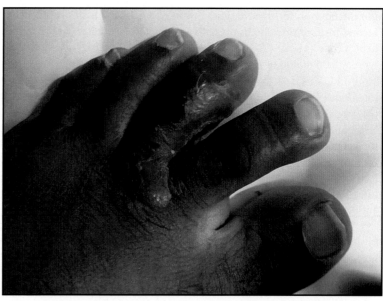

respond to this treatment should be referred to a physician for definitive diagnosis with a potassium hydroxide (KOH) stain or fungal culture and to receive systemic antifungals. Of note, recurrence of tinea cruris is common and may occur with tinea pedis or onchomycosis so treatment of these conditions need to be completed to prevent recurrence.

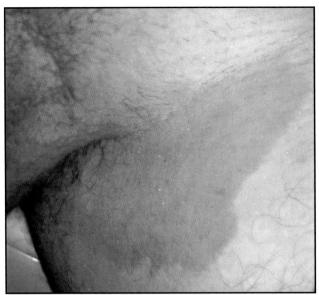

Figure 12-9. Tinea cruris. ("Tinea cruris" by Robertgascoin/used under CC BY-SA 3.0.)

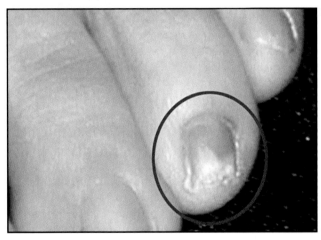

Figure 12-10. Tinea unguium.

Tinea Unguium

Tinea unguium is also caused by T. rubrum and affects the fingernails and toenails. Distal subungual onychomycosis is the most common form of this nail fungus and appears as a white, hyperkeratotic patch under the nail (Figure 12-10). The nail will also become thickened and discolored and will eventually separate from the nail bed. Proximal subungual onychomycosis occurs closer to the cuticle, with the fungus invading the proximal nail fold.

Trauma can predispose a nail for tinea unguium. Other predisposing factors include hyperhidrosis, diabetes mellitus, age, and poor venous and lymphatic drainage.[20]

Unlike other fungal infections, tinea unguium does not respond well to topical antifungals. Systemic antifungals such as itraconazole (Sporanox), terbinafine (Lamisil), and fluconazole (Diflucan) are commonly prescribed and usually will needs months of treatment along with nail hygiene to resolve. The presence of tinea unguium does not prevent an athlete from participating in their sport.

Figure 12-11. Tinea corporis. (Published in *Color Atlas of Dermatology*, 3rd ed, White G, 167, Copyright Elsevier [2004].)

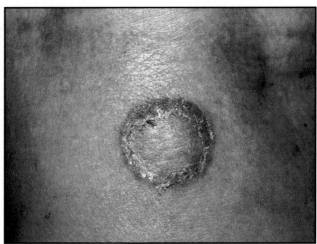

Tinea Corporis

Tinea corporis (ringworm) is most commonly caused by the T. rubrum dermatophyte. Because this fungal infection is highly prevalent in wrestlers, it is often referred to as *tinea gladiatorum*.[23,24] Tinea gladiatorum typically presents with a circular, erythematous, pruritic (itchy) plaque, with a raised edge, scaling, and central clearing (Figure 12-11).[5,23-26] On inspection, early lesions may have a similar appearance to dermatitis, with later lesions resembling psoriasis, or eczema. Tinea corporis can be differentiated from psoriasis by the central clearing of the tinea lesions. Some tinea corporis lesions may also be more papular and therefore resemble impetigo or early HSV lesions.[25,26] Individuals will usually complain of itching and burning.[23,24] Definitive diagnosis can be made by a physician using a KOH stain.

Tinea gladiatorum is spread through skin-to-skin contact and occurs most prevalently on the head, neck, and arms.[23,25-27] Wrestling mats or other equipment are not believed to be a factor in the spread of this skin condition.[24,27]

Athletes with tinea corporis gladiatorum should be treated with antifungal medications for at least 2 to 4 weeks, whereas the normal population may require only 1 to 2 weeks of treatment. Topical treatments such as clotrimazole (Lotrimin), miconazole nitrate (Micatin), and ketoconazole (Nizoral) are effective for noninflammatory cases.[23] These topical treatments, however, require consistent application to all lesions. In general, single lesions can be treated with topical medications, whereas 2 or more lesions should be treated with an oral medication such as griseofulvin (Grifulvin V, Fulvin-U/F, Gris-Peg), fluconazole (Diflucan), itraconazole (Sporanox), and terbinafine (Lamisil).[5,23,26] Oral antifungal medications are also recommended for lesions that fail to resolve with topical treatments. It is recommended that topical treatment be continued for 2 weeks after lesions have disappeared.

The NCAA requires athletes with tinea corporis gladiatorum to be withheld from practice and competition until they have received a minimum of 72 hours of topical antifungal treatment.[15] Once the athlete returns to practice or competition, the lesions should be covered until the flaking stops. The lesions can be covered with a gas-permeable dressing, prewrap, and elastic tape.[14,15] If the lesion cannot be covered, the athlete should be withheld from practice an additional 5 days. The NCAA recommends that dressings be changed after every match and that the routine for covering tinea corporis lesions include "selenium sulfide washing of lesion or ketoconazole shampoo (Nizoral), followed by application of naftifine gel or cream (Naftin) or terbinafine cream (Lamisil)."[15]

To prevent tinea corporis gladiatorum, athletes should shower immediately after practice and have their workout clothes laundered daily. Athletes should also report skin lesions as soon as they appear so that treatment can begin promptly. Athletic trainers should identify skin lesions requiring disqualification from competition or exclusion from practice.[5,23] Strict adherence to prevention

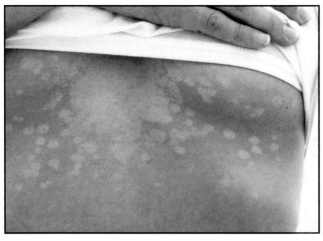

Figure 12-12. Tinea versicolor. (Image from Sarahrosenau/used under CC BY-SA 2.0.)

protocols has been shown to reduce the number of cases of tinea corporis in wrestlers.[28] Athletes with questionable lesions should be referred to a physician for confirmation of the lesion.

Tinea Versicolor

Tinea versicolor is a superficial fungal infection caused by the *Malassezia furfur* organism. It presents with macules or patches that have either a hypopigmented or hyperpigmented appearance and may also include a dust-like scale (Figure 12-12). This change in skin pigment produces variations in skin color from white to red to brown. The back, trunk, abdomen, and arms are the areas that are most commonly affected by the *M. furfur* organism.

Tinea versicolor occurs in approximately 2% to 8% of the population and is more commonly found in regions of the country with hot, humid climates. This condition is more noticeable in the spring and summer months since the involved areas do not tan like the adjacent skin areas do. Tinea versicolor is usually recognized by its unique clinical presentation; however, if necessary, a physician can confirm the diagnosis using an ultraviolet black (Wood) light or a KOH stain.

Tinea versicolor can be treated using topical or oral antifungal medications. The topical agents usually require that the cream or lotion be left on for as little as 10 minutes or as long as overnight before being rinsed off. For this reason, many patients prefer the oral antifungals for their convenience. The changes in pigment may take months to resolve after initiation of treatment. Regardless of the medication used, tinea versicolor has a high rate of recurrence, therefore, prophylactic dosing is recommended, particularly during the hot summer months. This condition is not contagious; therefore, it will not prevent participation in sports.

Parasitic Infections

Scabies

Scabies is a contagious parasitic infection caused by the *Sarcoptes scabiei*. It is spread through direct skin-to-skin contact. The most commonly affected sites include the finger and toe webs, flexor surfaces of the wrists, elbows, axillae, buttocks, breasts, and male genitalia. After transfer from the host, a pregnant mite will burrow into the epidermis to lay her eggs, although symptoms may not develop for 3 to 4 weeks after exposure. Initially, a vesicle or papule may develop; however, the extreme itching of the lesions often causes these to be removed. Severe itching, more common at night and out of proportion for skin changes, is the most common symptom.

Diagnosis of scabies infestation is made by scraping the lesion and placing the collected contents on a microscopic slide with mineral oil. The presence of mites, eggs, or feces represents a positive diagnosis.[22]

Scabies is treated with prescription-strength lotions or creams, such as lindane (Kwell), permethrin, and crotamiton, that are applied from the neck down and left on for 8 to 14 hours. The treatment should be repeated 1 week later to ensure that all newly hatched mites are killed. All people who have had contact with the infected individual (eg, teammates, family members, roommates, coaches) should also be treated, and clothing and bedding should be washed. Oral ivermectin may also be used as an alternative when topical therapy may be difficult to show compliance for.

Because scabies is very contagious, infected athletes should be withheld from contact sports during the treatment period. The NCAA guidelines require that wrestlers have a negative scabies test at the tournament in order to complete.

Pediculosis

Pediculosis refers to a parasite infestation with lice. The 3 most common sites affected include the head (*pediculus capitis*), body (*pediculus corporis*), and genital area (*pediculus pubis*). The lice are spread by direct skin-to-skin contact. Once infested, it may take up to 10 days for nits (eggs) to hatch. The newly hatched lice begin biting, causing 2 to 4 mm red papules and itching.

As with scabies, pediculosis can be diagnosed through microscopic examination of skin scrapings. A louse comb can also be used to identify and remove lice. Treatment requires 7 days of permethrin (Nix) lotion and lindane shampoo.[22] All individuals having had contact with the infected individual should also be treated and all clothing and bedding washed and dried. NCAA guidelines require that infected individuals complete treatment and show no signs of lice in order to compete.[15]

Inflammatory Skin Conditions

Most inflammatory skin conditions can be classified as either localized or of systemic origin. This chapter addresses 4 localized inflammatory conditions: acne vulgaris, contact dermatitis, chronic eczema, and psoriasis. The term eczema refers to a variety of inflammatory skin conditions. In many instances, the terms eczema and dermatitis are used interchangeably. This chapter will use dermatitis to refer to the acute conditions and eczema to refer to the chronic conditions.

Acne Vulgaris

Acne vulgaris is an inflammatory condition involving the sebaceous glands and hair follicles. Clinically, this condition presents as "blackheads" and pimples (pustules) that may progress to erythematous macules, papules, and cysts. The face, neck, upper back, shoulders, and thighs are the most common sites affected. Acne has familial tendencies and can also occur as a side effect of steroid use.

The sebaceous glands secrete an oily substance called sebum. When the hair follicles and sebaceous glands become blocked, sebum will accumulate and become inflamed. The body's immune system responds, which then leads to the development of pustules. If the wall of the pustules ruptures, the inflammation extends down into the dermis producing a deep, red, tender cyst or nodule.

Acne is graded according to severity. Mild acne is the term used to describe an outbreak with 3 to 10 lesions, while moderate acne consists of 10 to 30 lesions. Severe acne involves greater than 30 lesions. Acne is also classified as either noninflammatory, which includes cases with "blackheads" and pimples, or inflammatory, which involves cysts and nodules.

Treatment begins with educating the patient on the importance of washing acne sites twice a day and avoiding cosmetics and lotions that might lead to blockage of the sebaceous glands or hair follicles. Medical treatment involves the use of one or more of the following types of medications: (1) topical retinoids, (2) oral retinoids, (3) topical antibiotics, or (4) oral antibiotics. Mild acne usually responds to topical treatments with retinoids (adapalene, tazarotene, and tretinoin), antibiotics (erythromycin, tetracycline, clindamycin), or combinations of the 2 (zinc/erythromycin, benzoyl peroxide/erythromycin). Side effects of these medications include erythema, photosensitivity, pruritis, dryness, and peeling. Because of the photosensitivity, patients taking these medications should avoid excessive exposure to the sun and use liberal amounts of oil-free sunblock when planning to

Table 12-5. Common Allergens Associated With Allergic Contact Dermatitis

Rubber products (shoe insoles, wet suits, orthopedic appliances)	Epoxy (face gear)
	Leather sporting equipment
Topical creams (analgesics, antibiotics, antiseptics)	Fiberglass
Athletic tape (resin, adhesive backing)	

be outdoors. Moderate to severe acne is generally treated with a combination of systemic antibiotics and topical retinoids. Common oral antibiotics used to treat acne include tetracycline, erythromycin, doxycycline, minocycline, and trimethoprim-sulfamethoxazole. Acne vulgaris does not prevent patients from participating in competitive sports.

Contact Dermatitis

Acute allergic contact dermatitis is caused by exposure to or contact with a specific allergen. The rash produced by exposure to poison ivy is a classic example of contact dermatitis. The sap from the poison ivy leaves produces vesicles and papules that are usually very pruritic (itchy). There are a variety of allergens that can produce contact dermatitis; however, some individuals are hypersensitive to specific allergens. Table 12-5 lists several of the common allergens that are associated with allergic contact dermatitis. Changes in bath soap or laundry detergent can also cause contact dermatitis. Symptoms common to most cases of contact dermatitis include itching, erythema, clustered papulo-vesicles, and wet, weeping skin.[29,30] In some cases, symptoms may not take up to 7 days to develop. Symptoms may develop much sooner (after 1 day) when patients have been exposed to a particular allergen before.[29]

The clinical diagnosis of contact dermatitis is often made based on the history and the location and pattern of lesions. For example, acute inflammation from the substances within a neoprene knee sleeve will produce lesions in the localized area that was in contact with the sleeve. Differential diagnosis for contact dermatitis may include skin infections (bacterial, fungal, and viral) and atopic dermatitis.

The first step in treating contact dermatitis is to identify the irritant or allergen and eliminate exposure to it, although this is not always possible. Topical corticosteroid ointments are usually effective in reducing the itching caused by contact dermatitis. In severe cases, OTC antihistamines, such as diphenhydramine may also be used to relieve the discomfort of itching. When treating athletes with contact dermatitis, a second-generation antihistamine like loratadine (Claritin) or cetirizine (Zyrtec) should be used to avoid any sedative side effects. When individuals have a known sensitivity to specific allergens, efforts should be taken to prevent recurrent exposure. Individuals with persistent symptoms should be referred to a physician for further evaluation. Oral corticosteroid therapy may be used in cases such as poison ivy due to its ability to spread quickly.

Chronic Eczema

Contact dermatitis can become chronic as a result of cumulative exposure to an allergen. Chronic dermatitis is more frequently referred to as *eczema* and will usually present with slightly different symptoms than acute cases. Chronic eczema is associated with dry skin, thickening of the epidermis (lichenification), and fissure or cracks in the skin. Treatment is similar to that for acute contact dermatitis; however, the additional use of lubricants or non-alcohol-based skin moisturizers can help with the dry skin.

Figure 12-13. Psoriasis.

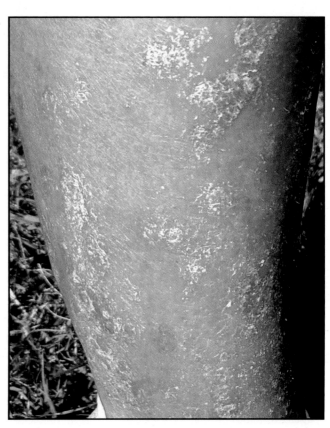

Neither acute contact dermatitis nor chronic eczema is contagious; therefore it is unnecessary to restrict athletes from participation. However, repeated scratching of these lesions can lead to secondary skin infections. Return-to-participation decisions in these cases would have to be made on an individual basis.

Psoriasis

Although there are several different forms of psoriasis, this chapter will focus on the most common form, plaque psoriasis. Plaque psoriasis is a chronic inflammatory skin condition commonly found on the extensor surfaces of the body (knees, elbows, knuckles). This T-cell-mediated disorder activates a cascade of inflammatory processes that lead to rapid growth of epidermal and vascular cells. The characteristic lesions appear as symmetrical, round, erythematous plaques with silver-colored scales (Figure 12-13).[31]

Treatment of plaque psoriasis usually involves a variety of topical and oral drugs used separately or in combination with each other. Because psoriasis is prone to recurrence, patients have to periodically change their treatment routines to include drugs from different classes or groups. Improving the moisture content of the skin is one of the primary goals of many topical treatments. Other topical treatments include coal tars, calcipotriene ointment, and corticosteroids. Most of the oral systemic treatments are associated with significant side effects and thus require regular medical follow-ups. Sunlight or artificial ultraviolet A (UVA) light is usually very effective in treating psoriasis. However, depending on the number and size of psoriasis lesions, many patients avoid sunlight because of their self-consciousness of the lesions.

The differential diagnosis for plaque psoriasis may include dermatophytosis (tinea infections) and eczema. Psoriasis is not contagious and does not prohibit an athlete from participating in sports activities.

Environmental Skin Conditions

Prolonged exposure to the environment, whether it is hot or cold, can cause adverse effects that can lead to skin damage. This chapter will address cold urticaria, frostnip, frostbite, sunburn, and skin cancer.

Cold Urticaria

Cold urticaria is caused by exposure to cold and is commonly associated with the application of therapeutic modalities such as ice massage, ice bags, or ice slush baths. Exposure to cold environmental temperatures may also cause this condition. Common symptoms include hives and itching, which usually develop shortly after contact with a cold agent or exposure to cold temperatures. Most cases involve local reactions only; however, in severe cases, individuals may develop a systemic reaction such as anaphylaxis. Patients should be screened for a history of cold urticaria before any cold modality is applied. Symptoms associated with localized reactions will usually resolve spontaneously without permanent injury.

Frostnip

Frostnip is a superficial skin injury caused by extended exposure to cold temperatures, and most commonly affects the exposed skin areas such as the face, nose, chin, and ears.[32] Frostnip generally produces transient blanching, numbness, throbbing or burning, and a blue-white tint to the affected area. Warming the area will usually return normal sensation and color fairly quickly. Individuals can return to play when their color and sensation are normal. Frostnip can be prevented by wearing multiple layers of clothes and covering exposed skin areas.

Frostbite

Frostbite involves deeper tissues and can, if not recognized and treated promptly, lead to damage of the subcutaneous tissue, muscle, and bone, which can also lead to limb loss.[33] With prolonged exposure, frostbite limited to the upper layers of the skin occurs as ice crystals form in extracellular spaces.[33-35] The skin appears waxy, dry, or cyanotic, and becomes hardened over the joints.[36] Ice in the tissues draws fluid from the cells, causing permanent damage to epithelial cells and blood vessels.[33] Once blood supply is disrupted, hypoxic necrosis occurs unless blood can be delivered through adjacent vessels. This tissue hypoxia is the primary cause of tissue damage in frostbite.[37]

Continued exposure progresses to deep frostbite, which involves freezing in the deep layers of skin and possibly muscle or other underlying tissues.[33] The mechanism of tissue damage is the same as superficial frostbite: ice formation and hypoxia from vascular destruction. The appearance of cyanosis, blood blisters, or completely frozen skin indicate extensive, irreversible tissue damage.[37]

Once frostbite is recognized, prompt removal from the cold should be undertaken. Weight bearing, pressure, or friction of the frostbitten area should be avoided to prevent further tissue damage.[34] Wet clothing can be removed if it is not frozen to the skin, and replaced with dry, soft blankets or other cloth. Superficial frostbite may be rewarmed simply and slowly by exposure to indoor temperatures, contact with another person's skin, or immersion in mildly warm water (98°F to 102°F [37°C to 39°C]).[34] Rapid rewarming of a more deeply frostbitten limb can be performed by immersion in warmer water (104°F to 108°F [40°C to 42°C]).[33,36,38,39] During rewarming, intense pain, bright erythema, edema, and eventually blistering occur as blood supply returns.[36] The area should not be thawed if refreezing is a possibility, since refreezing increases the extent of tissue damage.[34,38] With large regions of frostbite, urgent transport to a medical facility is required since 🆘 limb-threatening compartment syndromes and infection are common.

Dressing in layers can help maintain body heat and thus prevent frostbite.[32] Individuals suffering from frostbite should be removed from participation in outdoor activities. When treating frostnip or frostbite, evaluation and treatment for hypothermia is also required.

Sunburn

Extended exposure to UV rays, particularly during the peak times of 10 am to 2 pm, can cause sunburn. The degree of skin injury can vary based on a variety of factors, including total time of exposure, altitude (the intensity of the sun is greater at higher altitudes), and fairness of the skin. First-degree sunburns produce erythema, while second-degree burns will have erythema and blistering; third-degree burns will have erythema, blistering, and ulcerations.[40]

Cool compresses, lotions, and creams can be used to treat first-degree sunburns. Using nonsteroidal anti-inflammatory drugs alone or a combination of nonsteroidal anti-inflammatory drugs and topical corticosteroids can reduce the discomfort associated with mild sunburns. More serious burns may require oral corticosteroids.[40]

The best treatment for sunburn is prevention. Individuals should avoid the peak sun and ultraviolet light intensity times of 10 am to 2 pm and wear protective clothing such as a wide-brim hat and long sleeves. Water-proof or water-resistant sunscreens with a sun protection factor (SPF) of 30 or greater should always be worn when exercising outdoors. It is recommended that individuals working or exercising outdoors reapply sunscreen every 2 hours.[41] As mentioned previously, individuals who are taking medication for the treatment of acne are more susceptible to sunburn, and should therefore take extra precautions when outdoors.

Mild sunburn injuries do not require a restriction of athletic or recreational activity. However, sunburns involving blisters should be watched carefully and covered during participation to reduce the risk of secondary bacterial infections.

Skin Cancer

Skin cancer is the most common form of all cancers. There are 2 main types of skin cancer: nonmelanomas and melanomas. Nonmelanoma skin cancer occur most often, and typically involve the basal and squamous cells of the epidermis; whereas melanoma skin cancer occurs in the lower epidermis and is formed from melanocytes.

Approximately 2.2 million Americans are diagnosed with nonmelanoma skin cancer each year, with *basal cell carcinoma* making up about 80% of these new cases.[42] *Basal cell cancer* typically develops on skin areas that have the greatest sun exposure (eg, head and neck).[42] This type of skin cancer typically grows slowly and rarely spreads to other parts of the body. However, it is not uncommon for basal cell cancers to recur in the same place after treatment has been completed. Also, about 50% of patients with basal cell cancer will develop new skin cancer lesions within 5 years.[42]

Squamous cell carcinoma is the second leading form of nonmelanoma skin cancer. Like the basal cell carcinoma, this type of skin cancer also occurs most frequently on areas that receive the greatest sun exposure, such as the neck, face, lips, and ears.[42] The squamous cell cancer grows faster than its basal cell counterpart and is more likely to spread to other parts of the body, although to a much lesser degree than melanoma skin cancer.

Melanoma, also referred to as malignant melanoma, makes up only about 5% of the new skin cancer diagnoses each year; however, it accounts for more than 80% of skin cancer deaths.[41] The severity of melanoma is related to the fact that it commonly spreads to other parts of the body. Melanomas are typically brown or black, although they may also be pink, red, or white. The neck and face are common sites for melanomas, as well as the chest and back in men and the legs in women.[42] The prevalence of melanoma is about 20 times greater for whites than for Blacks. The lifetime risk for developing melanoma is also greater among Whites (1 in 50 or 2%) than Blacks (1 in 1000 or 0.1%) or Hispanics (1 in 200 or 0.5%).[42]

Risk Factors

Exposure to the sun and UV radiation is the number-one risk factor associated both with melanoma and nonmelanoma skin cancers (Table 12-6). There are 2 types of UV rays present in sunlight: UVA and UVB. Both types of UV rays can damage the DNA of skin cells, which in turn can lead

Table 12-6. Risk Factors for Skin Cancer

Exposure to sun and ultraviolet (UV) radiation[a]	Family history of skin cancer
Presence of numerous moles or large moles	Immune suppression
Fair skin, freckling, red or blond hair	History of severe sunburns during childhood or adolescence

[a] Risk reduced with use of sunscreen.

Table 12-7. Steps for Preventing Skin Cancer

Avoid being outside during the middle of the day (10 am to 2 pm) when UV light is at its peak intensity.

Wear protective clothing (long sleeve shirt and wide-brim hat).

Apply sunscreen (SPF 30 or greater) and lip balm (with SPF).

Wear sunglasses.

Avoid tanning beds and sun lamps.

Perform regular skin checks.

SPF = sun protection factor; UV = ultraviolet.

to skin cancer. The National Weather Service and the Environmental Protection Agency developed the *UV Index* to help people understand the intensity of UV rays in their area on any given day.[43] The UV Index, reported on a scale from 1 to 11+, describes the intensity of UV rays reaching the ground around the time period of 12 o'clock noon. The higher the UV Index, the more damaging the UV rays.

Individuals who work outdoors or spend a lot of time outdoors are at greater risk for UV-related skin damage. Other risk factors include living or vacationing at high altitudes and living or vacationing in tropical climates. Also, some medications can increase a person's sensitivity to the sun.

Prevention

There are a variety of steps that can be taken to prevent skin cancer as outlined in Table 12-7. The use of sunscreen is a very important part of any skin cancer-prevention plan; however, many people do not use it or they fail to use it correctly. Athletes and physically active individuals who participate in outdoor sports are at increased risk for melanoma and nonmelanoma skin cancers because of their chronic exposure to the sun and UV radiation.[44] Despite their increased risk, most athletes do not regularly use sunscreen.[45-47]

In the United States, the Food and Drug Administration regulates the manufacturing and labeling of OTC sunscreen products. In 2012, the Food and Drug Administration established new guidelines for the labeling of sunscreens in order to assist consumers in the selection of these products. As a result, sunscreens can be labeled as broad spectrum only if they provide protection against both UVA and UVB radiation. Since there is no evidence to support that SPF values higher than 50 provide any greater protection than SPF 50, the highest SPF value that can be printed on sunscreen labels is now SPF 50+. Also, manufacturers will no longer be able to make claims that their sunscreen is "waterproof" or "sweatproof."

The American Academy of Dermatology (AAD) recommends the use of a broad-spectrum sunscreen with an SPF of 30 or greater, that it be applied 15 minutes before going outdoors and that it be reapplied every 2 hours.[8] The AAD also recommends that, when possible, people should seek shade when outdoors during the hours of 10 AM and 2 PM, since this is when the sun's rays are

Table 12-8. ABCDE Rule for Detecting Skin Cancer

A	Asymmetry	One side of the mole does not match the other side.
B	Border irregularity	Mole has irregular or notched edges.
C	Color	Nonuniformity of color. Mole has shades of multiple colors: tan, brown, black, red, blue, or white.
D	Diameter	Mole is larger than the size of a pencil eraser (1/4 inch [6.3 mm]).
E	Evolving	Mole changes or evolves over time (eg, increases in size, changes color).

the strongest. In addition to wearing sunscreen, people should wear protective clothing, hats, and sunglasses when out in the sun. Lastly, the AAD recommends that people avoid using tanning beds.[8]

Early Detection and Diagnosis

As discussed in Chapter 5, early detection of cancer generally leads to the greatest outcome. The American Cancer Society recommends that individuals conduct regular self-exams of their skin. They promote the acronym ABCDE for recognizing skin changes that might be associated with skin cancer (Table 12-8). When inspecting a mole, you should look for asymmetry, border irregularity, nonuniformity in color, diameter greater than that of a pencil eraser, and evolving or changing of the appearance of a mole. The presence of any of these characteristics suggests a risk of skin cancer and requires referral to a physician (Figure 12-14).

A physician's diagnosis of skin cancer requires a thorough history, physical examination, and skin biopsy (incisional, excisional, shave, or punch). Once a diagnosis is made, the entire mole is removed and the lymph nodes are checked for cancer cells. Additional tests are then conducted to determine whether the cancer has spread to any other part of the body (see Chapter 5).

Treatment and Survival Rates

The treatment regimen chosen for patients with malignant melanoma depends on the size of the tumor and the stage of the cancer. Localized cases may be treated with surgical excision only. Skin cancer that has metastasized or spread to other parts of the body may be treated with chemotherapy, photodynamic therapy, or radiation therapy. Five-year survival rates for patients with melanoma vary depending on the stage of the cancer; however, in general, the lower the stage, the higher the survival rate (Stage I: 92% to 97%; Stage II: 70% to 81%; Stage III: 40% to 78%; Stage IV: 15% to 20%).[8]

SUMMARY

Common dermatological conditions encountered by the athletic trainer can range from minor rashes to infections and even cancer. Some of these conditions are contagious, such as impetigo, CA-MRSA infections, herpes gladiatorum, and MCV and, therefore, require early detection, proper treatment, and restrictions on sports participation in order to prevent spread from one individual to another. Although most skin conditions are relatively minor, others can be life threatening, such as skin cancer. All dermatological conditions should be taken seriously; therefore, athletic trainers should educate their patients to report all skin lesions when they are first noticed.

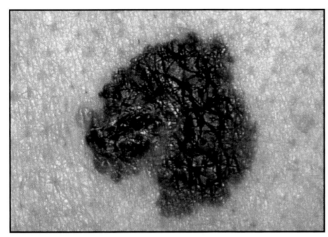

Figure 12-14. Skin cancer. (Published in *Color Atlas of Dermatology*, 3rd ed, White G, 249, Copyright Elsevier [2004].)

CASE STUDY

Last week, 4 football players at the high school where you work developed painful, draining boils. They have continued to participate in football practice with the areas covered. You have been treating them with twice-daily cleaning and antibiotic dressings, but the wounds seem to be getting worse rather than better. They have enlarged in size, increased in drainage, and become more painful. Today, another 2 players have come to you with similar-appearing lesions.

Critical Thinking Questions

1. What are some of the possible conditions that may be affecting these athletes? What is a likely explanation for the lesions worsening despite treatment?

2. What are the next reasonable steps in management of these 6 athletes? Include their participation status as well as any referrals, treatments, precautions, and instructions to the athletes and their parents.

3. What are some reasonable steps you may take to prevent other football players from developing the same problem?

REFERENCES

1. National Athletic Trainers' Association. *Athletic Training Education Competencies.* 5th ed. The Commission on Accreditation of Athletic Training Education; 2011.
2. Rogachefsky AS, Bergfeld WF, Taylor JS. Dermatology. In: Fu FH, Stone DA, eds. *Sports Injuries: Mechanisms, Prevention, Treatment.* 2nd ed. Lippincott, Williams & Wilkins; 2001:889-906.
3. Freiman A, Barankin B, Elpern DJ. Sports dermatology part 1: common dermatoses. *CMAJ.* 2004;171:851-853.
4. Pecci M, Comeau D, Chawla V. Skin conditions in the athlete. *Am J Sports Med.* 2009;37(2):406-418.
5. Dienst WL, Dightman L, Dworkin MS, Thompson RK. Pinning down skin infections: diagnosis, treatment, and prevention in wrestlers. *Phys Sportsmed.* 1997;25(12):45-56.
6. Schnirring L. MRSA infections. *Phys Sportsmed.* 2004;32(10):12-17.
7. National Athletic Trainers' Association. Official statement on community-acquired MRSA infections (CA-MRSA). Dallas, TX, National Athletic Trainers' Association Web site. Available at http://www.nata.org/publicinformation/files/ASTFstmt.pdf. Accessed September 4, 2005.
8. Liu C, Bayer A, et al. Clinical practice guidelines by the infectious disease society of America for the treatment of methicillin-resistant Staphylococcus aereus infections in adults and children. *Clin Infect Dis.* 2011;52(3):e18.
9. Adams BB. Sports dermatology. *Dermatol Nurs.* 2001;13:347-348, 351-348, 363.
10. Dhar AD. Cellulitis. In: Porter RS, Kaplan JL, eds. *The Merck Manual for Health Care Professionals.* Merck & Co.; 2012.
11. Lopez FA, Lartchenko S. Skin and soft tissue infections. *Infect Dis Clin North Am.* 2006 Dec;20(4):759-772,v-vi.

12. Cyr PR, Dexter W. Viral skin infections: preventing outbreaks in sports settings. *Phys Sportsmed*. 2004;23(7):33-38.

13. Stacey A, Atkins B. Infectious diseases in rugby players: incidence, treatment and prevention. *Sports Med*. 2000;29:211-220.

14. Zinder SM, Basler RSW, Foley J, Scarlata C, Vasily DB. National Athletic Trainers' Association position statement: skin diseases. *J Athl Train*. 2010;45:411-428.

15. NCAA Guideline 2j: Skin infections in athletics. *NCAA Sports Medicine Handbook*. National Collegiate Athletic Association; 2012:59-65.

16. Becker TM. Herpes gladiatorum: a growing problem in sports medicine. *Cutis*. 1992;50:150-152.

17. National Collegiate Athletic Association (NCAA). Skin infections (Appendix D). *NCAA Wrestling Rules and Interpretations*. National Collegiate Athletic Association; 2005:WA12-WA16.

18. Velasquez BJ. When is a skin rash more than just a rash? Sexually transmitted diseases: a dermatological perspective. *Athl TherToday*. 2002;7(3):16-23.

19. Stulberg DL, Hutchinson AG. Molluscum contagiosum and warts. *Am Family Phys*. 2003;67:1233-1240.

20. Trent JT, Federman D, Kirsner RS. Common viral and fungal skin infections. *Ostomy Wound Manage*. 2001;47:28-34.

21. Erbagci Z. Topical therapy for dermatophytoses: should corticosteroids be included? *Am J Clin Dermatol*. 2004;5:375-384.

22. Winokur RC, Dexter WW. Fungal infections and parasitic infestations in sports. *Phys Sportsmed*. 2004;32(10):23-33.

23. Kohl TD, Lisney M. Tinea gladiatorum: wrestling's emerging foe. *Sports Med*. 2000;29:439-447.

24. Kohl TD, Martin DC, Nemeth R, Evans DL, Berks County Scholastic Athletic Trainers' Association. Wrestling mats: are they a source of ringworm infection? *J Athl Train*. 2000;25:427-430.

25. Landry G, Chang C. Herpes and tinea in wrestling. *Phys Sportsmed*. 2004;32(10):34-42.

26. Landry G. Treating and avoiding herpes and tinea infections in contact sports. *Phys Sportsmed*. 2004;32(10):43-44.

27. Adams BB. Tinea corporis gladiatorum: a cross-sectional study. *J Am Acad Dermatol*. 2000;43:1039-1041.

28. Hand JW, Wroble RR. Prevention of tinea corporis in collegiate wrestlers. *J Athl Train*. 1999;34:350-352.

29. Fisher AA. Sports-related cutaneous reactions: part II. Allergic contact dermatitis to sports equipment. *Cutis*. 1999;63:202-204.

30. Smith A. Contact dermatitis: diagnosis and management. *Br J Community Nurs*. 2004;9:365-371.

31. Schnenberger DW. Curbing the psoriasis cascade. *Postgrad Med*. 2005;117(5):9-16.

32. Tlougan BE, Mancini AJ, Mandell JA, Cohen DE, Sanchez MR. Skin conditions in figure skaters, ice-hockey players and speed skaters. Part II: cold-induced, infectious and inflammatory dermatoses. *Sports Med*. 2011;41:967-984.

33. Grace TG. Cold exposure injuries and the winter athlete. *Clin Orthop Relat Res*. 1987;216:55-62.

34. Cappaert TA, Stone JA, Castellani JW, et al. National Athletic Trainers' Association position statement: environmental cold injuries. *J Athl Train*. 2008;43:640-658.

35. Seto CK, Way D, O'Connor N. Environmental illness in athletes. *Clin Sports Med*. 2005;25:695-718.

36. Thein LA. Environmental conditions affecting the athlete. *J Orthop Sports Phys Ther*. 1995;21(3):158-171.

37. Bracker MD. Environmental and thermal injury. *Clin Sports Med*. 1992;11:419-436.

38. DeFranco MJ, Baker CL 3rd, DaSilva JJ, Piasecki DP, Bach BR Jr. Environmental issues for team physicians. *Am J Sports Med*. 2008;36:2226-2237.

39. Noonan B, Bancroft RW, Dines JS, Bedi A. Heat- and cold-induced injuries in athletes: evaluation and management. *J Am Acad Orthop Surg*. 2012;20:744-754.

40. Snowise M, Dexter WW. Cold, wind, and sun exposure. *Phys Sportsmed*. 2004;32(12):26-32.

41. Dewald L. The ABCDs of skin cancer: a primer for athletic trainers and therapists. *Athl Ther Today*. 2002;7(3):29-32.

42. Basal and squamous cell. American Cancer Society. Accessed May 29, 2013.

43. American Cancer Society. American Cancer Society. Available at: http://www.cancer.org/cancer/cancercauses/sunanduvexposure/skincancerpreventionandearlydetection/skin-cancer-prevention-and-early-detection-what-is-u-v-radiation. Accessed May 30, 2013.

44. Harrison SC, Bergfeld WF. Ultraviolet light and skin cancer in athletes. *Sports Health*. 2009;1:335-340.

45. Dubas LE, Adams BB. Sunscreen use and availability among female collegiate athletes. *J Am Acad Dermatol*. 2012;67:876.e871-876.e876.

46. Hamant ES, Adams BB. Sunscreen use among collegiate athletes. *J Am Acad Dermatol*. 2005;53:237-241.

47. Wysong A, Gladstone H, Kim D, Lingala B, Copeland J, Tang JY. Sunscreen use in NCAA collegiate athletes: identifying targets for intervention and barriers to use. *Prev Med*. 2012;55:493-49.

CHAPTER 13

Neurological System

CHAPTER OUTLINE AND OBJECTIVES

Introduction

Review of Anatomy, Physiology, and Pathogenesis

◊ Describe the anatomy and physiology of the neurological system.

◊ Describe the pathophysiological mechanisms associated with injuries and illnesses involving the neurological system.

Signs and Symptoms

◊ Discuss the general signs and symptoms of neurological pathology.

Pain Patterns

◊ Identify the referred pain patterns associated with pathology of the central and peripheral nervous systems.

Medical History and Physical Examination Procedures

◊ Discuss medical history findings relevant to neurological pathology.

◊ Describe the clinical examination procedures relevant to neurological injuries, illnesses and diseases.

¤ Inspection

¤ Physical Examination

• Sensory Assessment

• Motor Assessment

• Assessment of Deep Tendon Reflexes

• Meningeal Irritation

• Cranial Nerve Assessment

Bhojani RA, O'Connor DP, Fincher AL. *Clinical Pathology for Athletic Trainers: Recognizing Systemic Disease, Fourth Edition* (pp 351-386).
© 2022 Taylor & Francis Group.

- Assessment of Cognitive Function
- Balance and Postural Stability

Pathology and Pathogenesis

◊ Discuss the signs, symptoms, management, medical referral guidelines, return to participation criteria, and prevention strategies for pathology involving the central nervous system.

- ¤ Stroke
- ¤ Cerebral Aneurysm
- ¤ Headaches
  - Migraine
  - Cluster
  - Toxic Vascular
- ¤ Brain Trauma
  - Concussion
  - Post-Concussion Syndrome
  - Second-Impact Syndrome
- ¤ Neurological Infections
  - Acute Bacterial Meningitis
  - Viral Meningitis
- ¤ Cerebral Palsy and Anoxic Brain Injury
- ¤ Epilepsy, Seizure, and Convulsion Disorders
- ¤ Spinal Cord Disorders
  - Spinal Cord Trauma
  - Spinal Bifida
- ¤ Multiple Sclerosis

◊ Discuss the signs, symptoms, management, medical referral guidelines, and return-to-participation guidelines for pathology involving the peripheral nervous system.

- ¤ Reflex Sympathetic Dystrophy
- ¤ Motor Unit and Neuromuscular Disorders
- ¤ Motor Neuron
  - Amyotrophic Lateral Sclerosis
  - Poliomyelitis
  - Postpolio Syndrome
- ¤ Axon
  - Peripheral Neuropathy
  - Guillain-Barré Syndrome
- ¤ Neuromuscular Junction
  - Myasthenia Gravis
- ¤ Muscle
  - Muscular Dystrophy
- ¤ Management of Neuromotor Diseases

Summary

Case Study

◊ Develop critical-thinking and clinical decision-making skills.

Online Resources

Content Area	Knowledge and Skills
This chapter addresses the following knowledge and skills from the *Athletic Training Education Competencies, Fifth Edition*[1]:
Content Area	**Knowledge and Skills**
Prevention and Health Promotion (PHP)	5, 17c
Clinical Examination and Diagnosis (CE)	1–3, 7, 13, 16–19, 20f, 21h, 22
Acute Care of Injuries and Illnesses (AC)	34, 36b, 36k

INTRODUCTION

Injury or illness can affect any portion of the neurological system (brain, brain stem, spinal nerves, or peripheral nerves). Many of these conditions are very serious and can result in permanent nerve damage, disability, or even death if not detected early. Although athletic trainers most commonly encounter sport-related injuries to the brain (concussions), spinal nerve roots, or peripheral nerves, they may also treat patients who suffer from progressive or degenerative neurological diseases. Recognition of the common signs and symptoms, as well as the indications for medical referral, is essential for the proper management of neurological pathology.

REVIEW OF ANATOMY, PHYSIOLOGY, AND PATHOGENESIS

The nervous system can be conceptually divided into 2 main functional components: the *central nervous system* (CNS), which includes the brain and spinal cord, and the *peripheral nervous system* (PNS), which includes the spinal nerve roots and peripheral nerves.[2] The brain is made up of 4 distinct regions, including the *cerebrum* (cerebral cortex, corpus collosum, and basal ganglia), *diencephalon* (thalamus, pineal body, and hypothalamus), *cerebellum*, and the *brainstem* (midbrain, pons and medulla oblongata) (Figure 13-1). The cerebrum, which controls cognitive function and memory, is divided into 2 paired (left and right) hemispheres separated by the longitudinal fissure. The left hemisphere receives input from and controls movements of the right side of the body. Likewise, the right hemisphere receives sensory input from and regulates movement of the left side of the body. The outer layer of the cerebrum is made up of the cerebral cortex (gray matter). The *hypothalamus* links the nervous system to the endocrine system and assists with homeostasis through the regulation of thirst, temperature, fluid balance, and blood pressure. The *thalamus* serves as the relay point for afferent sensory information, routing these signals to the appropriate segment of the brain. The cerebellum is located inferior to the cerebrum and functions to regulate fine motor coordination, balance, and posture. The *pons* serves as a bridge to connect the cerebellum to the brain stem. The *medulla oblongata* connects the brain to the spinal cord and serves to regulate heart rate, blood pressure, respiration, digestion, coughing, and vomiting. The *spinal cord* carries neural

Figure 13-1. Components of the central nervous system.

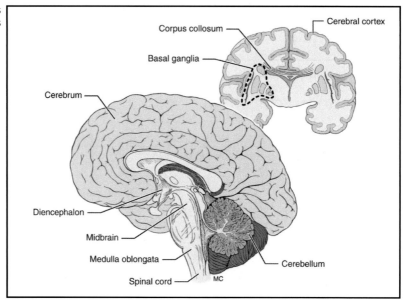

impulses back and forth between the brain and the body. Table 13-1 summarizes the functions of each section of the CNS.

Neurons are the cells in the nervous system. Figure 13-2 shows a typical neuron, including a cell body, dendrites (to receive electrochemical input), and axons (one or more to carry electrochemical impulses to other neurons). Neuron structure varies slightly according to its location and function in the nervous system.

Other types of cells serve different functions within the nervous system. *Astroglia*, for instance, adhere to blood vessels to form the *blood-brain barrier* (discussed later). In addition, astroglia assist in regulation of the electrochemical environment needed for proper neuron function. *Microglia* cells enter the nervous system from the blood to remove particles and microbes from the system. *Oligodendrocytes* bind the neuronal structures together and provide the myelin that surround and insulate axons. The astroglia, microglia, and oligodendrocytes are collectively known as "glial" cells.

Ependymal cells form connective tissues that line the cerebral ventricles and central spinal cord canal. These structures contain the *cerebrospinal fluid* (CSF), which bathes the CNS and transports nutrients, chemical messengers, and waste products. The CSF also supports and protects the brain by permitting it to float in the fluid rather than rest on the cranium. At various points, the CSF circulates into the subarachnoid space.

The entire CNS is covered with 3 connective tissue layers called the *meninges*. The innermost layer, the *pia mater*, lies directly on the brain and spinal cord and supports the blood vessels that supply the nerve cells and tissues. The *arachnoid mater* lies above the pia mater. Cerebral spinal fluid circulates in between the arachnoid mater and pia mater (the subarachnoid space), suspending the entire CNS in fluid. The outermost layer is the *dura mater*, a relatively tough membrane that isolates the CNS from the internal and external environments.

Blood vessels perfuse the brain, which is one of the most vascular organs of the body. Under normal circumstances, only certain compounds can pass from the blood into the brain. This blood-brain barrier is one of the most important protective mechanisms of the body. In general, lipid-soluble compounds can pass through the blood-brain barrier with greater ease than water-soluble compounds. As discussed in Chapter 3, pharmacologic agents that are designed to exert an influence on the CNS (eg, pain relievers, anti-seizure medications) must be engineered to pass through the blood-brain barrier. Some pathological conditions affect this barrier, subsequently letting toxic substances move into the CNS. In addition, the vessels within the barrier themselves are vulnerable to

Table 13-1. Functions of the Key Components of the Central Nervous System

STRUCTURE	MOTOR FUNCTION
Cerebrum (cerebral cortex, basal ganglia)	Motor function Cognition Memory Sensory perception (touch, pressure, pain, temperature) Special senses (sight, hearing, smell, taste)
Diencephalon (hypothalamus, thalamus, and pineal body)	Sensory relay and connection with the endocrine system Control of emotions (fear, anger) Regulation of body temperature and fluid balance
Cerebellum	Control of posture and movement Balance and coordination Fine motor movements
Brainstem (pons, medulla oblongata)	Regulation of the involuntary functions (heart rate, blood pressure, respiration, digestion) Coughing, vomiting
Spinal cord	Reflexes including stretch (myotatic), withdrawal, crossed extension, grasp

injury. Damage to these or other vessels within the brain can cause hemorrhage within the confined space of the cranium, resulting in compression of the brain.

The PNS begins where nerve roots exit the spinal cord at each vertebral level. Individual peripheral nerves branch out to every organ and system of the body. Much like the vascular system, virtually every cell of the body is connected to the nervous system.

The PNS is subdivided into the somatic nervous system and the autonomic nervous system. The *somatic nervous system* is responsible for voluntary control of the body, primarily through skeletal muscle contractions. This system receives input from the afferent (ascending) nerve pathways and then sends this input to the brain via afferent pathways within the spinal cord. Once this input is processed, the brain sends signals back to the spinal cord via efferent (descending) pathways where they are then sent to the corresponding muscles through other efferent pathways.

The *autonomic nervous system*, which regulates various body functions and behavior, is made up of 2 components: the sympathetic and parasympathetic systems. The *sympathetic nervous system* increases heart rate, respiratory rate, and neuromotor reaction, usually in response to physical stress, including exercise. The sympathetic system inhibits the gastrointestinal system to avoid diverting blood from working muscles. By contrast, the *parasympathetic nervous system* functions at rest to regulate basic metabolic processes, such as digestion. It assists recovery from sympathetic stimulation by slowing heart and respiration rates. The opposing, but balanced, output of these systems plays a major role in homeostasis. The sympathetic system responds to internal and external stresses, and the parasympathetic system restores and maintains basal function once the stress is removed.

The PNS includes 12 cranial nerves and 31 spinal nerves. The cranial nerves originate from the base of the brain or brain stem and exit from the base of the skull. These nerves are numbered as cranial nerve (CN) I through XII. Table 13-2 provides a listing of the cranial nerves, their functions,

Figure 13-2. General neuron and its structures.

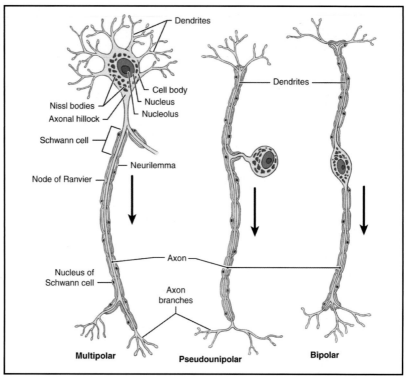

and the associated assessment procedures. Cranial nerve function can be impaired by a head injury or disease state that damages these nerves.

The peripheral nerves originate from the spinal nerves, which are formed by dorsal and ventral nerve roots branching off from the spinal cord. The *dorsal nerve roots* carry sensory fibers, while the *ventral nerve roots* carry motor fibers. Most peripheral nerves contain sensory and motor fibers from more than one spinal nerve. The spinal nerves are identified by their exit point from the spinal vertebrae and are grouped into 4 regions: cervical, thoracic, lumbar, and sacral. There are 8 cervical nerves (C1 to C8) that all exit the spinal column above their adjacent vertebrae. For example, C1 exits just above the first cervical vertebra and C8 exits just above the first thoracic vertebra. The thoracic (T1 to T12) and lumbar (L1 to L5) spinal nerves exit the spinal column just below their adjacent vertebrae (T3 exits just below the third thoracic vertebrae; L2 exits just below the second lumbar vertebra). Each spinal nerve is associated with a skin sensory pattern (*dermatome*) and muscle or muscle group (*myotome*). The sensory distribution of peripheral and spinal nerves is illustrated in Figures 13-3 and 13-4, respectively. Table 13-3 provides a summary of the spinal nerve roots with their corresponding dermatomes and myotomes as well deep tendon reflexes (DTRs). Testing sensory, motor, and reflex function forms the foundation for assessing neurological disorders.

Each nerve is covered with a sheath of myelin. *Myelin* is a protein-lipid structure that is created by Schwann cells, which reside along the length of the nerve. Myelin creates an insulating layer, similar to the covering on a wire, which keeps the electrical impulse from spreading outside of the nerve fiber. Loss of myelin results in delayed or blocked transmission of nervous impulses. Peripheral nerves may incur several types of injury. *Neurapraxia* is the disruption of nerve conduction without loss of axonal continuity. *Axonotmesis* is the disruption of nerve conduction with loss of axonal continuity, but preservation of the myelin sheath and other connective tissues. *Neurotmesis* is the loss of nerve conduction with loss of axonal continuity and damage to the connective tissues.

Table 13-2. Structure and Function of Cranial Nerves

CN	NAME	TYPE	FUNCTION
I	Olfactory	Sensory	Smell
II	Optic	Sensory	Vision acuity and peripheral vision
III	Oculomotor	Motor	Pupillary light reflex, eye movement (in toward nose, up and in, up and out, and down and out)
IV	Trochlear	Motor	Eye movement (down and in toward nose)
V	Trigeminal	Mixed	Sensory: face sensation Motor: clenching of teeth, side-to-side jaw movement
VI	Abducens	Motor	Eye movement (lateral)
VII	Facial	Mixed	Sensory: taste (anterior two-thirds of tongue) Motor: facial expressions
VIII	Vestibulocochlear (acoustic)	Sensory	Hearing, balance
IX	Glossopharyngeal	Mixed	Sensory: taste (posterior one-third of tongue), gag reflex Motor: swallowing
X	Vagus	Mixed	Sensory: gag reflex Motor: speech, voice quality
XI	Spinal accessory	Motor	Shoulder elevation
XII	Hypoglossal	Motor	Tongue movement

SIGNS AND SYMPTOMS

Syncope and Coma

Syncope (see Chapter 6), a brief loss of consciousness, occurs from a sudden compromise of the brain's vascular supply. *Coma*, however, is a relatively longer state of deep unconsciousness, during which the person cannot be aroused to a normal level of consciousness. A coma can last from hours to days or even years. Syncope can be the first sign of impending coma and may occur following head injury and intracranial bleeding.

Paresthesia

Pathology in the nervous system can cause a complete loss of sensation or alter the perception of tactile sensation, called *paresthesia*. Paresthesia may present as numbness, *hypoesthesia (decreased sensation)*, *hyperesthesia (increased sensation)*, tingling, or burning. The only body regions affected are those directly associated with the injured or diseased nerve or neurons.

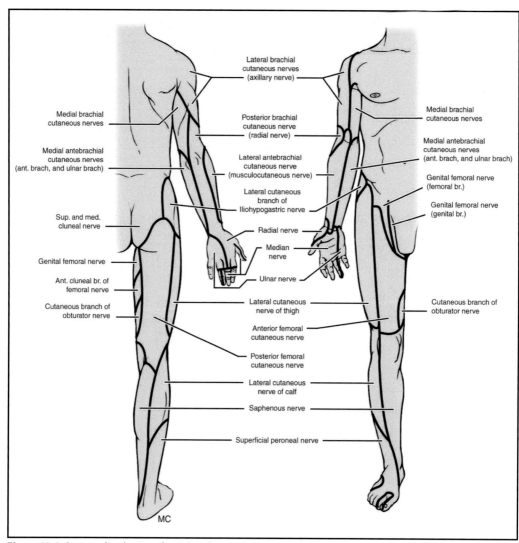

Figure 13-3. Sensory distribution of peripheral nerves.

Abnormal Motor Control, Coordination, or Tone

Decreased DTRs, paralysis, weakness, tremors, ataxia, and psychomotor agitation (a loss of coordination associated with changes in mood) can be signs of significant neurological system impairment.

Headache

Pain perceived in or around the head is an extremely common symptom associated with many pathological states. Musculoskeletal stress, vascular pathology, or common toxins such as alcohol and nicotine can cause benign headaches. An acute headache that persists for several hours is very common following head trauma. Chronic, recurrent, or severe headaches that are not associated with trauma or stress, particularly if increasing in intensity, frequency, or duration, can be a symptom of serious neurological pathology.

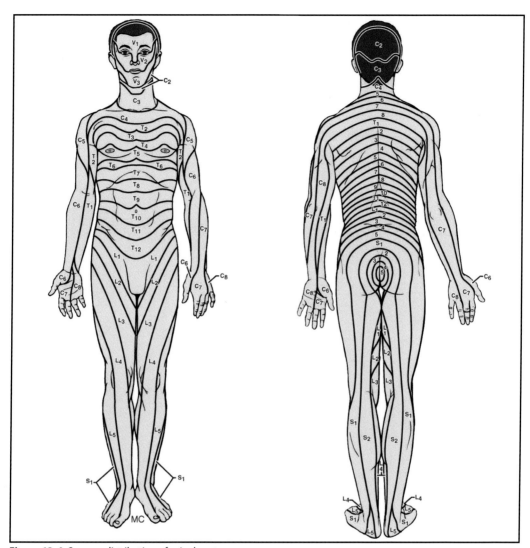

Figure 13-4. Sensory distribution of spinal roots.

Changes in Vision, Hearing, or Other Senses

The senses of smell, sight, hearing, taste, and facial sensation are all controlled by the cranial nerves. Injury or illness involving any of the 12 cranial nerves or brain stem can affect the normal functioning of these senses.

Changes in Mental Status

Cognitive changes occur with pathology of the cerebrum, which controls mental function, memory, and personality. Trauma, infection, degenerative or destructive neurological diseases, or biochemical toxicity may induce these changes.

Table 13-3. Spinal Nerve Roots and Their Sensory, Motor, and Reflex Distributions

NERVE ROOT	SENSORY	MOTOR	DEEP TENDON REFLEX
C1	None	Neck flexion	None
C2	Top of head	Neck extension	None
C3	Anterior and posterior neck	Lateral neck flexion	None
C4	Superior shoulders	Shoulder shrug	None
C5	Lateral upper arm	Shoulder abductors	Biceps
C6	Lateral forearm, thumb, and second finger	Elbow flexors or wrist extensors	Brachioradialis
C7	Middle finger	Elbow extensors or wrist flexors	Triceps
C8	Medial forearm, fourth and fifth fingers	Finger flexors	None
T1	Medial upper arm and elbow	Finger abductors	None
L1	Inguinal area; posterolateral hip	Hip flexion	None
L2	Proximal anterior thigh	Hip flexion	None
L3	Distal, anterior thigh; medial thigh	Knee extension	Patella
L4	Medial lower leg	Dorsiflexors	Patella
L5	Lateral lower leg, anterior lower leg and dorsum of the foot (second to fourth toes)	Great toe extension	Patella
S1	Lateral foot	Plantar flexion	Achilles
S2	Proximal, posterior lower leg	Knee flexion	Achilles

PAIN PATTERNS

Dorsal Spinal Columns

Light touch and proprioception neural impulses travel from the peripheral nerve receptors and nerves to ascend to the brain in the dorsal columns of the spinal cord. These pathways cross over to the opposite side (decussate) in the midbrain to the contralateral cerebrum.

Ventral Spinal Columns

Pain and temperature impulses travel from the peripheral receptors to pathways in the anterolateral (ventral) columns and decussate immediately on entering the spinal cord.

Peripheral Nerves

Specific peripheral nerves transmit sensation, autonomic function, and motor control to specific regions and structures. Figure 13-3 shows sensory distributions of selected peripheral nerves; testing these regions may indicate injury to a sensory peripheral nerve.

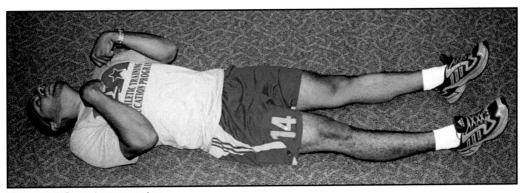

Figure 13-5. Decorticate posturing.

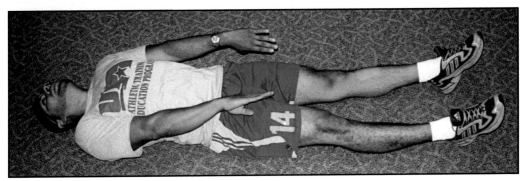

Figure 13-6. Decerebrate posturing.

Many neurological diseases affect a specific structure within the nervous system, but some produce lesions in several structures. The distribution of symptoms often aids physicians in preliminary diagnosis, which is confirmed by further clinical, laboratory, and imaging tests.

MEDICAL HISTORY AND PHYSICAL EXAMINATION PROCEDURES

Family and Personal History

Genetic factors contribute to the development of certain neurological conditions, such as epilepsy, muscular dystrophy, and some degenerative CNS disorders. A personal history of neurological pathology may affect the physical examination. For example, individuals with cerebral palsy or a history of stroke would not be expected to have "normal" reflexes or coordination in an affected limb. In addition, medications for such conditions should be noted since they often have many neuromotor side effects.

Inspection

Atrophy of certain muscles suggests peripheral nerve pathology. Certain CNS disorders can also cause tremors or affect gait and other gross movements. *Decorticate posturing*, in which the arms are rigidly flexed and the legs are fixed in extension (Figure 13-5), indicates interruption of neurological signals from the cerebral cortex. *Decerebrate posturing*, in which the arms and legs are both rigidly extended (Figure 13-6), indicates an interruption of neural signals from the cerebellum. The presence of blood or cerebral spinal fluid draining from the nose or ear indicates a possible skull

Figure 13-7. Two-point discrimination test.

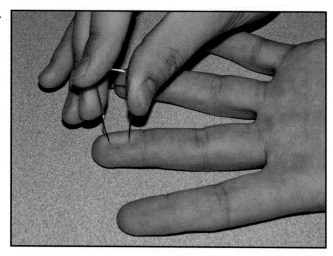

fracture. Other visual signs of a skull fracture include discoloration over the mastoid process (*Battle's sign*) or the eyelids and periorbital region (*raccoon sign*). Dilated and fixed pupils, unequal pupillary response (*anisocoria*), or involuntary rapid movement of the eyes (*nystagmus*) are all also associated with an injury to the CNS (ie, brain injury). Abnormal posturing, signs of a skull fracture, and pupillary signs of a brain injury are all considered to be medical emergencies and warrant immediate transportation to a medical facility.

Physical Examination

Sensory Assessment

Testing sensation on the entire body is usually unnecessary, so the physical examination concentrates around the symptomatic region. Touch sensation travels in bilateral spinal pathways to the brain and is a good quick test of peripheral and spinal nerve integrity. In general, athletic trainers use the dermatome patterns to assess sensory function (see Figure 13-4 and Table 13-3). Several levels of sensation (touch, pain, discrimination) can be tested depending on the symptoms and the assessment findings. *Light touch* sensation can be assessed using a cotton ball or a finger. With all of the sensory testing, assessment should be performed bilaterally for comparison. When comparing from side to side, the examiner can ask, "Can you feel this?" "Tell me when you feel something," or "Does this feel the same as this?" The ability to perceive pain can be tested using a straight or safety pin. Occasionally substitute the dull end of the pin for the sharp end in the assessment. Ask the patient, "Does this feel dull or sharp?" The pin stick should be enough to feel sharp but not enough to draw blood. To avoid the possibility of drawing blood, a wooden cotton-tipped swab can be broken in half, with the broken end used to test pain and the cotton-tipped end used to test touch and pressure. Two-point discrimination can be assessed using an open paperclip with the 2 ends placed approximately 5 mm apart or a specific 2-point discriminator device. With the patient's eyes closed, the 2 ends of the paperclip are lightly touched simultaneously to one of the patient's finger pads (Figure 13-7). Ask the patient if they feel 1 or 2 sticks. Alternate the use of one end with the use of 2 ends. If the patient is unable to differentiate the 2 points, the distance between points should be increased by approximately 1 mm and the test repeated. Pathology of the cerebral cortex will cause a widening of the space within which the patient can detect sensation at 2 different points.

Motor Assessment

Similar to the sensory examination, the motor examination is usually limited to the region of injury or symptoms. For non-emergency conditions involving the neck or back, test the upper extremities with suspected cervical problems and the lower extremities with suspected lumbar

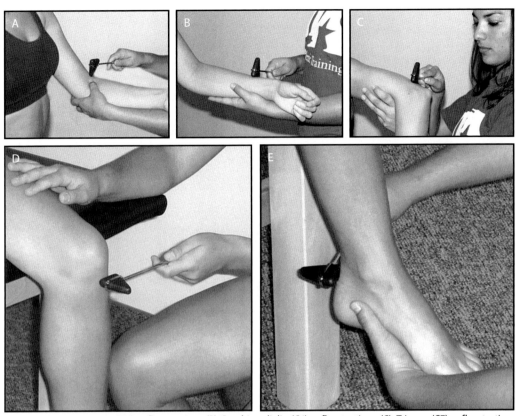

Figure 13-8. (A) Biceps (C5) reflex testing. (B) Brachioradialis (C6) reflex testing. (C) Triceps (C7) reflex testing. (D) Patellar (L2-L4) reflex testing. (E) Achilles (S1) reflex testing.

problems. The motor exam primarily involves testing for myotome weakness (see Table 13-3). The motor system is tested by asking the patient to contract specific muscle groups as the examiner provides resistance. Muscle strength can be tested through the entire range of motion or by using a break test. Weakness is noted by comparing to the same muscle on the contralateral, unaffected side.

Assessment of Deep Tendon Reflexes

An increase, decrease, or absence of DTRs (Achilles, patellar, biceps, brachioradialis, triceps) is associated both with injury and illness to the neurological system. These reflexes can be easily tested using a reflex hammer (Figure 13-8). Table 13-4 outlines the steps to follow when testing the upper and lower extremity DTRs and the normal response expected. If reflex testing fails to elicit a response bilaterally, instruct the patient to clench the teeth. Alternatively, when testing lower extremity reflexes, instruct the patient to clasp the hands in front and to try to pull them apart isometrically. Likewise, when testing upper extremity exercises, instruct the patient to cross the legs and perform isometric abduction. These procedures will enhance the reflex response. Asymmetries of reflex response, in either amplitude or delay, are important.

Athletic trainers document reflexes as "increased" or "decreased" in comparison to the contralateral limb. In acute spinal cord injury, a symmetric loss of reflexes distal to the injury is commonly present. Unilateral changes in these reflexes can occur with injury or illness to a nerve root or peripheral nerve. Increased reflexes are associated with CNS pathology, while decreased or absent reflexes suggest pathology involving the spinal nerve roots or peripheral nerves.

Disruption of the long motor tracts, the cerebral cortex motor neuron pathways, may be evaluated with the *Babinski test* (Figure 13-9) This test is performed with the patient laying supine. Using

Table 13-4. Assessment of Deep Tendon Reflexes

REFLEX (SPINAL LEVEL)	INSTRUCTIONS FOR ASSESSMENT	NORMAL RESPONSE
Biceps (C5)	1. Position the patient seated or standing. 2. Use 1 hand to support the patient's elbow in a position of 90 degrees of flexion, with the patient's forearm resting on your forearm (see Figure 13-8A). 3. Place the thumb of the hand supporting the patient's elbow over the biceps tendon near its insertion on the radius. 4. Using the pointed side of the reflex hammer's head, the examiner strikes their thumb. 5. Perform the test bilaterally for comparison.	Normally, the biceps contracts slightly, which can be observed and palpated.
Brachioradialis (C6)	1. Position the patient seated or standing. 2. Use 1 hand to support the patient's elbow in a position of 90 degrees of flexion, with the patient's forearm resting in a neutral position over your forearm (see Figure 13-8B). 3. Using the wide side of the reflex hammer's head, strike the brachioradialis tendon approximately 3 inches (7.6 cm) above the wrist. 4. Perform the test bilaterally for comparison.	Striking the brachioradialis tendon normally produces supination of the forearm.
Triceps (C7)	1. Position the patient seated or standing. 2. Support the patient's arm in approximately 30 degrees of shoulder extension with the elbow flexed approximately 3. 90 degrees (see Figure 13-8C). 4. Using the wide side of the reflex hammer's head, strike the triceps tendon just proximal to its insertion on the olecranon process. 5. Perform the test bilaterally for comparison.	Normally, the triceps should contract or twitch slightly.

(continued)

Table 13-4 (continued). Assessment of Deep Tendon Reflexes

REFLEX (SPINAL LEVEL)	INSTRUCTIONS FOR ASSESSMENT	NORMAL RESPONSE
Patellar (L2-4)	1. Position the patient seated on the edge of the table with the legs hanging off the edge. 2. Palpate the patellar tendon just distal to the inferior pole of the patella. 3. Using the wide side of the reflex hammer's head, strike the patellar tendon distal to the inferior pole of the patella (see Figure 13-8D). 4. Perform the test bilaterally for comparison.	The knee should move slightly into extension.
Achilles (S1)	1. Position the patient seated on the edge of the table with the legs hanging off the edge. 2. Palpate the Achilles tendon in the posterior ankle. 3. Lift the patient's foot into a neutral or slightly dorsiflexed position. 4. Using the wide side of the reflex hammer's head, strike the Achilles tendon just proximal to its insertion onto the calcaneus (see Figure 13-8E). 5. Perform the test bilaterally for comparison.	Normally, the foot should plantarflex slightly when the Achilles tendon is struck. The examiner should be able to palpate this response.

a blunt object, such as a pen or the end of reflex hammer, the bottom of the foot is stroked from the heel to the lateral border of the foot over the ball of the foot to the great toe. Normally, this test will cause the toes to flex. A positive Babinski sign (extension of the great toe with flexion and abduction of the other toes) indicates an upper motor neuron lesion (injury involving the brain or spinal cord). *Clonus,* another abnormal reflex, may be found at the ankle and occasionally the wrist. The test is conducted by quickly moving and maintaining the foot (or hand) into end-range dorsiflexion (or extension). A low-amplitude, involuntary oscillation of the foot or hand is abnormal and suggests an upper motor neuron disorder.

Cranial Nerve Assessment

Cranial nerve function indicates the status of the medulla oblongata and can be easily and quickly tested both in the athletic training facility and on a sports sideline. Any sign of cranial nerve impairment suggests injury or disease of the brain and requires urgent medical referral. If any cranial nerve functions are rapidly declining, the situation is a medical emergency (Box 13-1).

Assessment of Cognitive Function

Cognitive function (memory and attention) can be assessed through a variety of assessments, including individual screening exams; standardized, objective screening tools; and computerized or paper-and-pencil neurocognitive tests. These different types of cognitive assessment tests are described next.

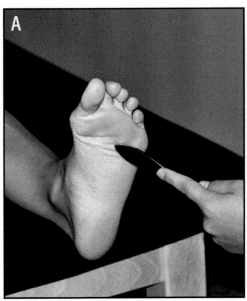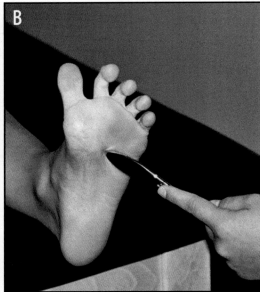

Figure 13-9. (A) Negative Babinski reflex. (B) Positive Babinski reflex.

Individual Cognitive Screening Tests

Simple serial tests, such as counting down from 100 by 7 (serial 7s) or 3 (serial 3s), can be used to evaluate a patient's ability to focus attention. Memory can be assessed by asking patients about events that occurred just prior to their head injury. Inability to remember these events indicates *retrograde amnesia*. Inability to recall events after the head injury suggests *anterograde amnesia* and can be assessed using tests such as the 3 or 5 object recall. To perform this test, the athletic trainer gives the patient a list of 3 to 5 unrelated words (eg, dog, cat, blue, summer, football). To test immediate recall, the athletic trainer immediately asks the patient to repeat the words. To test delayed recall, the athletic trainer should wait 2 to 3 minutes and then ask the patient to once again repeat the words. Inability to correctly list the given words represents a positive test and warrants medical referral.

Standardized Cognitive Screening Tools

There are also several standardized cognitive screening tools that have been developed for sideline and follow-up assessment of cognitive functioning following a sports-related concussion. The Standardized Assessment of Concussion (SAC)[3,4] and the Sport Concussion Assessment Tool (SCAT5)[4] are 2 commonly used standardized cognitive screening tests. The SAC is made up of 4 sections (orientation, immediate memory, concentration, delayed recall) that are each scored separately. The section scores are then combined for a total possible score of 30 points. The SCAT5 incorporates 8 sections that include a Glasgow Coma Scale, Maddock's Score (orientation assessment), symptom evaluation, cognitive and physical evaluation, neck examination, balance examination (which includes a modified Balance Error Scoring System [BESS]), coordination examination, and the SAC delayed recall score.

Neuropsychological Tests

Neuropsychological (NP) tests can provide an objective measure of a patient's cognitive impairment due to a sports-related concussion. There are 2 types of NP tests: paper-and-pencil and computerized. The paper-and-pencil NP tests are typically more expensive and take longer to administer, and require interpretation by a neuropsychologist.[5] There are many advantages of using the computerized NP tests, including: (1) they require less time for administration, (2) they are available in multiple forms for serial administration, which allows ease of monitoring athletes'

Box 13-1. Cranial Nerve Assessment

EYES

- Check vision (CN II). With pocket Snellen eye chart or comparable item (sports program, magazine, play book, etc) held approximately 14 inches (35.5 cm) from the patient, ask them to read a line of text.
- Check peripheral vision (CN II). Stand directly in front of patient. Ask patient to close right eye while you close left eye. Place your hand with raised finger equidistant between you and the patient, just out of peripheral view. Slowly move finger toward you and the patient. Finger should come into view for you and patient at the same time.
- Check pupillary reaction to light (CN III). Place hand along nose, between eyes, and perpendicular to the face. Shine penlight in right eye. Right pupil should constrict (direct response). Again shine penlight in right eye, but watch left eye. Left pupil should also constrict when light is shined in right eye (consensual response). Repeat test for left eye.
- Check eye tracking (CN III, IV and VI). Ask patient to follow movement of object (finger, penlight) with eyes only, without moving head. Move the object up, down, right, left, and inward toward the nose. Eye movements should be smooth and equal between eyes.

FACE

- Check sensation on forehead, checks and lateral jaw (CN V).
- Check facial expressions (CN VII). Ask the patient to raise the eyebrows, smile, frown, and puff out cheeks. Facial expressions should be symmetrical.
- Check jaw muscles (CN V). Ask patient to clench teeth. Ask patient to move jaw side to side.
- Check pharyngeal muscles (CN IX and X). Ask patient to swallow.
- Check tongue movement (CN XII). Ask the patient to stick out tongue. Movement should be smooth and straight along midline. Tongue should not deviate laterally.

EARS

- Check hearing (VIII). If the patient has been responding to your commands, then they are able to hear. If preferred, hearing can be checked further by snapping fingers beside each ear or whispering in each ear.
- Check balance and equilibrium (VIII). Instruct patient to perform Romberg test.

NECK AND SHOULDERS

- Check trapezius (CN XI). Ask patient to shrug shoulders against resistance.

OTHER

- Taste (CN VII and IX) and smell (CN I) are not typically tested in the field (sideline assessment). The loss of one or both of these senses will typically be reported by the patient prior to or during a clinical exam.

Table 13-5. Computerized Neuropsychological Concussion Tests

NAME OF TEST, MANUFACTURER, AND WEBSITE	DESCRIPTION
Immediate Postconcussion Assessment and Cognitive Testing (ImPACT) ImPACT http://impacttest.com/	Administered on desktop or laptop Designed specifically for sports-related concussions
Automated Neuropsychological Assessment Metrics (ANAM) Vista Life Sciences http://vistalifesciences.com/anam-intro	Administered on desktop or laptop Designed to evaluate cognitive functioning across multiple disease states and injuries, including sports-related injuries

cognitive functioning during recovery, and (3) they can be scored quickly, providing almost immediate feedback.[5] Table 13-5 provides a list of commonly used computerized NP tests used to assess sport-related concussions. Regardless of the type of NP test used, these assessments should be used as part of a comprehensive concussion assessment plan rather than used as a stand-alone tool. This is especially true when making return-to-play decisions.

Balance and Postural Stability

Balance and postural stability tests can be used to assess the extent of injury or recovery following a sports-related concussion. An athletic trainer may also document status of a known neuromotor disorder by using these tests. Balance and postural stability tests range from expensive, force-plate systems to simple clinical measures that can easily be performed on the sports sideline or in the athletic training facility.

The *Romberg test* is used to assess vestibular and postural control. The subject stands relaxed with feet together and eyes closed, with the examiner nearby for safety. Loss of balance or significant swaying suggests neurological impairment. A variation of this test can be performed with the arms positioned in 90 degrees of abduction.

The *BESS* is a clinical postural stability test that is made up of 6 20-second trials that include 3 stance positions (double leg, single leg, and tandem) and 2 surfaces (foam pad and firm surface) (Figure 13-10). Patients are instructed to perform each trial with their hands on their iliac crests and their eyes closed. They are further instructed to stand as motionless as possible and to try to minimize movement errors during each trial. Should they have a movement error, they are told to return to their original stance position as soon as possible. Lastly, patients are given a demonstration of each balance error and told how the test would be scored (Table 13-6). Patient's performance score on the BESS is determined by adding 1 point for every error performed during the 6 balance trials.

The NeuroCom Smart Balance System (Natus Medical Incorporated) is a computerized assessment system that incorporates both a stable and unstable surface as well as stable and dynamic visual environments (Figure 13-11). The NeuroCom's Sensory Organization Test (SOT) can be used to evaluate patients' ability to use their somatosensory, visual, and vestibular systems to maintain balance. When performing the SOT, patients complete 3 20-second trials for 6 different sensory conditions for a total of 18 trials. A composite equilibrium score is calculated based on the weighted average of all of the sensory condition scores. Research has shown that the NeuroCom SOT is effective in identifying balance deficits in patients following sports-related concussions[6]; however, it is recommended for use as part of a battery of concussion assessments (ie, combined with other assessments such as self-reported symptom scales and neurocognitive tests) rather than as an isolated test.[7,8]

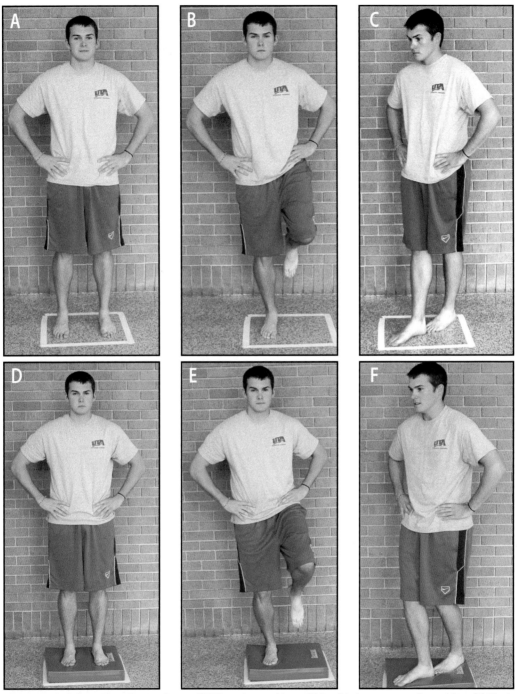

Figure 13-10. Balance Error Scoring System (BESS) testing positions. (A) Double leg stance on firm surface. (B) Single leg stance on firm surface. (C) Tandem stance on firm surface. (D) Double leg stance on foam surface. (E) Single leg stance on foam surface. (F) Tandem stance on foam surface.

Table 13-6. Errors Scored During Balance Error Scoring System Assessment

THE FOLLOWING ERRORS WILL RESULT IN 1-POINT DEDUCTION:

Patient removes hand off their hips

Patient opens eyes

Patient steps, stumbles, or falls

Patient moves weight-bearing hip(s) into more than 30 degrees flexion or abduction

Patient lifts foot or heel off the foam pad or firm surface

Patient falls out of or moves from the testing position for > 5 seconds

PATHOLOGY AND PATHOGENESIS

The cerebrum, midbrain, cerebellum, medulla (brain stem), spinal cord and associated structures (eg, thalamus, hypothalamus, basal ganglia, pons) may be damaged in several ways, including trauma, vascular compromise, anoxia, toxicity, and disease (eg, degeneration, cancer). Table 13-7 lists possible etiology and associated signs and symptoms by location for the CNS. Common neurological pathology is discussed next and is categorized as those conditions affecting the CNS, those affecting the PNS, and those that affect both systems simultaneously.

Central Nervous System Disorders

Cerebrovascular Events

Vascular injury (eg, stroke, aneurysm, trauma) in the CNS affects the structures supplied by the respective vessels. Signs and symptoms associated with these events appear from the neural region or structures that the vessels supply.

Strokes are the leading cause of brain injury in adults, with approximately 795,000 cases reported annually.[9] According to the 2016 statistics update from the American Heart Association, someone suffers a stroke in the United States every 40 seconds, and someone dies from a stroke every 4 minutes.[9] There are 2 main types of strokes: ischemic and hemorrhagic.[10] *Ischemic strokes* make up approximately 85% of all strokes[10] and occur when blood clots or plaque block a blood vessel in the brain, causing the blood flow to vital tissues to become blocked. *Hemorrhagic strokes* are caused by the bursting of blood vessels in the brain. The accumulation of blood increases pressure in the cranium and compresses the brain. The blood also stimulates an inflammatory response, causing secondary hypoxia in surrounding neural tissue, which leads to tissue necrosis. *Transient ischemic attacks* can occur when blood flow to a part of the brain is temporarily disrupted. The clinical presentation of these "mini"-strokes will be similar to those of a hemorrhagic or ischemic stroke; however, the duration of the signs and symptoms will be much shorter, sometimes lasting only 1 hour and always less than 24 hours. Recognition of transient ischemic attacks can prevent a major stroke by work-up and management changes.

The signs and symptoms of a stroke include severe headache, facial weakness or drooping, slurred speech, incoordination or weakness on one side of the body, poor balance, double vision, unilateral hearing loss, photophobia, nausea, vomiting, or loss of or altered consciousness. The American Heart Association promotes the "F.A.S.T." system as an easy way to remember the warning signs of a stroke. Table 13-8 outlines the F.A.S.T. system.

Early detection is the key to optimum treatment of strokes, therefore, anyone suspected of having a stroke should be immediately transported to the nearest emergency room. The initial

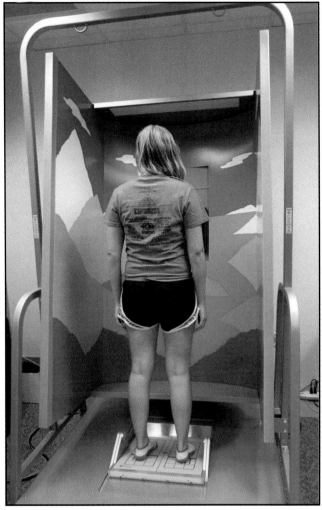

Figure 13-11. NeuroCom Smart Balance System (Natus Medical Incorporated).

treatment for a stroke is dependent on whether it is caused by a clot (ischemic) or bleeding (hemorrhagic). Diagnostic tests such as brain computed tomography (CT) scan or magnetic resonance imaging (MRI) can be used to identify bleeding within the brain caused by a hemorrhagic stroke. A CT arteriogram or magnetic resonance arteriogram can be used to visualize the blood vessels in the brain to identify blood clots.

Fibrinolytic (also referred to as thrombolytic) drugs can be administered to ischemic stroke victims to break up the clots that are blocking the blood flow to the brain. These drugs can significantly decrease the disability from a stroke and improve the quality of life; however, they must be administered within 3 hours of the onset of symptoms. Surgery may be required to stop the bleeding associated with a hemorrhagic stroke.

There are multiple risk factors for strokes, including a personal or family history of stroke, high cholesterol, hypertension, smoking, alcoholism, diabetes, and the use of cocaine or amphetamines.[11] Age and gender are also risk factors: Men have a greater risk for strokes than women and both genders have increased risk with age.[11]

Cerebral aneurysms are weak or thin spots within a blood vessel in the brain. Pressure within the vessel can cause bulging of a vessel wall, which can put pressure on the nerves within the brain. Aneurysms can also burst, causing bleeding within the brain. Unfortunately, in most cases, aneurysms do not present with neurological symptoms until they become very large or burst. If

Table 13-7. Central Nervous System Structure, Potential Pathogenesis, and Signs and Symptoms

STRUCTURE	POTENTIAL PATHOGENESIS	SIGNS AND SYMPTOMS
Cerebrum	Cerebral palsy/anoxia, vascular, cancer, trauma, degenerative	Altered cognition, disorientation, behavioral changes, difficulty initiating movements
Basal ganglia	Vascular, degenerative, cancer	Resting tremor or movements, rigidity, wild unintentional movements
Midbrain and medulla	Vascular, trauma, multiple sclerosis	Altered breathing and cranial nerve signs
Cerebellum	Vascular, degenerative, trauma	Ataxia, intention tremor, inability to move to target, inability to rapidly alternate movement, lack of coordination or balance
Spinal cord	Trauma, vascular, cancer, lateral sclerosis, multiple sclerosis, infection	Weakness/flaccidity, atrophy, hypertonia or hypotonia or both

Table 13-8. American Heart Association's F.A.S.T. System for Recognizing Warning Signs of Stroke

	SIGN/ACTION	ASSESSMENT	POSITIVE FINDING
F	Facial drooping	Ask the patient to smile.	Uneven smile (ie, one side going up, one side drooping down)
A	Arm weakness	Ask the patient to raise their arms.	Patient cannot hold both arms up; one arm drops or drifts downward.
S	Speech difficulty	Ask the patient to repeat a short, simple sentence, such as, "The grass is green."	Slurred speech; sentence repeated incorrectly.
T	Time to call 911	Note the time signs began.	

symptoms are present, they will include severe headache, pain above or behind the eye, vision changes, numbness or weakness of one side of the face, and dilation of pupils.[12]

    As with stroke, individuals suspected of having a cerebral aneurysm should be transported immediately to the nearest hospital. Prognosis is much better when aneurysms can be detected before they burst. Accurate detection will require medical imaging such as MRI, CT scan, or angiography (a dye test used to visualize arteries and veins).

Headaches

Headaches can be caused by several neurovascular problems. A *migraine headache* causes intense throbbing pain, usually unilaterally, with associated symptoms of nausea, vomiting, photophobia (aversion to light), and phonophobia (aversion to sound).[13] For many patients, migraine headaches are precipitated by an aura that will typically present with flashes of light or bright colored or white spots. Many who suffer migraines have a positive family history. The causes and mechanisms of migraine headaches are poorly understood but may be related to alterations in the neurotransmitter serotonin, inflammatory effects on the trigeminal nerve complex, or hormonal variations. Other triggers can include stress, lack of sleep, smoking, and the use of alcohol, particularly red wine. If the underlying mechanism of a patient's migraine headaches can be identified, avoidance of these triggers can help prevent future attacks. Medications are commonly used to treat migraine headaches. Many patients also find it beneficial to withdraw to a dark room and sleep.

A *cluster headache* is an intense, gnawing pain that is deep and non-throbbing in nature, occurring unilaterally around one eye. Unilateral autonomic symptoms, such as lacrimation (tearing), rhinorrhea ("runny nose") or nasal congestion, diaphoresis, unilateral pupillary constriction (miosis), ptosis (drooping eyelid), and psychomotor agitation, may also be present as a result of trigeminal nerve and parasympathetic involvement.[14] A cluster headache episode lasts 15 to 180 minutes and may recur on a daily basis; the defining characteristic is the recurrence of the headache across several days followed by a long period with no headache.[13] Common exacerbating factors include psychoemotional stress and alcohol or tobacco use. Similar to migraines, the etiology and pathophysiology of cluster headaches are not well understood, but may be related to neurovascular, hormonal, or autonomic nervous system abnormalities. Cluster headaches are most commonly treated with 2 types of medication: one to reduce the number of headaches and the second to reduce the severity of a headache when it occurs. Because cluster headaches come on very quickly, the pain-relieving medication may be administered via inhaler or injection to ensure quick action.

A *toxic vascular headache* presents diffuse, throbbing, severe pain over the entire crown of the head; this type of headache is never unilateral.[13] Etiology includes infection (usually accompanied by fever), caffeine abuse or withdrawal, alcohol abuse or withdrawal (hangover), hypoxia, hypoglycemia (low blood sugar), and metabolic disorders.[13]

People with vascular headaches are awake and alert, have no fever, and demonstrate a negative neurological examination.[13] Treatment consists of rest in a quiet, dark room and prescription medication if the headaches are recurrent and disabling. If other systemic signs occur simultaneously with a severe headache, emergency medical attention is required.

911

Concussion

A *concussion* is a brain injury that is caused by either a direct blow to the head or face or the transference of linear or rotational forces to the head from a blow to another part of the body. Sports-related concussions cause a transient impairment of neurological function, which in turn, produce the signs and symptoms that form the clinical presentation of this injury. At the cellular level, concussions involve a complex cascade of events that include disturbances in the normal ionic, metabolic, and physiological functions.[4,5]

Table 13-9 outlines the general signs and symptoms that are associated with sports-related concussions. These signs and symptoms can be categorized into 6 main domain areas: symptoms (somatic, cognitive, and/or emotional), physical signs, cognitive impairment, behavioral changes, balance impairment, and sleep-related disturbances. In the majority of cases, these signs and symptoms will resolve within

7 to 10 days; however, children and adolescents may take longer to fully recover.[4] Also, it is important to note that some signs or symptoms of concussions can be delayed in their presentation, or gradually deteriorate over time. In rare instances, acute brain trauma can cause a seizure that lasts from seconds to several minutes. Because of the evolving nature of brain trauma, any athlete suspected of having a sports-related concussion should be re-assessed at regular intervals for several

Table 13-9. Signs and Symptoms of a Concussion

DOMAIN	SIGN OR SYMPTOM
Physical	Headache
	Nausea and/or vomiting
	Dizziness or lack of balance
	Decreased coordination
	Vacant stare
	Blurred or double vision
	Change in pupil reaction to light
	Unequal pupils
	Sensitivity to light
	Athlete appears dazed
Cognitive	Confusion or disorientation
	Decreased concentration
	Feeling "foggy" or out of it
	Retrograde amnesia (memory of events prior to head injury)
	Anterograde amnesia (memory of events after a head injury)
Behavioral	Change in behavior or personality
	Change in emotions (feeling irritable or sad)
Sleep-related	Insomnia
	Sleeping more than usual
	Waking during sleep

911 days. Parents should be made aware of the signs and symptoms to watch for that would warrant immediate referral to the closest emergency medical facility (Table 13-10).

Concussion assessment should incorporate a multifaceted approach that adequately addresses the multiple domains of this complex injury. The National Athletic Trainers' Association (NATA) has published a position statement regarding the management of sport-related concussions.[16] The assessment should include tests to rule out a cervical spine injury. Sideline concussion assessment should include a symptoms checklist as well as an evaluation of the cranial nerves, cognitive functioning, and balance.[5,17] As previously described, there are a number of standardized assessment tools that can be used for sideline assessment. The Sideline Concussion Assessment Tool 5 (SCAT5) incorporates the Glasgow Coma Scale, Maddock's orientation questions (which are more pertinent to athletes than the standard orientation questions), a symptoms checklist, cervical spine assessment, the SAC, and a modified BESS assessment. The SCAT5 is appropriate for evaluating individuals 13 years of age or older. The Child SCAT5 is available for evaluating children 12 years of age or younger. There are several sideline assessment findings that would warrant activation of the emergency action plan and immediate transport of the athlete to the nearest emergency facility. These findings include a deterioration of mental status, a Glasgow Coma score less than 15, a potential cervical spine injury, and any worsening symptoms or the development of any new neurologic symptoms.

There are more than 25 different grading scales that have been used throughout the years to quantify the severity of a concussion. Many of these scales have been based on the loss of

Table 13-10. Delayed Concussion Signs and Symptoms Warranting Emergency Transport

Worsening headache	Repeated vomiting
Deteriorating mental status	Deteriorating balance
Development of seizures	Slurred speech
Increased drowsiness, difficulty in waking the individual	Weakness or numbness in arms or legs
	Unable to recognize people or places
Increased confusion and/or irritability	

consciousness and/or the presence of amnesia.[18] Current guidelines recommend against the use of grading scales in favor of a comprehensive assessment and management plan that can be individualized for each athlete based on their clinical and cognitive signs and symptoms.[4,18] The comprehensive plan should include the assessment and monitoring of multiple domains, including clinical symptoms, physical signs, cognitive impairment, behavioral changes, balance impairments, and sleep disturbances.[4] It is also recommended that neuropsychological testing be incorporated into the comprehensive plan; however, current evidence does not support routine baseline testing for all athletes.[4]

Athletes diagnosed with a concussion during an on-field or sideline assessment should not be allowed to return to play that same day.[5] The initial recovery period following a concussion requires both physical and cognitive rest (ie, avoidance of cell phones, computers, video games). During this time period, student athletes may also need accommodations at school (eg, reduced workload and extra time for assignments).[5] Often cognitive functioning may continue to be impaired beyond the point when the physical symptoms have subsided. Of note, after the initial recovery period, it is imperative to start a return to learn and modified physical activity if symptoms are tolerated.[5]

A graduated return to play protocol can be initiated once the athlete is completely symptom free.[4] Table 13-11 outlines the 6-step progression from rest through full return to play. Each step must be separated by a 24-hour period. In order to advance to the next step, the athlete must be symptom free. If the athlete experiences symptoms at any step, they must return to the previous step and wait 24 hours to proceed with the protocol.

Epidural or Subdural Hematoma

Rupture of cranial or brain blood vessels can cause epidural and subdural hematomas. Bleeding from a damaged vessel occurs either outside of the dura mater (epidural) or between the dura mater and arachnoid mater (subdural). As the hematoma expands in the limited space of the cranium, the brain tissue can become compressed.

Epidural hematomas are formed by arterial bleeding and therefore may occur within hours of the head injury. Although individuals with a developing epidural hematoma may initially have been knocked unconscious or show signs and symptoms of concussion (see Table 13-9), they will usually also have had a short period of very lucid (mentally clear) consciousness. This period of lucidness can be misleading and remove suspicion of a serious head injury. For this reason, all individuals who suffer a head injury should be monitored closely for the first few hours after their head injury. As the pressure of the hematoma builds within the cranium, the individual may report a headache with increasing intensity. The individual may also present with new signs and symptoms, including signs of cranial nerve impairment, or experience a deterioration of existing signs and symptoms. Epidural hematomas represent life-threatening emergencies, therefore, individuals should be **911** referred immediately.

Table 13-11. Graduated Return-to-Play Protocol

REHABILITATION STAGE	FUNCTIONAL EXERCISE AT EACH STAGE OF REHABILITATION	OBJECTIVE OF EACH STAGE
1. No activity	Symptom-limited physical and cognitive rest.	Recovery
2. Light aerobic activity	Walking, swimming or stationary cycling keeping in-tensity < 70% maximum permitted heart rate. No resistance training.	Increase heart rate
3. Sport-specific exercise	Skating drills in ice hockey, running drills in soccer. No head impact activities.	Add movement
4. Non-contact training drills	Progression to more complex training drills (eg passing drills in football and ice hockey). May start progressive resistance training.	Exercise, coordination, and cognitive load
5. Full-contact practice	Following medical clearance participate in normal training activities.	Restore confidence and assess functional skills by coaching staff
6. Return to play	Normal game play	

Reproduced with permission from McCrory P, Meeuwisse W, Aubry M, et al. Consensus statement on Concussion in Sport—the 4th International Conference on Concussion in Sport held in Zurich, November 2012. *J Sci Med Sport.* 2013;16(3):178-189.

Subdural hematomas involve venous bleeding and therefore may take several days before signs of deterioration begin. Parents, family members, or roommates of patients who experienced loss of consciousness, prolonged amnesia, or who continued to have symptoms at bedtime should be instructed to check the person's orientation and level of consciousness throughout the night. The athletic trainer or physician should reassess the patient the following morning. Any individual who has lost consciousness should be withheld from strenuous activity until neurological testing by a physician has been performed.

Post-Concussion Syndrome

Post-concussion syndrome (PCS) is a spectrum of signs and symptoms that appear or persist for an extended period of time following a concussion (Table 13-12).[19] The etiology of PCS is highly debated, with some researchers attributing it to microdamage in the CNS while others believing the origin is primarily psychological. Symptoms include headache, dizziness, attention deficits, and changes in mood. Neurological testing should be conducted to document residual deficits in cranial nerve function, reflexes, balance, coordination, and mental function, and this information should be passed to the treating physician. Vigorous physical activity should be avoided until the symptoms resolve completely. Chronic symptoms without relief in severity, frequency, or duration should be referred to a physician for medical testing.

Table 13-12. Criteria for Diagnosis[a] of Post-Concussion Syndrome

Diagnosis requires symptoms from at least 3 of the following categories within 4 weeks of the concussion injury:

- Headache, dizziness, fatigue, noise intolerance
- Irritability, depression, anxiety, emotional lability
- Patient reported cognitive deficits (ie, concentration, memory, mental processing); does not require neuropsychological evidence of cognitive impairment
- Sleep disturbance (insomnia)
- Reduced tolerance to alcohol or stress
- Preoccupation with aforementioned symptoms and fear of brain damage, with hypochondriacal concern and adoption of a sick role

[a] The International Classification of Diseases (ICD)-10.

Reproduced with permission from Khurana VG, Kaye AH. An overview of concussion in sport. *J Clin Neurosc.* 2012;19(1):1-11.

Second-Impact Syndrome

Although rare, *second-impact syndrome* can occur when an individual receives a second blow to the head while he is still symptomatic from his initial concussion.[19] This second blow may be very minimal in force or even involve a minor contrecoup injury, such as might occur from a tackle or fall. The second blow is thought to disturb the brain's normal autoregulation of blood flow, causing vasodilation and increasing intracranial pressure.[19] Individuals suffering from second-impact syndrome will deteriorate very quickly (within 2 to 5 minutes) following the second blow, demonstrating both general concussion signs and symptoms and progressing signs of cranial nerve impairment. Loss of consciousness may occur very quickly. Second-impact syndrome is associated with a 50% rate of mortality; therefore, prevention is the key. Individuals should not be returned to activity when they still show any signs or symptoms of a concussion.

Neurological Infections

Bacteria and viruses can cause inflammation of the meninges, called *meningitis*. These organisms may enter the CNS through the bloodstream, the cranial sinuses, or after surgical or traumatic wounds that expose the meninges. The CNS has relatively few immune defenses, so bacteria replicate rapidly. As the concentration of bacteria increases, fluid is drawn into the cranium and cranial blood vessels. Intracranial pressure increases rapidly, causing compression and ischemia of the brain. In addition, the inflammatory response increases the permeability of the blood-brain barrier, allowing inappropriate substances into the brain and further increasing pressure. In response to the increasing cranial pressure, the blood pressure drops rapidly and death may occur from either shock or cerebral ischemia.

Acute bacterial meningitis, caused by *Streptococci*, *Haemophili*, or *Meningococci* species, can be fatal within hours of infection. An intolerable headache, very stiff or rigid neck, violent vomiting, and a rapidly rising fever occur and worsen in only a few hours. Altered cognition, syncope, seizures, and coma may also occur. Emergency transport for hospitalization and aggressive antibiotic and corticosteroid therapy is the course of treatment. Bacterial meningitis is highly contagious and can become epidemic in schools, the military, athletics, and other environments in which people spend extended time in close physical contact. Exposure to a person who has bacterial meningitis requires a course of prophylactic antibiotics and medical monitoring. Vaccines that are effective against the more common of the Meningococci species are available and may be useful in preventing the disease in at-risk populations.

Viral meningitis is most commonly caused by mumps, coxsackievirus, Epstein-Barr, and herpes simplex type II viruses. Viral meningitis causes the same signs and symptoms as bacterial meningitis, but less severe. It is less threatening than bacterial meningitis and typically requires only supportive and symptomatic treatment. Viral meningitis is also less contagious than the bacterial form.

Other organisms, including drugs, lead poisoning, and parasites, cause less severe forms of meningitis. Differentiating the type of meningitis requires medical procedures and laboratory tests performed by a physician. When presented with history, signs, and symptoms consistent with meningitis, the athletic trainer should document the person's vital signs, particularly body temperature, and make an emergency medical referral. Return-to-play decisions for athletes with meningitis will depend on the type of meningitis, the degree of complications, and the time frame necessary for symptom resolution.

Cerebral Palsy and Anoxic Brain Injury

Cerebral palsy (CP) refers to a group of neurological disorders that occur during birth or early childhood and are caused by an anoxic, metabolic, or ischemic brain injury.[20] The resulting neurological deficits are not progressive, not communicable, and cannot be transmitted genetically. The most evident and common consequences involve posture and voluntary movement, although sensory, perceptual, or mental disturbances may also occur.

Impairment in CP depends on the cerebral regions that are damaged. Motor disorders can involve one limb (*monoplegia*), the unilateral upper and lower extremities (*hemiplegia*), only the lower extremities (*diplegia*), or the entire body (*tetraplegia*).[2,21] The major type of CP is spastic and presents with hypertonicity (constant spasm). Other types, comprising less than 25% of all cases, include ataxic and dyskinetic (*athetoid*).[20]

Athletic trainers may encounter persons with mild or moderate CP in athletics or participating in other physical activities. Adults with CP may have a history of multiple corrective surgeries, or sustain overuse injuries, weakness, and impairment of range of motion at affected joints. Rehabilitation to address CP specifically is usually provided by physical, occupational, and speech therapists.

Epilepsy, Seizure, and Convulsion Disorders

Seizures result from a sudden electrochemical discharge in the brain that temporarily interrupts normal brain function.[22] They can be partial, affecting only a portion of the brain, or generalized, affecting the majority of the brain.[23,24] The first of the 2 major types of seizures is the *petit mal* or *absence* seizure, during which the person briefly loses cognitive awareness and may lose postural control. These seizures often last only seconds and the affected person may not realize a seizure has occurred. During conversation, observers may notice the person taking a long pause in between words or sentences or having a blank stare.

The second major type of seizure, the *grand mal* or tonic-clonic seizure, causes a sudden, complete loss of consciousness and postural control. The person usually falls to the ground and exhibits extreme postural rigidity (*tonic phase*) followed by convulsive-type contractions (*clonic phase*) involving the entire body.[23,24] In the period immediately following the seizure, called the *postictal phase*, the person may regain consciousness immediately or remain unconscious for some time after the seizure stops.[23] Seizures are most often associated with epilepsy, but may also be caused by chemical toxicity, hypoxia, head injury, and other pathological disorders. In either type of seizure, the person may experience an aura, such as a hallucinatory smell, sound, or vision, that precedes the onset of the seizure.[24] Not all people with epilepsy experience an aura, and auras may also occur with conditions such as migraine headache.

Many people experience a seizure at some time during their life, but do not develop a seizure disorder.[25] Recurrent seizures are called *epilepsy*, which has a prevalence of 3% across the population.[26] Most people with epilepsy experience seizures before 30 years of age.[24,26] If an athlete reports a history of epilepsy, the athletic trainer should note the medications used and their side effects, the frequency of seizures, and the nature of the seizures (petit mal, grand mal, does the athlete typically experience auras). Common side effects associated with anticonvulsant medications include nausea, vomiting, drowsiness, dizziness, and other balance disturbances.

Although many people with epilepsy do not participate in competitive sports, there is no medical reason they could not do so. People with epilepsy are, in general, not at higher risk for injury than their peers. Exercise may actually inhibit seizures, since most seizures occur at rest rather than during activity.[26] Persons with a seizure disorder who choose to swim or scuba dive require close supervision to avoid accidental drowning. Motor sports are contraindicated for individuals who experience one or more seizures per year.[26] Collision and contact sports, however, pose no particular increased risk.

Participation in sports or regular group physical activity may provide psychological benefits. People with epilepsy often feel excluded because of their condition and are at increased risk for emotional disturbances and suicide. Being accepted as part of a team or peer exercise group may help allay feelings of exclusion.[26] The athletic trainer should educate coaches and peers as necessary, including the nature of seizures, how to respond to a seizure (see next), and reasonable precautions during activity.

Management of a seizure is first concerned with protecting the person from harm.[24,25] Removing equipment, furniture, and bystanders from the immediate vicinity to avoid head or limb injury may be necessary. Towels or pillows can protect the person's head. Nothing should be inserted into the mouth, nor should the mouth be forced open.[24] The person may bite their tongue, become incontinent, or produce copious saliva ("foam at the mouth"). Turning the person to their side may prevent blocking the airway by these fluids. Once the clonic stage of the seizure ceases, assess airway, respiration, and other vital signs. If clear, begin a secondary evaluation of face, tongue, head, and joints to identify injuries. On recovery of consciousness, the person will be confused and fatigued, and should therefore be moved to a quiet area to rest and be reassured.

A first seizure or a seizure lasting more than 2 to 5 minutes, depending on the individual's seizure duration history, requires activation of the emergency action plan and transport to the nearest medical facility.[25] Other indications for emergency transport include a seizure that does not fit into the individual's pattern of previous seizures or repeated seizures without return to normal mental status. Any injury incurred during a seizure should be appropriately stabilized and referred to a physician as usual. In adolescents, noncompliance with epilepsy medication is often the precipitating factor for a seizure.

Spinal Cord Disorders

Spinal Cord Trauma

Traumatic spinal cord injury can be complete, which disrupts all ascending and descending tracts, or incomplete, disrupting only some of the spinal tracts. With complete lesions, all voluntary and autonomic neural functions controlled by spinal neurons distal to the injury are immediately and permanently lost. Function is partially preserved with incomplete lesions depending on the exact site and extent of damage. In addition to the initial structural damage, secondary tissue damage from contusion, inflammation, neurapraxia, and compression within the spinal cord follows the acute injury. After the acute injury and cessation of neural function distal to the injury (spinal shock), deep tendon reflexes return and spasticity develops. Clonus develops and most autonomic reflexes return, including bowel and bladder function, although sensation and voluntary movement do not.

The assessment, management, and prevention of spinal cord injury are covered extensively in most orthopedic assessment texts, and thus are not addressed in this chapter. We encourage athletic trainers to consult an orthopedic assessment text and review this information regularly.

Spina Bifida

Spina bifida is a congenital defect that is caused by incomplete formation of the neural tube (vertebral arch and meninges). The severity of this condition can range from mild, with little to no disability (*spina bifida occulta*), to severe, with significant neurological disability (*myelomeningocele*). *Meningocele* is associated with herniation of the meninges through the spinal column defect. Myelomeningocele includes herniation of the spinal cord as well as meninges. Both of these conditions result in impairment distal to the defect and varying degrees of disability. They are both usually diagnosed at birth and require surgical intervention.

Spina bifida occulta is associated with an incomplete formation of the posterior vertebral arch but without herniation of meninges or the spinal cord.[27] This condition is often discovered when the person has an X-ray for complaints of back pain. Occasionally, skin abnormalities, such as a skin discoloration called a port wine mark because of its color or a patch of hair called a fawn's beard, are present over the site of the defect. One or more spinous processes are absent on palpation. Neurological function (sensation, reflex, motor) is usually preserved.

Athletic trainers working with able-bodied patients or athletes may encounter only individuals with spina bifida occulta. Treatment for symptomatic cases may require trunk strengthening or, in rare cases, surgical stabilization. Athletic trainers who work with disability sport athletes will very likely encounter individuals with meningocele or myelomeningocele forms of spina bifida. These athletes must regularly inspect the skin on their low back, hips, and lower extremities because of the potential for abrasions and contusions related to wheelchair usage.[28] Because of the lack of sensation to these areas, minor skin conditions can easily go undetected until they become serious infections. Also, individuals with spina bifida may have shunts that have been surgically inserted to drain CSF from their brains into their stomachs for pickup by the lymphatic system. Occasionally these shunts can become blocked or infected. Signs and symptoms related to shunt complications include possible seizures, headaches, cognitive and behavioral changes, and vision disturbances.[28] Any suspicion of shunt complications would warrant immediate referral to the treating physician.

Multiple Sclerosis

Most commonly appearing in early adulthood, *multiple sclerosis* (MS) is a degenerative autoimmune disease that forms regions of intermittent inflammation ("plaques") in the CNS. These plaques cause demyelination of surrounding neurons and usually affect several regions within the CNS simultaneously (cerebral cortex, cerebellum, motor and sensory tracts), following no standard pattern.[29] The plaques lapse and recur, with each recurrence affecting new regions of the CNS. Eventually, demyelination causes irreversible neuronal degeneration.

Initial signs and symptoms vary depending on where plaques occur in the CNS, but commonly include visual disturbances (diplopia—double vision—or a spot in the visual field), peripheral paresthesia, and weakness or clumsiness in a leg or hand.[29] Other early symptoms can include stiffness or fatigue in a limb, minor gait dysfunction, vertigo, and bladder control issues.[29] As the disease progresses, patients will develop bilateral lower extremity muscle weakness.

The etiology of MS is unknown, although immunologic factors may have a role and it occurs twice as often in women than men. Diagnosing MS is difficult and no specific test provides a definitive diagnosis. When MS is suspected, physicians will typically order an MRI, which might reveal lesions within the brain. Other diagnostic tests include a spinal tap to examine cerebral spinal fluid, an electroencephalogram and electromyogram. No cure for MS currently exists. Most cases of MS are classified as relapsing-remitting, with acute attacks being followed by complete or partial recovery. Treatment is focused on reducing the frequency of attacks and managing symptoms. Self-injections of interferon are one example of a drug therapy used to reduce the frequency of acute episodes in cases of relapsing-remitting MS. Another form of this disease, progressive MS, is associated with more significant disability. Counseling, activity modification to avoid fatigue, exercise to preserve function, and speech therapy when needed are also essential elements in any treatment plan for MS. Heat seems to exacerbate the symptoms of MS and should therefore be avoided (eg, hydrocollator packs, heated aquatic therapy, outdoor exercise on hot days). Life span is not usually affected, except in the severely progressive forms of MS, but impairment and disability may become profound.[29]

An athlete's ability to participate in competitive sports will depend on the type of MS and the degree of disability. At one time, exercise was viewed as a contraindication for MS patients; however, it is now viewed as a vital component for managing the disease.[30] Current evidence demonstrates that MS patients can benefit from aerobic and resistance exercise.[30-32]

Peripheral Nervous System (and Combined Central-Peripheral) Disorders

Complex Regional Pain Syndrome

Complex regional pain syndrome (CRPS), previously referred to as *reflex sympathetic dystrophy*, usually occurs in the distal extremities when the CNS produces continuous sympathetic stimulation of that limb.[33] Recall that the sympathetic nervous system is activated in response to stress. The activity of small-fiber pain receptors from a chronic injury may contribute enough physical stress to cause CRPS. Joint injury, limb trauma, lengthy immobilization, disorders affecting nerve roots, and peripheral neuropathy increase the risk of developing CRPS.[33,34] In an athletic setting, CRPS most commonly occurs after a severe injury or fracture is followed by immobilization and non-weight bearing.

CRPS causes symptoms across several peripheral nerve distributions.[33] Symptoms include pain that is disproportional to the injury, skin hypersensitivity (even to clothes or bed sheets), and extreme reluctance to move the joint or bear weight.[33] Clinical signs include swelling, decreased range of motion, increased skin temperature, and atrophic skin, hair, and nail changes of the affected limb.[33,34] As the syndrome progresses over several weeks, atrophy and poor peripheral vascular control, as indicated by cyanosis, intolerance to cold, and pallor, develops.[33] After several months, sympathetic activity decreases and the entire limb (skin, muscle, and bone) becomes atrophic, cool, pale, and so hypersensitive it is no longer functional.[33,34]

Recognition and treatment of CRPS may be very difficult.[33] CRPS may be prevented by encouraging movement, particularly at uninjured joints, and weight bearing (if not contraindicated) after an injury. Rehabilitation for CRPS consists of rhythmic weight bearing, gentle joint distraction, active range of motion, desensitization techniques, and joint mobilization.[33] Transcutaneous nerve stimulation units may be prescribed for pain relief. Analgesic medications and anesthetic injections to block the sympathetic impulses may also be used in resistant cases.[33] Persistent and aggressive treatment increase the probability of a successful outcome.

Motor Unit and Neuromuscular Disorders

The motor unit is composed of a single motor neuron, its axon and axon branches (the peripheral nerve), and the muscle fibers controlled by the motor neuron. Motor units operate on the "all or none" principle: either the motor neuron discharges and all of the associated muscle fibers contract, or the neuron fails to discharge and no contraction occurs. Motor unit diseases can affect the motor neuron body, the axons, the neuromuscular junction where the axon joins the muscle fiber, or the muscle directly.[35] Table 13-13 outlines the neurological pathology that affects the various parts of the motor unit.

Motor Neuron

Amyotrophic Lateral Sclerosis

The etiology of *amyotrophic lateral sclerosis* (ALS or "Lou Gehrig's disease") is unknown. Toxic and autoimmune responses have been suggested. The disease degenerates nerve fibers and neurons

Table 13-13. Neuromuscular Disorders

STRUCTURE	POTENTIAL PATHOLOGY
Motor neuron	Amyotrophic lateral sclerosis (ALS; Lou Gehrig's disease)
	Poliomyelitis and post polio syndrome
Axon	Peripheral neuropathy
	Guillain-Barré syndrome
Neuromuscular junction	Myasthenia gravis
Muscle	Muscular dystrophy (MD)
	Myopathy, polymyositis, dermatomyositis

and progresses from distal to proximal. Gradual, progressive weakness appears, often noticed first in the hands and arms. Spasticity, hyperactive reflexes, and tics develop as the disease progresses, followed by dysarthria and difficulty swallowing (*dysphagia*). Cognition is unaffected.

ALS occurs in adulthood, most commonly in middle age. Treatment is supportive to maintain function as long as possible, including mobility, speech, feeding, and breathing. ALS currently has no cure and half of individuals with ALS die within 3 years of onset; up to 10% will live 10 years. Complications of respiratory failure usually cause death.

Poliomyelitis

The poliovirus destroys motor neurons in the anterior spinal cord, producing the disease called polio. Development of effective vaccines and immunization programs has virtually eliminated polio in the United States, although it still occurs in developing countries. The athletic trainer may occasionally encounter someone who recovered from childhood polio. Recovery depends on the amount of motor neuron destruction and strengthening of unaffected motor units.

Postpolio Syndrome

Postpolio syndrome is common among polio survivors who contracted the disease before widespread vaccination. This syndrome is characterized by the appearance of symptoms 2 to 3 decades after the initial infection.[36] Arthralgia, myalgia, weakness, atrophy, and unusual muscle fatigue (and, of course, a history of poliovirus infection) define postpolio syndrome.[36] The syndrome progresses slowly and is treated symptomatically, with assistive devices and activity modification as necessary.

Axon

Peripheral Neuropathy

Peripheral neuropathy is a "catch-all" term describing many disorders of the nerve fiber. Motor and sensory changes can occur, as well as loss of vasomotor control. Sensory changes can range from numbness or mild tingling to painful hypersensitivity. Many different conditions can produce peripheral neuropathy, including diabetes mellitus, trauma, toxicity, infection, or demyelinating disease. Treatment and prognosis for recovery depend on the underlying disorder. Hence, identification of the underlying disorder is paramount.

Guillain-Barré Syndrome

An autoimmune response to a viral infection is thought to cause *Guillain-Barré syndrome*, an acquired demyelinating polyneuropathy—meaning that it affects many nerves. In this disease, a sudden, disabling symmetric weakness of both legs occurs, progresses to the arms, and is accompanied by loss of the DTRs. Cognitive function is maintained, although the ability to speak may be affected. Guillain-Barré progresses rapidly and may lead to loss of respiratory control. Anyone presenting with bilateral weakness or numbness in the legs should be referred immediately to avoid respiratory failure. Weakness peaks about 3 weeks after onset, but a full recovery may take months. In some individuals, residual weakness may persist for years and neuropathies may recur.

Neuromuscular Junction

Myasthenia Gravis

Myasthenia gravis is an autoimmune disorder of the neuromuscular junction, where the motor neuron connects to muscle fibers. The autoimmune response destroys postsynaptic acetylcholine receptors at the neuromuscular junction. When acetylcholine is released, the decrease in receptors results in a lower than normal change in electrical potential. The decreased potential translates into inefficient muscle contraction, clinically manifested as weakness and fatigability.

Extreme muscle fatigue, double vision (*diplopia*), and *ptosis* (sagging eyelids) develop suddenly and progressively worsen over several hours or days. Respiratory muscles may be affected, and dysarthria (difficulty speaking), dysphagia (difficulty swallowing), and dyspnea may occur. DTRs are not affected. Medical treatment consists of corticosteroids and drugs that act at the neuromuscular junction. No cure exists, although most functional ability can be restored and maintained with careful medical management.

Muscle

Muscular Dystrophy

Muscular dystrophy (MD) describes a class of genetic disorders that affect muscle fiber structure. In the most common type, Duchenne muscular dystrophy, muscle fibers progressively degenerate and are replaced by non-contractile connective tissue. The proximal, limb-girdle muscles of the shoulder and pelvis are affected first, producing a wide-base gait, difficulty with stairs, frequent falls, and difficulty rising from the floor. The disease appears in early childhood and wheelchair use is necessary by about 10 years of age. Eventually the respiratory muscles are affected, causing death usually before the age of 20.

Other forms of MD are less disabling and allow a normal life span. No cure for MD exists, although gene therapy has shown promise. Corticosteroids may counter the inflammation accompanying muscle fiber destruction. Moderate exercise to maintain function and nutritional counseling to avoid obesity (which increases demand on muscles) are recommended. Intense activity damages muscle tissue and should be avoided.

Management of Neuromotor Diseases

Virtually all diseases of the motor unit adversely affect strength, endurance, and flexibility.[37] Incoordination of posture and voluntary movements may also occur and reflex responses may increase or decrease. Many neuromotor diseases cause progressive weakness and paralysis. Weakness produces limited movement and often leads to secondary problems such as obesity, joint stiffness or contracture, and skin lesions, all of which further inhibit motion and compound the effects of the underlying disease.[37] As a result, metabolic demands of movement and activity increase significantly and may cause fatigue. Aerobic capacity or strength may not increase with rehabilitation exercises, but functional tasks may become easier or more effective after conditioning.[37]

For a person with a neuromotor disease, the qualification for participation in sports is made on a case-by-case basis, depending on the nature and stage of the disease, the desired activity and level of competition, the approval of the attending physician, and the person's (or parents') goals. Adaptive sports or activities may be appropriate to protect the participant from injury and allow a rewarding experience. Many of these neuromotor conditions prevent participation in competitive athletics, but may occur among physically active individuals.

SUMMARY

Neurological disorders can be obvious or subtle, but nearly always affect physical performance. Pathology can occur in any region of the nervous system, including the brain, brain stem, spinal cord, and peripheral nerves. Signs and symptoms depend on the location and extent of the disorder, but often include paresthesia, weakness, change in reflexes, incoordination, dysarthria, dysphagia, or dyspnea. Head trauma (concussion, PCS, and second-impact syndrome), spinal trauma, and seizure disorders (eg, epilepsy) are the neurological disorders most likely to be encountered among athletes. Many individuals with neurological disorders participate in regular physical activity. Athletic trainers should therefore be aware of the basic types of neuromotor disorders and their effects.

CASE STUDY

Barry is a 15-year-old male who has epilepsy. His physician has cleared him for participation in soccer. Barry had his first seizure when he was 12 years old, and he has been prescribed medication that he takes on a daily basis.

Critical Thinking Questions

1. What further information would be useful to know about Barry's seizure history, type of seizure, and postictal phase?
2. What education might you provide to Barry's coaches and teammates?
3. What is your plan for seizure management if Barry should have a seizure during practice or a game? What other individuals need to be informed of the management plan?

REFERENCES

1. National Athletic Trainers' Association. *Athletic Training Education Competencies.* 5th ed. The Commission on Accreditation of Athletic Training Education; 2011.
2. Gould BE. Neurologic disorders. *Pathophysiology for the Health-Related Professions.* W.B. Saunders Company; 1997:320-376.
3. McCrea M. Standardized mental status testing on the sideline after sport-related concussion. *J Athl Train.* 2001;36:274-279.
4. McCrory P, Meeuwisse WH, Jvorak J, et al. Consensus statement on concussion in sport: the 5th International Conference on Concussion in Sport, Berlin, October 2016. *Br J Sports Med.* 2017;51:838-847.
5. Harmon KG, Clugston JR, Dec K, et al. American Medical Society for Sports Medicine position statement: concussion in sport. *Br J Sports Med.* 2019;53:213-225.
6. Guskiewicz KM, Ross SE, Marshall SW. Postural stability and neuropsychological deficits after concussion in collegiate athletes. *J Athl Train.* 2001;36:263-273.
7. Broglio SP, Ferrara MS, Sopiarz K, Kelly MS. Reliable change of the sensory organization test. *Clin J Sport Med.* 2008;18:148-154.

8. Broglio SP, Macciocchi SN, Ferrara MS. Sensitivity of the concussion assessment battery. *Neurosurgery.* 2007;60:1050-1057.

9. Mozaffarian D, Benjamin EJ, Go AS, et al. Executive summary: heart disease and stroke statistics—2016 update: a report from the American Heart Association. *Circulation.* 2016;133:447-454.

10. Centers for Disease Control and Prevention. Types of stroke. Available at: http://www.cdc.gov/stroke/types_of_stroke. htm. Accessed June 10, 2013.

11. Giraldo E. Overview of stroke. The Merck Manual for Health Care Professionals. Available at: http://www.merck-manuals.com/professional/neurologic_disorders/stroke_cva/overview_of_stroke.html?qt=stroke&alt=sh. Accessed June 21, 2013.

12. National Institute of Neurological Disorders and Stroke. Cerebral aneurysm fact sheet. Available at: http://www.ninds. nih.gov/disorders/cerebral_aneurysm/detail_cerebral_aneurysms.htm. Accessed June 30, 2013.

13. Dimeff RJ. Headaches in athletes. *Clin Sports Med.* 1992;11:339-349.

14. Garten CE. Headaches and athletes. *Athl Ther Today.* 2005;10:28-29.

15. McCrory P, Johnston K, Meeuwisse W, et al. Summary and agreement statement of the 2nd International Conference on Concussion in Sport, Prague 2004. *Br J Sports Med.* 2005;39:196-204.

16. Broglio SP, Cantu RC, Gioia GA et al. National Athletic Trainers' Association Position Statement: Management of Sport-Related Concussion. *J Athl Train.* 2014;49(2):245-265.

17. Putukian M, Raftery M, Guskiewicz K, et al. Onfield assessment of concussion in the adult athlete. *Br J Sports Med.* 2013;47:285-288.

18. Halstead ME, Walter KD, Council on Sports Medicine and Fitness. American Academy of Pediatrics. Clinical report—sport-related concussion in children and adolescents. *Pediatrics.* 2010;126(3):597-615.

19. Khurana VG, Kaye AH. An overview of concussion in sport. *J Clin Neurosci.* 2012;19:1-11.

20. McBride MC. Cerebral palsy (CP) syndromes. The Merck Manual for Health Care Professionals. Available at: http://www.merckmanuals.com/professional/pediatrics/neurologic_disorders_in_children/cerebral_palsy_cp_syndromes. html?qt=cerebral%20palsy&alt=sh. Accessed July 4, 2013.

21. Perin B. Physical therapy for the child with cerebral palsy. In: Tecklin JS, ed. *Pediatric Physical Therapy.* J.B. Lippincott Company; 1989:68-105.

22. Adamolekun B. Seizure disorders. The Merck Manual for Health Care Professionals. Available at: http://www.mer-ckmanuals.com/professional/neurologic_disorders/seizure_disorders/seizure_disorders.html?qt=epilepsy&alt=sh. Accessed July 5, 2013.

23. Fuller KS. Epilepsy. In: Goodman CC, Boissonnault WG, eds. *Pathology: Implications for the Physical Therapist.* W.B. Saunders Company; 1998:785-790.

24. Parks ED. Seizure disorders in athletes. *Athl Ther Today.* 2006;11:36-38.

25. Dimberg EL, Burns TM. Management of common neurological conditions in sports. *Clin Sports Med.* 2005;24:637-662.

26. Cantu RC. Epilepsy and athletics. *Clin Sports Med.* 1998;17:61-69.

27. Gould BE. Congenital and genetic disorders. *Pathophysiology for the Health-Related Professions.* W.B. Saunders Company; 1997:97-107.

28. Naugle K, Stopka C, Brennan J. Common medical conditions in athletes with spina bifida. *Athl Ther Today.* 2007;12:18-20.

29. Apatoff BR. Multiple sclerosis. The Merck Manual for Health Care Professionals. Available at: http://www.merckman-uals.com/professional/neurologic_disorders/demyelinating_disorders/multiple_sclerosis_ms.html?qt=Multiple%20 Sclerosis&alt=sh. Accessed July 4, 2013.

30. Padgett PK, Kasser SL. Exercise for managing the symptoms of multiple sclerosis. *Phys Ther.* 2013;93:723-728.

31. Huisinga JM, Filipi ML, Stergiou N. Elliptical exercise improves fatigue ratings and quality of life in patients with multiple sclerosis. *J Rehabil Res Dev.* 2011;48:881-890.

32. White LJ, Dressendorfer RH. Exercise and multiple sclerosis. *Sports Med.* 2004;34:1077-1100.

33. Kasdan ML, Johnson AL. Reflex sympathetic dystrophy. *Occup Med.* 1998;13(3):521-531.

34. Rosenthal AK, Wortmann RL. Diagnosis, pathogenesis, and management of reflex sympathetic dystrophy syndrome. *Compr Ther.* 1991;17(6):46-50.

35. Homnick DN, Marks JH. Exercise and sports in the adolescent with chronic pulmonary disease. *Adolesc Med.* 1998;9(3):467-481.

36. Smith MB. The peripheral nervous system. In: Goodman CC, Boissonnault WG, eds. *Pathology: Implications for the Physical Therapist.* W.B. Saunders Co; 1998:811-837.

37. Small E, Bar-Or O. The young athlete with chronic disease. *Clin Sports Med.* 1995;14:709-726.

ONLINE RESOURCES

◊ **Concussion Clinical Toolkit**
  ¤ http://www.cattonline.com/
◊ **NATA Position Statement: Management of Sport Related Concussion**
  ¤ http://www.nata.org/sites/default/files/MgmtOfSportRelatedConcussion.pdf
◊ **NATA Position Statement: Preventing Sudden Death in Sports**
  ¤ http://www.nata.org/sites/default/files/Preventing-Sudden-Death-Position-Statement_2.pdf
◊ **National Institutes of Neurological Disorders and Stroke**
  ¤ www.ninds.nih.gov

Please visit www.routledge.com/9781630917234
to access additional material.

CHAPTER 14

Psychological Conditions

CHAPTER OUTLINE AND OBJECTIVES

Introduction

Signs and Symptoms

◊ Discuss medical history findings relevant to psychological disorders.

◊ Identify signs and symptoms of psychological disorders.

¤ Change in Sleep Pattern

¤ Change in Cognitive Status or Function

¤ Weight Loss and Loss of Appetite

¤ Emotional Lability and Change in Affect (Mood)

¤ Inexplicable or Uninterpretable Symptoms

Pain Patterns

Medical History and Physical Examination Procedures

◊ Perform physical examination tasks relevant to psychological disorders.

Pathology and Pathogenesis

◊ Describe the common mental health professionals (eg, psychiatrists, psychologists, counselors, social workers) and the role they may play in treating psychosocial disorders.

◊ Describe basic psychological concepts such as behavior, mood, orientation, and perception.

◊ Identify risk factors associated with common psychological disorders.

◊ Identify and describe the signs, symptoms, interventions and, when appropriate, the return-to-participation criteria for the common psychological disorders.

¤ Substance Abuse

¤ Eating Disorders and Disordered Eating

Bhojani RA, O'Connor DP, Fincher AL. *Clinical Pathology for Athletic Trainers: Recognizing Systemic Disease, Fourth Edition* (pp 387-403).
© 2022 Taylor & Francis Group.

- ¤ Mood Disorders
- ¤ Anxiety Disorders
- ¤ Somatoform Disorders
- ¤ Personality Disorders
- ¤ Psychoses

Pediatric Concerns

- ◊ Child Abuse
- ◊ Behavioral or Conduct Disorders

Summary

Case Study

- ◊ Develop critical-thinking and clinical decision-making skills.

Online Resources

This chapter addresses the following knowledge and skills from the *Athletic Training Education Competencies, Fifth Edition*[1]:

Content Area	Competency #
Prevention and Health Promotion (PHP)	3, 5, 46, 47, 48, 49
Clinical Examination and Diagnosis (CE)	16, 17, 18, 22
Acute Care of Injury and Illness (AC)	36n, 41
Psychosocial Strategies and Referral (PS)	11, 12, 13, 14, 15, 16
Clinical Integration Proficiencies (CIP)	5, 8

INTRODUCTION

This chapter discusses several general categories of psychological disorders. Disordered eating and substance abuse are the most common psychological conditions encountered by athletic trainers. Psychological issues can also affect the course of treatment or the outcome for a musculoskeletal injury. Control of behavior, mood, personality, and cognitive function reside exclusively in the brain. Consequently, pathology in the brain can affect psychological status. Psychological disorders may also simulate or mask symptoms from pathology of other organ systems.

SIGNS AND SYMPTOMS

Change in Sleep Pattern

Psychological disturbance can affect sleep patterns, either increasing or decreasing sleep duration and quality. It can also affect the ability to fall asleep, stay asleep, or both.

Change in Cognitive Status or Function

Cognitive changes may be noted by the affected person's acquaintances. Increased passivity (apathy) or aggressiveness, memory problems, inattention or indifference to environment, disorientation in familiar surroundings, or difficulties with ordinary daily tasks (eg, misplacing or losing things, forgetting to turn off appliances) suggest a possible psychological disorder.

Weight Loss and Loss of Appetite

Psychological conditions such as depression and eating disorders can cause significant weight gain, weight loss, or loss of appetite.

Emotional Lability and Changes in Affect (Mood)

Emotional lability refers to frequent, dramatic shifts in mood, such as uncontrollable laughter one minute and crying the next, and can be a sign of a psychological condition. By contrast, mood disorders such as depression are relatively stable, lasting days or weeks. Relatives or friends often report these changes rather than the affected person, who may not recognize changes in their own mood. People with depression, however, often report "feeling depressed" if specifically asked. The athletic trainer may notice these subtle changes in mood if they are familiar with the person or around them on a daily basis.

Inexplicable or Uninterpretable Symptoms

People with disabling psychological disorders may be unable to describe their perceptions in logical, reasonable terms. This does not mean that symptoms or injuries are imaginary. Occasionally, extreme psychological stress, such as physical or emotional abuse, unstable home environment, extreme emotional or social pressures, causes symptoms that do not correspond with physical examination results. If the clinical presentation is not interpretable, referral to a physician with a report of history and physical examination findings is indicated.

PAIN PATTERNS

A person who has a somatoform or psychosomatic disorder may report symptoms that do not match any known referral pattern or nerve distribution. Symptoms of pathology in the major organ-systems may be exaggerated, misinterpreted and inaccurately reported, or ignored by someone who has a psychological condition.

MEDICAL HISTORY AND
PHYSICAL EXAMINATION PROCEDURES

Family and Personal History

Some psychological conditions, such as depression and substance abuse, have genetic components. A family history positive for a diagnosed psychological condition is significant if behavior or mood changes are noticed. It is recommended that during the pre-participation physicals to ask if there is a first-degree relative with psychological conditions.

Known or reported abuse and/or social disturbances within the immediate family are major warning signals for psychological disorders. As an allied health care professional, the athletic trainer is obligated to report suspected abuse to state authorities to protect the abused person. An athletic trainer should be familiar with their state laws regarding responsibilities and process for health professionals reporting abuse. Obtaining legal evidence of abuse is often difficult since abused

Table 14-1. Mental Status Questions

MENTAL FUNCTION	QUESTION	ACCEPTABLE ANSWERS OR INTERPRETATION
Judgment	If you found a wallet in the lobby of an office building, what should you do with it?	Turn it in to security, or any other logical answer
Orientation	(Person) What is your name?	The correct name; inability to identify self indicates a serious mental impairment
	(Place) Where are you now?	The correct place; disorientation to place occurs with serious injury or impairment
	(Time) What quarter/half are we in? What day of the week is it?	The right answers; orientation to time may be affected even with relatively mild injury or impairment
Cognitive	Subtract backwards from 100 by 7 (or from 50 by 3)	Should be correct for at least several consecutive subtractions
Memory	List 3 objects (for example, elephant, hubcap, and pencil) for subject to repeat immediately and at the end of examination	Remembering any less than all 3 objects indicates a memory deficit

individuals often deny the situation or that they are in danger. Indicators of child abuse are discussed later.

Many psychotropic medications have physical side effects and substantially affect athletic performance. These medications may affect fine motor coordination and cause weight gain/loss, both of which decrease athletic performance. Furthermore, many of these drugs cause dehydration and hyperthermia,[2] so exercise intensity and duration and fluid intake need to be closely monitored during physical activity.

Physical Examination

Physical examination findings may be inconclusive, confusing, inconsistent, or illogical when a psychological disorder exists. A person's behavior may be the best indicator of their psychological status. People with significant mental or emotional impairment may behave erratically, such as walking in circles or muttering the same phrase over and over, or appear confused or disheveled.[3]

Mental Status Examination

Table 14-1 lists basic screening questions that can be used to examine mental status.[3,4] Inappropriate responses warrant referral for medical examination.

PATHOLOGY AND PATHOGENESIS

The most prevalent psychological issues among athletes are substance abuse and disordered eating.[2,5] Other disorders may arise, either as primary (depression, anxiety, behavioral, and affective disorders) or secondary (following brain trauma) conditions. Table 14-2 outlines the general

Table 14-2. Categories of Psychological Disorders

CATEGORY	SPECIFIC DISORDERS
Substance abuse	Prescription or illegal drug abuse, alcoholism
Disordered eating	Anorexia nervosa, bulimia nervosa
Mood disturbances	Depression; bipolar disorder; seasonal affective disorder
Anxiety disorders	Phobias; panic disorders; generalized anxiety; obsessive-compulsive disorder; post-traumatic stress and dissociative disorders
Somatoform disorders	Somatization; hypochondria; conversion disorder; malingering; Munchausen's syndrome; chronic pain syndrome
Personality disorders	Antisocial behavior; borderline personality
Psychoses	Schizophrenia; delusional disorders; organic brain syndrome
Child abuse	May coexist with spousal abuse or substance abuse

categories of psychological pathology and specific disorders within those classes that are discussed in this chapter. Other than medication side effects or significant disability (eg, requiring hospital or institutional care), most psychological conditions do not disqualify someone from participation in sports. Recognition of these disorders in their athletes or patients would warrant referral to a mental health professional. For this reason, athletic trainers should be familiar with the network of mental health professionals in their area. Table 14-3 identifies the common mental health professionals and the role they may play in treating psychosocial disorders.[6]

Substance Abuse

Substance abuse and addiction crosses all gender, socioeconomic, ethnic, and geographical boundaries.[2,5,7] *Substance abuse* is a pattern of chemical use that interferes with normal physiological, social, psychological, or emotional function, or the use of a chemical substance for other than its intended purpose. Any substance that can act biochemically has the potential to be abused, including hallucinogenic, stimulants (eg, methamphetamine, ephedrine, caffeine, phenylpropanolamine), depressants, anabolic steroids, analgesics, narcotics, cocaine, marijuana, caffeine, and over-the-counter medications, and otherwise beneficial substances such as vitamins, minerals, and amino acids.[8] Table 14-4 lists some signs indicative of potential substance abuse.

Alcohol and tobacco are the most frequently used and abused drugs in the United States.[5,9] Population health effects of alcohol abuse, including drunk driving accidents, and tobacco abuse, including several pulmonary and oral diseases, are far greater societal problems than abuse of all other substances combined.[7] Of note, the increasing use of marijuana and CBD oils may pose future abusive health effects on the population.

Of all drugs, alcohol is the most destructive in terms of prevalence of abuse, social and economic consequences, and medical complications. Anyone drinking alcohol during or before classes, work, or athletic workouts needs immediate intervention and counseling. Such behavior is a sign of uncontrolled alcohol abuse that may lead to alcoholism. *Alcoholism*, the syndrome of alcohol addiction, is treated with abstinence and counseling programs, but has a very high rate of reoccurrence. Medical problems due to chronic alcohol abuse are many, affect nearly every organ system, and are attributable to the combined effects of cellular toxicity and malnutrition. There are several screening tools used to screen for unhealthy alcohol use, including single-item screening, AUDIT-C, AUDIT, and CAGE questionnaires. The athletic trainer should familiarize themselves with one or more of these screening tools such as the single-item screening and the AUDIT-C. These 2 questionnaires are short, easy to ask, and can give insight into the risk of unhealthy use.

Table 14-3. Mental Health Care Professionals

PROFESSIONAL	ROLE	TYPICAL WORK SETTING	COMMON CONDITION/ DISORDER TREATED
Psychiatrist (MD)	Psychotherapy; prescribe medications for treating mental illness	Hospitals; independent or group practices	Depression; manic-depression; panic disorders; anxiety disorders' obsessive-compulsive disorder; schizophrenia
Clinical psychologist (PhD or PsyD)	Psychotherapy; research (may have specialization in health psychology, neuropsychology, geropsychology); administer diagnostic tests	Counseling centers; independent or group practices; hospitals	Assist individuals with mental and emotional disorders adjust
Counselor psychologist (PhD or PsyD)	Psychotherapy; administer and interpret standardized, diagnostic psychosocial tests	University counseling centers, hospitals, individual and group practices	Personal well-being; stress related concerns; crisis resolution
Social Work Counselor (LCSW)	Psychotherapy	Private or clinical practice	Assist individuals with confronting serious illness, disability, domestic abuse, neglect, and substance abuse; assist with functioning within family, friends, and community
Sports psychologist (PhD or MS/MA)	Consultation	One-on-one with athletes or small groups of athletes	Sports performance enhancement; competition-related stress

Adapted from Lemberger ME. Issues and processes related to psychosocial referrals for athletic trainers. In: Mensch JM, Miller GM, eds. *The Athletic Trainer's Guide to Psychosocial Intervention and Referral.* SLACK Incorporated; 2008:79-84.

Abuse of nicotine in all of its forms (cigarettes, cigars, chewing tobacco, snuff) is also a major health concern. Although direct health effects of nicotine are relatively moderate (acting as a mild stimulant), health risks are greatly increased by chronic exposure to the carcinogens introduced by the methods of delivery, which are typically inhaled smoke or prolonged contact of processed tobacco leaves with the oral or nasal epithelium. In addition, since use of most tobacco products is socially acceptable and conveniently available, nicotine is abused much more frequently than most other drugs other than alcohol. The frequency of use greatly increases the number of exposures over time, which increases the risk of developing disease. In addition to cancers of the lung, throat, esophagus, and pancreas, tobacco use increases the risk of emphysema, atherosclerosis, thrombo-angiitis obliterans, and stroke.

Anabolic steroids, the chemical analogs or precursors of the male hormone testosterone, receive frequent media attention for their abuse among athletes. Many steroid abusers in the American population are actually young males who use them to enhance their physical appearance rather

Table 14-4. Behavioral Signs Potentially Related to Substance Abuse

Expresses a feeling or need to limit substance use.

Annoyed by criticism of substance use.

Expresses guilty feelings related to their substance use.

Uses substances in morning (eg, for hangover).

Uses substances in socially inappropriate situations (eg, during class, practice, work).

Displays consistent irresponsible behaviors (eg, missed classes, practices, or appointments).

Increasing academic or legal troubles (eg, declining grades, substance-related arrests).

Injury as a result of substance use.

than their athletic performance.[10,11] Medically, anabolic steroids are used to maintain body weight among people with chronic, wasting illnesses. Since no legitimate uses exist for healthy individuals, any use is, by definition, abuse.

Testosterone acts on the tissues of the body by increasing protein synthesis (anabolism) and inhibiting protein catabolism. A primary role of testosterone is spermatogenesis, which is regulated through a complex hormonal feedback system that depends on circulating testosterone levels. Regular anabolic steroid abuse produces muscle mass and strength gains, but also causes side effects including infertility, testicular atrophy, gynecomastia (feminization of the male breast), aggressive behavior, increased libido, and enlargement of the clitoris in females.[2,7,9,12] Chronic abuse causes premature epiphysis closure in children, a variety of severe liver disorders, heart disease, increased blood lipids, and atherosclerosis.[2,7,12,13] Some of the health effects of steroid abuse during adolescence persist into adulthood, including increased risk of cardiac pathology and psychiatric disorders, although the extent and severity of all of the long-term consequences remain poorly understood.[10]

A rapid gain of lean body mass that is inconsistent with normal growth and the typical responses to resistance training is the most obvious physical sign of anabolic steroid abuse.[12] Striae (discolored stripes in the skin), hirsutism, severe acne, hypertension, frequent nose bleeds, and needle marks on the thighs or buttocks may also be observed.[7,12] Anabolic steroid abusers may take several such drugs at one time in very large doses and may add other substances such as human growth hormone or other hormones in an effort to achieve maximum gains.[11] This practice is inherently dangerous since the source and quality of the substances and the understanding of how these drugs interact pharmacologically are often unknown to the user. The use of anabolic steroids is also discussed in Chapter 3.

Some athletes abuse stimulants (eg, caffeine, ephedrine, amphetamine, nicotine) to increase physiological excitement during competition.[7,9] These drugs act by stimulating the same receptors as epinephrine (adrenaline). The National Collegiate Athletic Association (NCAA) and International Olympic Committee maintain strict guidelines regarding the use of these agents and specify allowable dosage during athletic competition. Stimulants increase energy and elevate mood, but various side effects can occur such as hypertension, tachycardia, hyperpnea, arrhythmia, irritability, hyperthermia, convulsions, coma, and even death.[2,7] Many stimulants are widely available as over-the-counter cold and flu medications, various caffeinated beverages, most "energy drinks," and certain "health" or "energy" supplements. In high enough doses, any of these substances can be toxic and most also act as diuretics.

Diuretics increase urine volume, emetics induce vomiting, and laxatives increase defecation. Athletes in sports requiring weight classification (eg, wrestling), that involve attention on the body's physical form (eg, gymnastics, dance), or individuals with eating disorders may abuse these substances to lose weight.[14,15] Abuse of these substances can produce dehydration, electrolyte imbalances, and malnutrition, and can lead to a medical emergency.[2,15]

Abuse of prescription drugs is also frequent. Opioids (narcotics), which are chemical opium derivatives such as heroin, codeine, and morphine, depress the central nervous system. Opioids are often prescribed as analgesics following an injury or surgery. Abusers of opioids seek the feelings of euphoria (pleasant relaxation) that can occur with these drugs. Acute opioid overdose is a medical emergency due to severe slowing of cardiac and respiratory function.[7] Chronic use increases tolerance to opioid drugs, which requires the person to take a higher dose to achieve the same effects, and results in physical addiction. Both of these effects are a result of repeated stimulation of opioid receptors in the body that decreases their sensitivity to the drug. More stimulation is then needed to produce the same effect (tolerance), and removal of the drug produces a physical reaction as the receptors react to the lack of stimulus (physical addiction). Sudden cessation after chronic use leads to withdrawal syndromes that can also be life threatening.

Other depressants, such as barbiturates, sedatives, and sleeping pills, cause effects similar to opioids. Low doses produce intoxication, and overdose causes depressed breathing, falling blood pressure, and shock. Tolerance, addiction, and withdrawal also occur with abuse of these drugs.

Abuse of illegal drugs, such as marijuana, hallucinogens, cocaine, and heroin, may also be encountered. Heroin is an opioid. Marijuana produces mild intoxication and hallucination, as well as euphoria, tachycardia, and hypertension.[7] Other hallucinogens, such as lysergic acid diethylamide, are also frequently abused. The relative toxicity of these drugs is generally low (ie, require large doses for a toxic effect), but their purity may be questionable, as with any drug bought illegally, so medical problems may arise from the other substances that are mixed with the drug. Hallucinogens affect behavior and cognitive processing, which can increase risk of accidents when performing activities requiring coordination or judgment.

Cocaine, extracted from the coca leaf, is a mild topical anesthetic, but acts as a stimulant when ingested. It can be absorbed through oral (chewed leaves) or nasal (snorted powder) membranes, intravenous injection, or through the alveoli by inhalation of cocaine smoke vapor.[7] Cocaine ingestion causes hypertension, tachycardia, irritability, seizure, cardiac arrhythmia, and coronary artery spasm, sometimes leading to acute myocardial infarction.[7] Smoking marijuana, cocaine, heroin, or most any substance, can also lead to inflamed, obstructed airways, similar to cigarette smoking.

Risk of cardiac death during exercise is greatly increased by drug abuse, such as cocaine, anabolic steroids, and alcohol.[16-20] Specifically, cocaine can induce cardiac arrhythmia or coronary artery spasm and anabolic steroids can cause hypertrophic cardiomyopathy.[17,20] Drug abuse can also cause myocardial ischemia, inflammation, or fibrosis, as well as a host of other medical complications in many organ-systems.[16,19]

Table 14-5 lists the general signs of intoxication, overdose, and withdrawal. Most cases of mild intoxication, depending on the drug, can be treated by removal to a quiet room, reassurance to calm the person, and rest to allow the drug to metabolize. If changes of vital signs occur, immediate emergency medical care is needed. Overdose, indicating acute toxicity (poisoning), of any drug is a medical emergency. Withdrawal, a condition with physical and psychological effects, occurs with stopping use of a physically addicting substance after a period of chronic abuse. Withdrawal from physically addictive drugs (ie, alcohol, opiates, sedatives, and barbiturates) can be life threatening and should be medically supervised. Treatment of substance abuse requires substantial and sustained physical and psychological intervention and social support.

Eating Disorders and Disordered Eating

A distinction exists between a medically diagnosed *eating disorder* and the syndrome of *disordered eating*.[21] Many athletes display behaviors that can be described as disordered eating, including restrictive diets (fad or extreme diets), or occasional binge-eating (excessive intake of food) and purging (self-induced vomiting or excessive laxative use).

Risk of disordered eating is higher in females (10 to 1 female-to-male ratio) and increases with perfectionist personality, abnormal attention to body image, participation in sports emphasizing a thin body (eg, gymnastics, figure skating, dance), sports associating low body fat with success

Table 14-5. General Signs of Intoxication, Overdose, and Withdrawal

INTOXICATION	Euphoria, decreased voluntary motor control; decreased reflex motor control (pupil, tendon reflexes), behavioral changes (stupor to raging), odor (alcohol, smoke, unusual body odor), poor judgment
OVERDOSE (TOXICITY)	Hypopnea, syncope, stupor, coma, pinpoint pupils, vomiting, shock
WITHDRAWAL	Tremors, headache, nausea, insomnia, irritability, low-grade fever, diaphoresis

(eg, running, swimming), or sports that classify participants by weight category (eg, wrestling, boxing, martial arts),[2,21-24] although it does not appear that prevalence of disordered eating is higher in female athletes than in non-athletes.[25] Long-term dieting (particularly during adolescence), significant emotional trauma (injury, family problems, etc), and substantial increases in training have also been identified as factors in disordered eating among elite female athletes.[24] Other psychosocial factors are often associated with disordered eating, such as a conflicted family environment, physical or sexual abuse, inability to handle stress, low self-esteem, and various personality disorders.[21,24,26]

Disordered eating often begins as a seemingly harmless change in diet, such as eliminating meat or "fattening foods" to lose weight. Over time, as disordered eating develops, a self-imposed "forbidden foods" list is created.[21] Simultaneously, self-directed exercise increases to excessive levels, often consuming several hours a day. The person may openly criticize other people's eating habits or begin to purge (induce vomiting) in addition to restricting their diet. Alternately, the person may binge (consume large quantities of food) in reaction to severe hunger, then purge in response to feelings of guilt.[21]

Weight loss, dry skin, brittle nails, intolerance to cold, menstrual disorders, orthostatic hypotension, dizziness, and constipation may be early signs of disordered eating. Although the person may not be observed purging, indications of frequent vomiting, such as fatigue, sore throat, abdominal pain, edematous face, and sour breath, may be noticed.[21] Dehydration and inadequate caloric intake from these behaviors increase the risk of injury or illness.[14]

If the disordered eating behaviors persist or progress, the probability of developing an eating disorder increases dramatically. The most common eating disorders among active people are anorexia nervosa and bulimia nervosa.[21,22,26]

Anorexia nervosa, the refusal to maintain a normal healthy body weight,[9] has been noted in 5% to 15% of young females who have amenorrhea and approximately 1% of all females. The reported mortality rate is alarmingly high, between 10% and 20%.[23,26] The hallmark signs of anorexia nervosa are a severely underweight appearance, inability to recognize self-emaciation, and refusal to maintain body weight within an acceptable range for height and gender.[14,26] Avoidance of weight gain becomes an obsession and a substantial distortion of body image develops. In girls and women, the chronic malnourishment eventually results in amenorrhea (see Chapter 9).[14,23,26]

Anorexia nervosa is often episodic (ie, cycles of remission and recurrence), with severity of behavior increasing in each successive episode.[21] People with anorexia nervosa may purge, use laxatives, or use diuretics to avoid weight gain. Despite multiple metabolic crises, individuals with anorexia often continue to exercise excessively.[21,26] Anorexia nervosa, if untreated, causes electrolytic imbalances, dehydration, endocrine dysfunction, cardiovascular disorders, metabolic collapse, and eventually death from either starvation or cardiac failure.[14]

Bulimia nervosa is characterized by "binge and purge" cycles recurring at least twice a week for 3 consecutive months.[9,23] Binge-eating involves bouts of rapid and massive food intake, up to 10,000 or 15,000 calories in less than 2 hours.[21,26] To avoid weight gain, purging occurs shortly after a

Table 14-6. Warning Signs for Eating Disorders

Obsession with calories and body weight

Expression of "being fat" when clearly not overweight

Consuming inappropriate amounts of food, high or low

Compulsive exercise

Expresses excessive concern with other peoples' eating habits

Greater than 5% change in body weight in 4 weeks

Sudden changes in mood or personality

binge-eating episode. Most commonly, purging manifests as self-induced vomiting. Other purgative behaviors include laxative and diuretic abuse (neither actually affects caloric absorption), excessive exercise, or self-imposed fasting.[14,21,23,26] Purging is associated with many complications, including electrolyte imbalances, gastrointestinal disturbance, renal complications, and seizures.[14,27]

In contrast to anorexia nervosa, people with bulimia nervosa often have normal body weight and do not develop amenorrhea. They express concern about their "lack of control" over eating or food, whereas individuals with anorexia exhibit very strict control of their eating habits. An estimated 1% to 3% of young women have bulimia nervosa, and the mortality rate is considerably lower than that of anorexia nervosa.

Abrasions or lacerations on the back of the hand or knuckles ("Russell's sign") may be the most obvious physical sign of bulimia nervosa.[27] These lesions are created during self-induced vomiting by placing fingers in the throat as the upper incisors cut into the dorsum of the hand.[27] Associated physical findings are erosions of the posterior surface of the frontal teeth and inflamed parotid glands (anterior and inferior to the ears).[14,27]

Treatment of eating disorders has 2 components: recognition and intervention.[23] Recognizing eating disorders may be difficult unless behaviors are directly observed. Table 14-6 lists warning signs of disordered eating syndromes.[21,23,28,29] Intervening when disordered eating is suspected can also be difficult, requiring expression of a desire to understand rather than accuse.[21] Presenting evidence of the behaviors and stating a concern for the person's health are appropriate first interventions.[21] Involving family members or friends in a non-confrontational manner may be necessary. If an eating disorder is suspected, prompt referral to a physician and a multidisciplinary treatment program are required.[23,26,30]

Prevention programs, particularly among young female athletes, may be useful. Effects of disordered eating on health and athletic performance should be presented to athletes at least annually.[22] In addition, education of coaching staff to avoid comments or behaviors that may inadvertently reinforce disordered eating may be appropriate, such as daily weigh-ins, unrealistic expectations for weight loss, and inappropriate weight loss plans.[23] The American College of Sports Medicine and the NCAA provide information for such programs.[31,32]

Mood Disorders

Mood disorders include depression, bipolar disorder, and seasonal affective disorder.[9]

Depression

Prevalence of depression, properly termed major depression disorder, a medical condition wherein feelings of grief or sadness impair physical and social function, is estimated to be between 10% and 20%.[33] Signs and symptoms include a loss of pleasure, changes in body weight (gain or loss), disturbed sleep pattern, fatigue, inability to concentrate, and suicidal thoughts or expressions.[9,33]

Table 14-7. Signs of Increased Suicide Risk

Depression
Previous suicide attempt
Family history of suicide
Social isolation
Substance abuse
Recent personal loss
Expression of hopelessness
Impulsive or secretive behavior

Behavioral manifestations include isolation from family and friends, sudden changes in academic or athletic performance, interpersonal conflicts, and increased complaints of medical problems.[33] Depression is a major risk factor for suicide and requires medical referral for treatment. Table 14-7 lists other suicide risk factors.[34-36]

Depression has been linked to a relatively low level of the neurotransmitter serotonin in the brain. Current pharmacological treatment focuses on increasing the activity of serotonin. Counseling and behavioral interventions may also be indicated.

Bipolar Disorder

Recurrent cycles of depression and elation ("mania"), both severe enough to impair normal daily life, characterize bipolar disorder.[3] The signs and symptoms of the depression phase are similar to those listed above. The elation or "manic" phase produces hyperactive motor and speech patterns, and insomnia. During the manic phase the person may be very productive and successful in work and activities. Eventually, however, this over-stimulated state interferes with judgment and impairs social interactions.[3]

The etiology of bipolar disorder is unclear, but may be related to serotonin or dopamine action in the brain, genetics, and environmental factors. Treatment involves mood-stabilizing medication to control both the manic and the depressive phases, psychotherapy, and behavioral interventions.

Seasonal Affective Disorder

Seasonal affective disorder describes depression that occurs only during particular seasons, most commonly winter.[9,37,38] The relative decrease in sunlight affects the body's internal metabolic rhythm (circadian rhythm) and the production of serotonin, which works in the mood centers of the brain. The condition completely resolves in the other seasons. Increased sleep, food intake, weight gain, irritability, and mild physical fatigue occur in seasonal affective disorder.[37,38] Four times more common among females, seasonal affective disorder occurs most often in early adulthood and decreases with age. It often occurs in the more northern latitudes because of the pronounced seasonal sunlight and weather changes. As with depression, seasonal affective disorder may affect performance.[37]

Depression, seasonal or otherwise, requires referral to a physician or psychological health consultant. Artificial light exposure of a certain intensity and duration is often used as treatment, although medication or psychotherapy may be used to augment treatment.[37,38]

Anxiety Disorders

Perceived physical, mental, or emotional stress can cause a normal reaction called anxiety, a state of intense worry. Pathological anxiety, however, changes behavior or interferes with normal social function. Some types of anxiety disorder are: phobias, obsessive-compulsive disorders, and dissociative disorders.[3]

Phobias

An abnormal fear of a specific object or situation that does not cause anxiety in the average person is called a phobia.[3] Phobias are thought to result from adverse experiences during growth or stressful or emotional periods of life. For example, athletes may experience performance anxiety, where the phobia becomes so intense that performance is impaired or avoided. Other common phobias include fear of darkness, heights, strangers, closed or crowded spaces, and germs or dirt. Clinical indications of a phobia (other than anxiety) may include physical avoidance of a situation or object, increased psychoemotional stress on mention or thought of a situation or object, or an unusual attachment to a "protective" person or place.[33] Treatment involves counseling, gradual, controlled exposure to the precipitating factor, and medication.

Generalized anxiety disorder, another example of phobia, is characterized by incessant worry about future events, self-conscious mannerisms, a perfectionist attitude, and a desire for constant reaffirmation from others.[33] Panic attacks, episodes of frequent and intense anxiety, impair daily life.

Obsessive-Compulsive Disorder

Recurrent thoughts that focus on an irrational or unreasonable fear constitute an obsession. Compulsions are behaviors that are ritually repeated, sometimes hundreds of times a day.[9,39] People with obsessive-compulsive disorder display related obsessions and compulsions, such as a compulsion to recheck the lock on a door because of an obsession with being robbed. When these behaviors interfere with daily life, the condition may require treatment with medication and counseling. Depression often coexists in individuals with obsessive-compulsive disorder.[39]

A deficiency of serotonin may be related to development of obsessive-compulsive disorder, although the etiology is thought to be multifactorial. Treatment involves psychotherapy to modify behaviors and medication to increase serotonin levels. Family involvement in therapy is recommended.

Dissociative Disorders

Dissociative disorders occur when a person's identity or behaviors suddenly change so radically that "association," or memory, of their "former self" is temporarily lost.[34] People with dissociative disorders often have no awareness of their various identities. Dissociative disorders can be induced by extreme physical-behavioral stress such as prolonged physical or mental abuse, severe injury, or extreme emotional states, thus constituting a form of post-traumatic stress syndrome.[40]

In such situations, the mind separates intolerable thoughts and experiences from the primary identity by forming alternate identities. The alternate identities experience and remember the situation, thus sparing the primary identity. Complete amnesia for a single event or period of time may exist, or entirely separate personalities may develop if the offending experiences are recurrent or unresolved (eg, physical or sexual abuse, overwhelming debt). Treatment of dissociative disorder is complex, involving medication and extensive psychotherapy in order to reintegrate the personalities into a single identity. Addressing the experiences that led to dissociation is a focus of treatment.[40]

Somatoform Disorders

Somatoform disorders are perceived or imposed physical disorders that are produced by mental or emotional disturbances. The person unconsciously seeks attention and comfort for an imagined, exaggerated, or artificially imposed physical problem. Complaints are often vague, exaggerated, inconsistent, and recurrent.[33] A stressful family or home environment may be a factor in these syndromes. Risk factors include overprotective spouse or parents, frequent but unresolved family conflicts, a major life event (divorce, death of a family member), or physical or sexual abuse.[33] An athletic trainer should never assume a somatoform disorder exists. If the person's comments or behavior suggest a psychological issue may be complicating clinical decision making, a medical referral with complete documentation is indicated.

Personality Disorders

Personality disorders may appear as recurrent antisocial behaviors, such as violence or crime.[33] Often the behavior continues to escalate in frequency and severity despite disciplinary efforts. One type of personality disorder is "borderline" personality, or abnormal dependence on other people for personal psychoemotional stability. Similar to other major psychological illnesses, an unstable or abusive family environment can contribute to development of an unstable personality. Many personality disorders are thought to be a result of inherited traits and psychosocial factors, such as abuse or neglect. Treatment involves psychotherapy. Medications are less effective because, to date, no consistent biochemical changes that may respond to pharmacological intervention have been identified.

Psychoses

Psychoses are disorders of orientation to physical surroundings. The ability to perceive and interpret experiences and surroundings is impaired. People who have psychotic disorders may hallucinate (visual, auditory, or sensory) or display a complete lack of logical order to their thoughts and actions. Psychoses are extremely disabling and may be caused by a number of medical conditions, neurotoxicity, drug toxicity or withdrawal, increased electrical activity in the brain, or abnormally high levels of dopamine. Treatment is focused at eliminating the underlying cause.

PEDIATRIC CONCERNS

Child Abuse

Child abuse is a familial or social disorder, meaning that the entire family is affected. Any behavior that interferes with a child's development, particularly when that behavior changes the child's personality, is child abuse.[3] In many cases, an abused child acts more like an adult and becomes a "caretaker" for other family members.[3] Aggressive behavior appears and increases in the abused child, but they may seem unaware of, or indifferent to, the effects of violence.[3] The family in which abuse occurs often isolates itself socially and physically, avoiding contact with other relatives and authority figures. The parents often express very high expectations for the child, effectively relying on the child to provide them with emotional support in a reversal of social roles.[3,41] Conflict arises when the expectations are not met.

Various manifestations of child abuse include physical, sexual, emotional, or neglect (withholding physical and emotional support), with neglect being the most commonly reported. Neglect is associated with parental substance abuse or depression, which affects the parent's ability to care both for themselves and their family.[41]

The family dynamic can be very complex in the case of an abused child, usually including one abusive parent and one who "looks the other way," is abused themselves, or is completely passive in family interactions. More than one sibling may be abused, and often the abusive parent was abused as a child and consequently failed to develop emotionally.[41] In addition, an abused child may be hyperactive, impulsive, or handicapped, thus requiring more emotional support than the parents are capable of providing. The abusive parent resents the dependency of the disabled child, which reinforces the abusive behavior.

Identifying child abuse is complicated. Suspicion should be raised under certain circumstances. A parent or child unable or unwilling to report how an injury occurred, or an injury that is inconsistent with the reported history may be early indications.[41] Signs of abuse include skin injuries (cuts, bruises, burns) hidden under clothing, abdominal trauma, face and head trauma, or a fracture without a reasonable history. Multiple injuries in various stages of healing is highly suggestive of abuse.[41] Signs of neglect include malnutrition, fatigue, poor hygiene, poor school attendance, and trouble with peer social interactions.[41]

In cases of suspected abuse, discussions with the child and parents should be calm and supportive, attempting to elicit information and expressing concern for injuries rather than making accusations.[41] Treatment may involve medical treatment of injuries, removing the child from the family, family counseling, and long-term family therapy.[41]

Health care workers are required by law to report suspected abuse to local child and family protection agencies, but may feel reluctant to do so without "hard evidence." Careful documentation is essential, including history, physical examination findings, and notes of parental meetings or discussions if possible. State and local laws outline the reporting of child abuse. These regulations include what required information and specific situations obligate reporting to a protective agency.

Behavioral or Conduct Disorders

Behavioral or conduct disorders among children and adolescents may be indicative of psychological or social disturbances.[3,33] Recurrent, escalating violent or antisocial behavior (fighting, vandalism, setting fires, stealing, etc) may be a result of an unstable or abusive home environment, poor adult role models, lack of parental empathy or contact, or substance abuse by the family or child.[3,33]

The child with behavioral or conduct disorders develops a limited sense of responsibility or consequences of their behavior and a decreased ability to learn from experience.[33] When confronted, the child may blame their behavior on others (eg, "he left me no choice except to punch him").[33] Medication is prescribed to decrease aggressive behavior. Various psychosocial interventions, including family psychotherapy, peer groups programs, and counseling, address other contributing psychosocial issues.[33]

SUMMARY

Psychological disorders, while relatively common, may be difficult to detect and may or may not interfere with physical health and performance. Mental or emotional impairment is often as disabling as physical impairment. Understanding psychological disorders may assist athletic trainers when they work with persons who have these conditions. Changes in mood or behavior may accompany onset of a psychological disorder. Unstable family or home life also contributes to development of many psychological conditions. Disordered eating, substance abuse, and child abuse are psychological conditions that may be encountered in the practice of athletic training.

CASE STUDY

The university where you work has had several recent cases of drug overdoses and injuries related to intoxication. One of the injuries was a basketball player who jumped from a second-story balcony during a party while drunk. As part of a university-wide program, you have been asked to present a lecture to the athletes and coaches on how to recognize potential signs of substance abuse. The university would also like you to include how to recognize potential abuse of performance-enhancing drugs in your presentation to the athletes.

Critical Thinking Questions

1. What types of substance abuse will you review? Alcohol? Nicotine? Why? What types of performance-enhancing drugs might you include?

2. What signs will you tell the athletes and coaches to look for? What types of behavioral or other problems might be related to substance abuse?

3. What will you advise the athletes and coaches to do if they suspect someone is abusing drugs?

4. What other steps or actions might you take to assist the athletic department and university to eliminate substance abuse from its campus?

REFERENCES

1. National Athletic Trainers' Association. *Athletic Training Education Competencies*. 5th ed. The Commission on Accreditation of Athletic Training Education; 2011.
2. Macleod AD. Sport psychiatry. *Aust N Z J Psychiatry*. 1998;32(6):860-866.
3. Good WV, Nelson JE. *Psychiatry Made Ridiculously Simple*. 4th ed. MedMaster; 2005.
4. Goldberg S. *The Four-Minute Neurologic Exam*. 2nd ed. MedMaster; 2011.
5. Blood KJ. Non-medical substance use among athletes at a small liberal arts college. *Athl Train*. 1990;25:335-338.
6. Lemberger ME. Issues and processes related to psychosocial referrals for athletic trainers. In: Mensch JM, Miller GM, eds. *The Athletic Trainer's Guide to Psychosocial Intervention and Referral*. SLACK Incorporated; 2008:79-84.
7. Felter RA, Fitzgibbon J. Drug-related emergencies in athletes. *Clin Sports Med*. 1989;8:129-138.
8. Zadik Z, Nemet D, Eliakim A. Hormonal and metabolic effects of nutrition in athletes. *J Pediatr Endocrinol Metab*. 2009;22:769-777.
9. Reardon CL, Factor RM. Sport psychiatry: a systematic review of diagnosis and medical treatment of mental illness in athletes. *Sports Med*. 2010;40:961-980.
10. Kanayama G, Hudson JI, Pope HG Jr. Long-term psychiatric and medical consequences of anabolic-androgenic steroid abuse: a looming public health concern? *Drug Alcohol Depend*. 2008;98:1-12.
11. Rogol AD. Drugs of abuse and the adolescent athlete. *Ital J Pediatr*. 2010;36:19.
12. Potteiger JA, Stilger VG. Anabolic steroid use in the adolescent athlete. *J Athl Train*. 1994;29:60-64.
13. Neri M, Bello S, Bonsignore A, et al. Anabolic androgenic steroids abuse and liver toxicity. *Mini Rev Med Chem*. 2011;11:430-437.
14. Stephenson JN. Medical consequences and complications of anorexia nervosa and bulimia nervosa in female athletes. *Athl Train*. 1991;26:130-135.
15. Roerig JL, Steffen KJ, Mitchell JE, Zunker C. Laxative abuse: epidemiology, diagnosis and management. *Drugs*. 2010;70:1487-1503.
16. Basilico FC. Cardiovascular disease in athletes. *Am J Sports Med*. 1999;27:108-121.
17. Franklin BA, Fletcher GF, Gordon NF, Noakes TD, Ades PA, Balady GJ. Cardiovascular evaluation of the athlete: issues regarding performance, screening and sudden cardiac death. *Sports Med*. 1997;24:97-119.
18. Futterman LG, Myerburg R. Sudden death in athletes: an update. *Sports Med*. 1998;26:335-350.
19. Maron BJ. Cardiovascular risks to young persons on the athletic field. *Ann Intern Med*. 1998;129:379-386.
20. O'Connor FG, Kugler JP, Oriscello RG. Sudden death in young athletes: screening for the needle in a haystack. *Am Fam Physician*. 1998;57:2763-2770.
21. Johnson MD. Disordered eating in active and athletic women. *Clin Sports Med*. 1994;13:355-369.
22. Dick RW. Eating disorders in NCAA programs. *Athl Train*. 1991;26:136-147.
23. Grandjean AC. Eating disorders: the role of the athletic trainer. *Athl Train*. 1991;26:105-112.
24. Sundgot-Borgen J. Risk and trigger factors for the development of eating disorders in female elite athletes. *Med Sci Sports Exerc*. 1994;26:414-419.
25. Coelho GM, Soares Ede A, Ribeiro BG. Are female athletes at increased risk for disordered eating and its complications? *Appetite*. 2010;55:379-387.
26. Johnson C, Tobin DL. The diagnosis and treatment of anorexia nervosa and bulimia among athletes. *Athl Train*. 1991;26:119-128.
27. Daluiski A, Rahbar B, Meals RA. Russell's sign: subtle hand changes in patients with bulimia nervosa. *Clin Orthop Relat Res*. 1997;343:107-109.
28. Teitz CC, Hu SS, Arendt EA. The female athlete: evaluation and treatment of sports-related problems. *J Am Acad Orthop Surg*. 1997;5(2):87-96.
29. West RV. The female athlete: the triad of disordered eating, amennorrhea, and osteoporosis. *Sports Med*. 1998;26:63-71.
30. Woscyna G. Nutritional aspects of eating disorders: nutrition education and counseling as a component of treatment. *Athl Train*. 1991;26:141-147.

31. Otis CL, Drinkwater B, Johnson M, Loucks A, Wilmore J. American College of Sports Medicine position stand. The Female Athlete Triad. *Med Sci Sports Exerc.* 1997;29:i-ix.

32. NCAA Committee on Competitive Safeguards and Medical Aspects of Sport. *Guideline 2F: nutrition and athletic performance.* National Collegiate Athletic Association, 2002.

33. Post D, Carr C, Weigand J. Teenagers: mental health and psychological issues. *Prim Care.* 1998;25:181-192.

34. Bilkey WJ, Koopmeiners MB. Screening for psychological disorders. In: Boissonnault WG, ed. *Examination in Physical Therapy Practice: Screening for Medical Disease.* 2nd ed. Churchill Livingstone; 1995:277-301.

35. Schapira K. Suicidal behavior. In: Beers MH, Berkow R, eds. *The Merck Manual of Diagnosis and Therapy.* 17th ed. Merck Research Laboratories; 1999:1544-1549.

36. Smith AM, Milliner EK. Injured athletes and the risk of suicide. *J Athl Train.* 1994;29:337-341.

37. Rosen LW, Smokler C, Carrier D, Shafer CL, McKeag DB. Seasonal mood disturbances in collegiate hockey players. *J Athl Train.* 1996;31:225-228.

38. Saeed SA, Bruce TJ. Seasonal affective disorders. *Am Fam Physician.* 1998;57:1340-1346.

39. Goodman CC. Biopsychosocial concepts related to health care. In: Goodman CC, Boissonnault WG, eds. *Pathology: Implications for the Physical Therapist.* W.B. Saunders Co; 1998:9-43.

40. Kluft RP. Dissociative disorders. In: Beers MH, Berkow R, eds. *The Merck Manual of Diagnosis and Therapy.* 17th ed. Merck Research Laboratories; 1999:1519-1525.

41. Sayre JW. Child abuse and neglect. In: Beers MH, Berkow R, eds. *The Merck Manual of Diagnosis and Therapy.* 17th ed. Merck Research Laboratories; 1999:2300-2303.

ONLINE RESOURCES

◊ **Alcoholics Anonymous**
   ¤ http://www.aa.org/

◊ **Cocaine Anonymous**
   ¤ http://www.ca.org/

◊ **Drug Free America Foundation Inc**
   ¤ http://www.dfaf.org/

◊ **Mental Health Foundation**
   ¤ http://www.mentalhealth.org.uk/

◊ **Narcotics Anonymous**
   ¤ http://www.na.org/

◊ **National Association of Anorexia Nervosa and Associated Disorders (ANAD)**
   ¤ Referrals to treatment and information (847) 831-3438
   ¤ http://www.anad.org/

◊ **National Eating Disorders Association**
   ¤ www.nationaleatingdisorders.org/

◊ **National Eating Disorder Referral and Information Center**
   ¤ (858) 481-1515
   ¤ http://www.edreferral.com/

◊ **The National Center for Drug Free Sport Inc**
   ¤ http://www.drugfreesport.com/

◊ **National Suicide Prevention Lifeline**
   ¤ http://www.suicidepreventionlifeline.org/ (also provides a link for hotlines in each state)

◊ **NCAA Banned Drug List**
   ¤ http://www.ncaa.org

◊ **NCAA Personal Welfare**
   ¤ http://www.ncaa.org

◊ **Suicide Hotlines (National)**
- ¤ (800) 784-2433
- ¤ http://www.suicide.org/suicide-hotlines.html

◊ **Toll-Free Resources**
- ¤ National Adolescent Suicide Hotline (800) 621-4000
- ¤ National Foundation for Depressive Illness Inc (800) 248-4344
- ¤ National Youth Crisis Hotline (reporting child abuse and help for runaways) (800) 448-4663
- ¤ Nationwide Crisis Hotline (800) 333-4444
- ¤ United Way Helpline (800) 233-HELP (1-800-233-4357)

Please visit www.routledge.com/9781630917234 to access additional material.

GLOSSARY

Phonetic pronunciations of medical terms are in [brackets]. Dashes (-) indicate separation of syllables. CAPS indicate the syllable(s) that is stressed in speech. Some of the very common medical terms do not include phonetics. For unfamiliar terms, practice pronunciation by reading the phonetic syllables slowly, then repeating them more rapidly until they sound like a single word.

allergy: Localized, cell-mediated immune reaction to a toxin (ie, an antigen).

alopecia: [al-oh-PEE-she-ah] Lack of hair in a body region that normally has hair.

amenorrhea: [a-MEN-o-REE-uh] Lack of menstruation for 3 consecutive months, or less than 3 menstrual cycles per year; primary amenorrhea occurs when menarche (ie, initiation of menstruation) has not occurred by the age of 16 years.

anaphylaxis: [ann-uh-fuh-LACK-sis] Generalized inflammatory response, including vascular, pulmonary, and dermatologic systems.

anasarca: [ann-uh-SAR-kah] Generalized edema; fluid in the interstitial spaces.

anemia: [a-NEE-mee-uh] A condition defined as a very low number of circulating red blood cells relative to a person's gender and age group.

angina: [ann-JIY-nuh] Distinctive type of chest pain that radiates to the arm, neck, jaw, or back, usually lasting 2 to 10 minutes.

anorexia: [ann-oh-RECK-see-uh] Loss of appetite; occurs with a number of physical, medical, or psychological conditions.

anoxia: [ann-OCK-see-uh] Lack of oxygen.

antigen: A foreign substance that initiates an immune response upon contact with tissue.

anuria: [ann-oo-REE-uh] Absence of urination.

anxiety: A state of intense worry.

arachnodactyly: [uh-rack-no-DACK-tee-lee] Long, thin fingers ("spider-like").

arrythmia: [ah-RITH-mee-uh] Interruption of the heart's electrical system, causing an irregular heartbeat.

arteriosclerosis: [ar-TEER-ee-oh-skleh-ROH-sis] Hardening of the arteries.

arthralgia: [ar-THRAL-jee-uh] Joint pain.

ascites: [ah-sy-TEEZ] Abnormal accumulation of fluid in the peritoneal space of the abdomen.

Bhojani RA, O'Connor DP, Fincher AL. *Clinical Pathology for Athletic Trainers: Recognizing Systemic Disease, Fourth Edition* (pp 405-413). © 2022 Taylor & Francis Group.

ataxia: [uh-TACK-see-uh] Inability to control voluntary movements.

atelectasis: [at-uh-LECK-ta-sis] Complete removal of air of a segment of lung tissue.

atherosclerosis: [ATH-er-oh-skleh-ROW-sis] Lipid deposits on interior of blood vessels causing a narrowing of the vascular lumen.

atopy: [AT-o-pee] Allergy producing symptoms upon exposure to an offending antigen.

atrophy: [AT-row-fee] Decrease in cell and tissue size, caused by a decrease in metabolic supply or metabolic demand.

auscultation: [AWS-kuhl-TAY-shun] Use of a stethoscope to listen for sounds originating in, or conducted by, the body.

benign: [beh-NINE] Mild, relatively harmless (opposite of malignant).

bioavailability: The amount of a drug that is available to the body's tissues, which is typically less than the ingested dose.

blood-brain barrier: Impermeable membrane of the brain's vascular system that prevents diffusion of certain compounds into the central nervous system.

bradycardia: [brayd-ee-KAR-dee-uh]Heart rate relatively slower than normal, usually less than 60 beats per minute; may occur at rest in healthy athletes as a result of training.

bronchiectasis: [brahng-kee-ECK-tah-sis] Abnormal increase in diameter of bronchus and consolidation of smaller bronchi due to disease process.

bronchophony: [brahng-KOFF-oh-nee] Abnormal auscultation; spoken sounds are clearly heard.

bruit: [BREW-ay] Abnormal sound upon auscultation, particularly one detected over an artery.

cancer: Proliferation of undifferentiated cells replacing normal cells at a high rate of division; malignant dysplasia.

carcinogen: [KAR-sih-noh-jin] Substances known to cause cancer in human tissue.

cardiac hypertrophy: Abnormal enlargement of all or part of the heart structures.

cardiac output: The product of stroke volume and heart rate; the amount of blood ejected by the heart in 1 minute.

catabolism: Metabolic breakdown of cells and tissues.

cerumen: [sih-ROO-min] Waxy substance secreted in the external auditory canal.

chief complaints symptoms: Causing an injured or ill person to seek medical attention.

cilia: [SIHL-ee-uh] Small hair-like projections, particularly on cells lining the airway.

claudication: [KLAW-dih-KAY-shun] Impairment of gait (ie, limping) caused by vascular pathology.

clinical decision making: Determining the best medical course of action for a patient, based on history, signs, and symptoms.

clinical diagnosis: The identification of an injury, illness, or disease based primarily on medical history and physical examination, without laboratory tests or imaging studies.

clinical pathology: The medical practice of pathology as it pertains to the care of patients.

clonus: [KLOH-nus] Abnormal reflex elicited by sudden flexion or extension of a distal joint and demonstrated by rapid oscillations.

coexisting condition: A medical condition in addition to the one for which the patient is seeking care (see also comorbidity).

colic: [KAH-lick] A very sudden attack of severe abdominal pain, characteristic of spasm of an obstructed abdominal organ (adj. colicky).

coma: [KOH-ma] A complete, profound, and persistent loss of consciousness from which a person cannot be aroused (compare with lethargy).

communicable: Describes a disease that can be passed directly from person to person, person to animal, or animal to person.

comorbidity: The simultaneous existence of 2 or more pathological conditions in one person (see also coexisting condition).

concussion: Collision of the brain with the cranium, causing temporary interruption of neural function.

contagious: [kon-TAY-jus] Describes a disease that can be directly passed from person to person.

contrecoup: Concussion occurring opposite to the side of impact to the head.

cor pulmonale: [KOR PUL-moh-NAHL-ee] Right ventricular hypertrophy resulting from increased pulmonary tension, eventually leading to congestive heart failure.

coryza: [koh-RIH-zah] "Common cold" or rhinitis; accompanied by nasal drainage, sore throat, sneezing, sinusitis.

cough: Forceful, often involuntary expiratory effort, usually to clear the airway of sputum or other substances or objects.

croup: [kroop] High, resonant cough, often described as "barking," accompanied by loud, labored breathing, usually associated with laryngeal obstruction.

cyanosis: [sigh-ah-NO-sis] Bluish tint to the skin; characterized as either peripheral (in the extremities) or central (present throughout the body, particulary the lips, tongue, and face); caused by insufficient oxygenation of the blood.

dermatome: Area of cutaneous sensation supplied by one spinal nerve root.

diagnosis: Definitive identification of an injury, illness, or disease.

diagnostic reasoning: Identifying and interpreting signs and symptoms to obtain a diagnosis.

diaphoresis: [DIE-uh-four-EE-sis] Profuse sweating not caused by physical exertion.

diarrhea: [die-uh-REE-uh] More than 3 bowel movements per day, or an unexpected increase in frequency of bowel movements.

diastole: [die-AS-toe-lee] Passive filling phase of the cardiac contraction cycle.

differential diagnosis: Determination of which specific disease a patient has.

differentiation: Sorting and interpretation of signs, symptoms, and other information.

diplopia: [die-PLOH-pee-uh] Blurred or "double" vision.

disease: Disruption of homeostasis caused by cellular damage or abnormal organ function.

dysarthria: [dis-AR-three-uh] Difficulty speaking.

dyspareunia: [dis-pa-RUE-nee-uh] Painful intercourse.

dysphagia: [dis-FA-jee-uh] Difficulty swallowing.

dysplasia: [dis-PLAY-zee-uh] Change of normal cells to several abnormal types with increased rate of division.

dyspnea: [DISP-nee-uh] Difficulty breathing or "shortness of breath."

dysuria: [dis-YOU-ree-uh] Painful or difficult urination.

ecchymosis: [EK-ee-MO-sis] Very dark red, blue, or black discoloration of the skin, caused by blood cells in the interstitial space; a "bruise."

edema: [uh-DEE-muh] Collection of fluid in a body cavity or interstitial space.

egophony: [eh-GOF-oh-nee] Abnormal auscultation; spoken sound is transmitted in a high pitch.

embolism: [EM-bo-liz-im] Sudden obstruction of a blood vessel by an embolus.

embolus: [EM-bo-lis] An abnormal particle or object (eg, air bubble, blood clot) freely floating in the blood.

emesis: [EM-eh-sus] Vomiting.

endocardium: Connective tissue sac that surrounds and invests the structures of the heart.

endothelium: Cells lining the cardiovascular system, including the heart, arteries, and veins (see also epithelium).

enteric coating: A protective covering on a pill that delays medication release until the pill reaches the small intestine.

epistaxis: [ep-uh-STACK-sis] Nosebleed.

epithelium: Cells lining the interior cavities and exterior surfaces of the body (see also endothelium).

erythema: [er-ih-THEE-mah] Reddening of the skin, usually a result of inflammation.

etiology: [eh-tee-AHL-oh-jee] The study of pathogenesis, including theories of illness and disease.

euphoria: [yew-FOH-ree-uh] A sensation of pleasant relaxation or well-being.

exacerbated: [EKS-as-ur-BAY-tihd] Increase in intensity or severity of a disease.

fatigue: State of metabolic imbalance that occurs when energy demands exceed energy supply.

fever: Systemic increase in body temperature; "low-grade" fever is less than 102°F; "high-grade" fever is equal or greater than 102°F.

glucosuria: [glue-koh-SUE-ree-uh] Presence of glucose in the urine.

goiter: [GOY-tur] An abnormally enlarged thyroid gland.

gonads: Organs of reproduction.

gynecomastia: [GUY-nih-coh-MASS-tee-ah] Feminization of the female breast, including development of mammary glands.

heart failure: Inability of the heart to maintain normal cardiac output.

hematemesis: [HEE-mih-TIM-ee-sis] Bloody vomitus.

hematochezia: [HIM-ah-toh-KEE-zee-ah] Presence of blood in the feces or during defecation.

hematoma: [HEE-mah-TOH-mah] Collection of blood outside the vascular system.

hematuria: [HEE-muh-TUR-ee-uh] Blood in the urine, in either microscopic or grossly visible amounts.

hemoglobinuria: [HEE-moh-gloh-bih-NEW-ree-uh] Hemoglobin in the urine, producing a reddish tint.

hemoptysis: [hih-MOP-tih-sis] Coughing or spitting bloody sputum.

hemorrhage: [HIM-ih-ridj] Sudden loss of blood (either internally or externally) resulting from damage to the vascular system.

hemorrhoids: [HIM-ih-roydz] Varicose veins in the rectum or on the anus.

hemospermia: [HIM-uh-to-SPERM-ee-uh] Blood in the male ejaculate.

hemostasis: [HEE-mo-stay-sus] A vascular response to control blood loss after injury.

hepatomegaly: [hih-PAT-uh-MEG-uh-lee] Pathologic enlargement of the liver.

hernia: [HER-nee-ah] A condition in which an organ or part of an organ protrudes through a defect in the wall of the body cavity that normally contains that organ.

hirsutism: [HIR-sue-tiz-um] Appearance of course hair on the chest and face of females, caused by abnormal concentrations of androgens from endocrine disorders or anabolic steroid abuse.

homeostasis: [HOH-mee-oh-STAY-sis] A healthy state of biochemical dynamic equilibrium within the body's internal environment.

host: An organism harboring an infectious agent.

hydrocele: [HI-droh-seel] Fluid-filled sac in the scrotum.

hypercapnia: [hi-pur-KAP-nee-uh] Increased carbon dioxide levels in the blood.

hyperhidrosis: [hi-pur-hi-DRO-sis] Excessive global or localized sweating (eg, the palms of the hands).

hyperlipidemia: [hi-pur-lip-ih-DEEM-ee-ah] Excessive fat (lipids) in bloodstream.

hyperplasia: [hi-pur-PLAY-see-ah] Increase in the total number of cells in a given tissue.

hyperpnea: [hi-PERP-nee-uh] Rapid ventilation rate.

hypertension: High blood pressure; usually systolic over 140 mm Hg or diastolic over 90 mm Hg.

hyperthermia: Central body temperature above 105°F or 39°C.

hypertrophy: [hi-PUR-tro-fee] Increase in cell size, causing an associated increase in tissue size, resulting from increased metabolic demand.

hyperventilation: Increase in ventilatory rate without an increase in ventilatory depth.

hypervolemia: [HI-pur-voh-LEE-mee-ah] Abnormally high retention of fluid in the bloodstream; eventually produces hypertension.

hypotension: Low blood pressure; usually systolic below 95 mm Hg or diastolic below 60 mm Hg.

hypothermia: Central body temperature below 94°F or 34.4°C.

hypoxemia: [HI-pock-SEE-mee-ah] Reduced oxygen saturation in arterial blood.

hypoxia: [hi-POK-see-ah] Reduced availability of oxygen to the tissues.

icterus: [ICK-tur-us] Yellow discoloration of the sclera, skin, and mucous membranes (see also jaundice).

idiopathic: [ID-ee-oh-PATH-ick] Without a known etiology; occurring spontaneously.

ileus: [ILL-ee-us] Paralyzed section of bowel, usually a result of obstruction or infarction.

impotence: [IM-poh-tense] Also called erectile dysfunction; inability to achieve or maintain an erection.

incontinence: Loss of the ability to control either urination or defecation.

incubation: Time interval between infection and appearance of symptoms.

insidious: Very gradual and unnoticeable progression of disease.

inspection: Careful observation of a patient to detect signs of pathology.

interstitial space: Space between cells containing extracellular fluid.

ischemia: [iss-KEE-mee-ah] Loss of blood flow to a tissue.

jaundice: [JAWN-dis] Yellow discoloration of the sclera, skin, and mucous membranes (see also called icterus).

lability: [lah-BILL-ih-tee] Instability, unsteadiness, particularly used to refer to mood.

lethargy: [LETH-ar-jee] A profound sleep or extreme fatigue accompanying or following disease state; differentiated from coma in that the person can be aroused.

leukocytes: [LEW-koh-siyts] White blood cell (eg, phagocytes, eosinophils).

libido: [lih-BEE-doh] Normal hormonal and emotional sex drive.

lipolysis: [liy-POLE-eye-sis] Metabolic breakdown of stored fat in response to energy demand (eg, during exercise).

lymphadenitis: [LIM-fad-ih-NIH-tiss] Swelling of the lymph nodes.

lymphadenopathy: [lim-fad-ih-NOP-ah-thee] Enlargement of the lymph nodes; a sign of possible infection.

malaise: [mah-LAYZ] General discomfort; "not feeling well."

malignant: [mah-LIG-nant] Severe and harmful; resistant to treatment; highly invasive and pervasive.

medical history: The status of the person, past and present, related to the current illness.

melena: [mel-EE-nah] Black stools with the consistency of tar.

menarche: [meh-NAR-kee] First menses.

meninges: [meh-NIN-jeez] Protective layers of connective tissue surrounding the central nervous system.

menses: [MEN-seez] Sloughing of endometrial lining, consisting of mucous and blood, from uterus through the vagina.

metabolism: Interrelated biochemical functions and processes of the organ-systems.

metaplasia: [met-ah-PLAY-zee-ah] Replacing of one cell type by another.

metastasis: [mih-TASS-tah-sis] Migration of malignant cells to organs and systems other than those of origin.

myalgia: [my-AL-jee-ah] Muscular aching.

myocardial infarction: Ischemic damage to the myocardium; a "heart attack."

myocardium: muscle tissue which comprises the heart, as distinct from striated (skeletal) and smooth (organ) muscle.

myoglobulinuria: [MY-oh-GLOHB-oo-lin-OO-ree-ah] Myoglobin in the urine, a result of excessive exercise and muscle breakdown.

myotomal: [my-oh-TOH-mal] Refers to groups of muscles controlled by a single nerve root.

necrosis: [nih-KROH-sis] Metabolic death in a group of cells.

neoplasm: [nee-oh-PLAH-zum] Tumor; abnormal cell proliferation.

nociceptor: [no-see-SEP-tur] A receptor that responds to potentially harmful (painful) stimuli.

nocturia: [nock-TOO-ree-ah] Unusual urgency to urinate, waking the victim from sleep.

occult: [oh-KULT] Hidden, undetected, or undiagnosed.

oligomenorrhea: [AHL-ee-goh-men-oh-REE-ah] Three to six menstrual cycles per year, with cycles in excess of 35 days.

oliguria: [AHL-ee-GOO-ree-ah] Very infrequent urination.

orthopnea: [or-thop-NEE-ah] Dyspnea (ie, shortness of breath) exacerbated when the trunk is upright (as in sitting or standing).

overdose: Ingestion of toxic amounts of a chemical compound, usually used to indicate poisoning as a result of drug use or abuse.

ovulation: [oh-voo-LAY-shun] Release of an ovum from the ovary; part of the menstrual cycle.

pain: A sensory and emotionally unpleasant symptom, usually associated with tissue damage.

pallor: [PAL-or] General paleness of skin caused by vasoconstriction of fever or vascular collapse.

palpation: Manual touch or manipulation conducted during the physical examination.

palpitation: [pal-pih-TAY-shun] Uncomfortable sensation of forceful, rapid, or fluttering heartbeats.

paresthesia: [pair-es-THEE-zee-ah] Abnormal cutaneous sensation, including numbness, tingling, burning, etc.

pathogenesis: The cause of a particular disease or morbid process.

pathology: Medical science concerned with all aspects of disease; the structural and functional changes that result from disease.

pathophysiology: The physiology of disease.

pectus carinatum: [kar-NAY-tum] Abnormal convexity of the sternum and anterior ribs; also called "pigeon-chest."

pectus excavatum: [ex-kah-VAH-tum] Abnormal concavity of the sternum and anterior ribs; also called "funnel-chest."

percussion: Striking to cause vibration in the internal structures of the body.

pericardium: A double-walled sac of connective tissue which surrounds the heart and its great vessels; contains the pericardial fluid; attaches endocardium to thorax.

peritoneum: [PAIR-ee-toh-NEE-um] Connective tissue lining the abdomen and abdominal organs.

peritonitis: [pair-EE-toh-NIH-tis] Inflammation of the peritoneum, usually a result of infection (primary) or trauma (secondary).

phagocyte: [FAHG-oh-siyt] White blood cells that destroy and ingest foreign microorganisms and cell debris.

phagocytosis: [FAHG-oh-siy-TOH-sis] Process of ingesting foreign microorganisms and cell debris.

piles: Hemorrhoids; varicose veins in the rectum or on the anus.

pleura: [PLOOr-ah] The sacs of connective tissue lining the thorax and the surface of the lungs; contain fluid to reduce the friction between the inspiring lung and the chest wall.

pleurisy: [PLOOR-ee-see] Pain resulting from inflammation of the pleura; sharp and localized, occurring over the affected region.

pleuritic pain: Pain similar to that caused by pleurisy; pain over the affected pleural region of that worsens during respiration.

pneumoconiosis: [NEW-moh-coh-nee-OH-sis] Lung disease resulting from chronic inhalation of insoluble or semisoluble particles causing fibrous scarring within the lung.

pneumothorax: Air or gas in the pleural space (between visceral and parietal pleura of the lung) causing widespread collapse of the alveoli.

polydipsia: [pahl-ee-DIP-see-ah] Excessive thirst, usually a result of dehydration or loss of blood volume.

polyphagia: [pahl-ee-FAY-jee-ah] Excessive intake of food.

polyuria: [pahl-ee-OO-ree-ah] Excessive frequency or volume of urine.

postprandial: [post-PRAN-dee-ahl] Relating to the period following a meal.

prandial: [PRAN-dee-ahl] Relating to the period during a meal.

preparticipation examination: Physical screening, survey medical history, and review of systems conducted before allowing participation in athletics.

prodromal: [pro-DROH-mal] Relating to a symptom preceding onset of an illness.

prognosis: Predicted outcome of injury, illness, or disease.

prostatitis: [prahs-tah-TIY-tis] Inflammation of the prostate gland.

proteinuria: [pro-tay-ee-NOO-ree-ah] Presence of protein in the urine.

pruitis: [proo-RIY-tis] Severe itching.

ptosis: [TOH-sis] Sagging of the upper eyelids as a result of muscle or nerve dysfunction.

purulent: [PYEW-roo-lent] The presence of a thick fluid (ie, pus) containing leukocytes, dead cells, and other tissue debris.

rales: [rahlz] Also called crackles; abnormal auscultation of a series of distinct pops during inspiration.

rebound tenderness: Pain elicited upon sudden release of a manually depressed abdomen.

relapse: Recurrence of active disease that was previously in remission.

remission: Absence of detectable or active disease in a person who previously demonstrated the disease; often used to refer to recovery from cancer.

renin: [REE-nin] Hormone secreted by the kidneys; renin increases vasoconstriction and thus raises blood pressure.

respiration: Exchange of oxygen and carbon dioxide between the circulatory system and the atmosphere; occurs in the alveoli of the lung.

review of systems: Screening examination of each major organ system; usually conducted by survey or during the medical history.

rhonchi: [RON-ky] Abnormal auscultation of continuous rumbling during inspiration and expiration.

rigidity: "Splinting"; protective muscular spasm, particularly of the abdominal wall.

sanguineous: [san-GWIN-ee-us] Describes bloody discharge or drainage of body fluid.

seizure: Sudden electrochemical discharge in the brain causing interruption or alteration of normal cerebral activity.

septicemia: [sep-tih-SEE-mih-ah] Presence of an infectious organism in the blood.

septum: A wall of tissue that divides an organ, such as the heart, into chambers or sections.

serosanguineous: [SEE-roh-san-GWIN-ee-us] Describes a combination of watery and bloody discharge or drainage of body fluid.

serous: [SEER-us] Describes watery discharge or drainage of body fluids.

shock: Sudden and severe impairment of the life-sustaining functions of the body; signs include tachycardia, hypotension, diaphoresis, and altered level of consciousness.

sign: Any indication of pathology observed by the clinician.

smooth muscle: Muscle tissue of various internal organ systems, such as the gastrointestinal system.

spasm: Involuntary continuous contraction of skeletal or smooth muscle.

spirometer: [spir-AHM-a-tur] Instrument used to measure ventilatory volumes.

splenomegaly: [SPLEH-noh-MEG-ah-lee] Pathological enlargement of the spleen.

sputum: [SPYOO-tum] Fluid expelled from the mouth during spitting, coughing, or sneezing.

stool: Feces.

stria: [STRY-ah] Longitudinal cutaneous discolorations caused by a constant stretch on the skin, such as occurs during pregnancy.

striated muscle: Muscle tissue which moves the bony skeleton.

stridor: [STRY-dur] Raspy sound upon inspiration, usually indicative of a partially obstructed airway; usually detectable without auscultation.

stroke volume: Amount of blood ejected into the aorta during a single ventricular contraction.

symptom: Any departure from normal function, appearance, or sensation experienced and reported by the patient.

syncope: [SIN-koh-pee] Complete loss of consciousness and postural tone, caused by a sudden reduction in blood supply to the brain.

systole: [SIS-toh-lee] Active contraction phase of the cardiac cycle.

tachycardia: [tack-ee-KAR-dee-ah] Rapid heart rate, usually in excess of 100 beats per minute.

tachypnea: [tack-ip-NEE-ah] Rapid respiration rate; may be in excess of 20 breaths per minute.

thrombosis: Formation of a blood clot in a blood vessel.

thrombus: A clot of blood attached to the wall of a blood vessel.

triage: [TREE-ahj] Initial examination of a patient to determine the severity of their condition.

tumor: Neoplasm; abnormal cell proliferation.

tympanites: [TIM-pah-NEE-teez] Abnormal air or gas within the abdomen.

urinalysis: [yu-rih-NAL-ee-sis] Laboratory analysis of the chemical composition of urine.

urolithiasis: [YU-roh-lih-THI-ay-sis] Kidney stone.

urticaria: [UR-tree-KAR-ee-uh] Hives; lesions of the skin characterized by red, raised regions, usually widespread in reaction to anaphylactic or allergic reaction.

varices: [VAR-ih-seez] Pathologically dilated veins; "varicose veins."

varicoceles: [VAR-ih-koh-seel] Varicose veins in the scrotum.

varicose: [VAR-ih-kohss] Describes permanently dilated veins.

vector: An organism, usually an insect or animal, that passes an infectious organism from one host to another without being affected.

ventilation: Physical movement of air into and out of the lungs.

verrucae: [veh-ROO-kah] Warts; tumorous skin lesion caused by papillomavirus.

virulence: [VEER-yu-lint] The relative severity, progression, noxiousness, or toxicity of a disease.

vital signs: Heart rate, respiration rate, blood pressure, and body temperature.

wheals: [wheelz] Hives; inflammed, raised areas of skin, generally in reaction to an immune response.

whispered pectoriloquy: [peck-toh-RIL-oh-kwee] Abnormal auscultation; whispered sound is clearly heard.

withdrawal: Physical and psychological condition produced by the cessation of chronic use of a physically addicting substance.

APPENDIX

Normal Lab Values

Most laboratory reports highlight low and high values, and provide normal ranges, which may vary between laboratories. Results should be interpreted using the ranges provided by the laboratory. The values in the following table are an example of typical reference ranges.

BLOOD CHEMISTRY	NORMAL (REFERENCE) RANGE
pH	7.35 to 7.45
Bicarbonate	22 to 26 mEq/L
Red blood cells	3.6 to 5.4 million/µL
White blood cells	5000 to 10,000/µL
Platelets	150,000 to 350,000/µL
Hemoglobin	Males: 14 to 18 g/dL Females: 12 to 16 g/dL
Hematocrit	Males: 40% to 50% Females: 37% to 47%
Sodium	135 to 142 mEq/L
Potassium	3.8 to 5.0 mEq/L
Calcium	4.0 to 5.0 mEq/L
Magnesium	3 mEq/L
Chloride	95 to 102 mEq/L
Total protein	6.0 to 8.6 g/dL
Albumin	3.2 to 4.5 g/dL
Glucose (fasting)	70 to 110 mg/dL
Total iron	60 to 150 µg/dL
Total lipids	400 to 800 mg/dL

(continued)

Bhojani RA, O'Connor DP, Fincher AL. *Clinical Pathology for Athletic Trainers: Recognizing Systemic Disease, Fourth Edition* (pp 415-416).
© 2022 Taylor & Francis Group.

BLOOD CHEMISTRY (CONT.)	NORMAL (REFERENCE) RANGE (CONT.)
Cholesterol	150 to 250 mg/dL
Triglycerides	75 to 160 mg/dL
High-density lipoproteins	>40 mg/dL
Low-density lipoproteins	<180 mg/dL
Bilirubin (direct)	0.1 to 0.4 mg/dL
Creatinine	0.6 to 1.2 mg/dL
Uric acid	Males: 2.4 to 7.4 mg/dL
	Females: 1.4 to 5.8 mg/dL
URINALYSIS	**NORMAL (REFERENCE) RANGE**
pH	4.5 to 8.0
Hemoglobin or cells	0
Sodium	75 to 200 mg/24 hours
Potassium	25 to 100 mEq/L
Protein	0 to 150 mg/24 hours
Glucose	0
Bilirubin	0
Creatinine	1.0 to 2.0 g/24 hours
Uric acid	0.6 to 1.0 g/24 hours
Urea	25 to 35 g/24 hours
Ammonia	20 to 70 mEq/L
Acetone	0

INDEX